MOVEMENT

THEORY AND PRACTICE

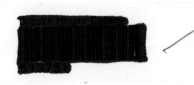

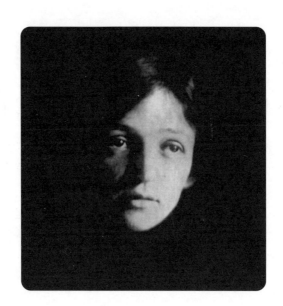

Jarmila Kröschlová

MOVEMENT
THEORY AND PRACTICE

Jarmila Kröschlová

Translated from the Czech by Olga Malandris
with Zora Šemberová

Foreword by Jiří Kylián

CURRENCY PRESS
Sydney

Translated by Olga Malandris
with artistic and technical advice from Zora Šemberová

English translation copyright © Olga Malandris and Zora Šemberová 2000
Appendix 1 and original manuscript copyright © Eva Kröschlová
Anatomical diagrams first published in *Principles of Anatomy for Physical Training Instructors*, London: Her Majesty's Stationery Office, 1957.
© Reproduced by kind permission.
Main text figure drawings © Jo Williams
Appendix figure drawings © Alena Kavanová

National Library of Australia – CIP Data

Kröschlová, Jarmila, 1893– .
[Nauka o pohybu. English]
Movement theory.

ISBN 0 86819 577 4.

1. Human mechanics. 2. Dance. I. Title. II. Title: Nauka o pohybu. English.

Cover design by Susan Mikulic.
Cover photograph: Rachel Jenson, of Leigh Warren and Dancers, Adelaide.
Photo by Alex Makeyev.
Typeset by Post Pre-press Group
Printed by Hyde Park Press

Publication of this title was assisted by the Government of South Australia through Arts South Australia.

CONTENTS

Foreword

It seems strange that since the discoveries and innovations of Isadora Duncan which revolutionalised our perception and understanding of dance, the dance world has never been given a study which scientifically analyses the principles of human motion with such precision and gravity as the book lying before you.

This book is a summary of life-long experiments, studies and their application of everyday praxis. It should be understood that this work is not intended as a source of knowledge only for people of the dance world; it carries invaluable information for everyone who cares about his or her physical well-being, or physicality in general.

Studying this book can bring about different and more efficient training methods for dance teachers or sports coaches. It will enable physiotherapists to guide their patients to exercise correctly and consequently achieve better results. By following the teaching of Jarmila Kröschlová, stage artists (dancers, actors, singers) will be able to use their kinetic abilities in a way which will ultimately give their performance a more natural and more convincing impact. Even parents, if they follow her advice, will be able to teach their children correct posture and natural movement, which could prevent the development of physical deformation in older age.

This book was written by a woman who was greatly appreciated by her contemporaries and who widened and deepened the horizon of her art through her love, dedication, persistence and integrity.

Last but not least, it should be said that the person who has initiated the translation of this book is of equal stature to the author: Zora Šemberová is a greatly respected dance teacher and senior lecturer. Now in her mid-eighties, she has inspired scores of dancers, teachers, musicians and other artists through her uncompromising commitment to the *truth* in art and in life.

I wish the readers of this book much pleasure living with it, as life is movement and movement is life.

Jiří Kylián
Den Haag, The Netherlands

Acknowledgements

We extend our gratitude to Her Majesty's Stationery Office, London, for their kind permission to allow reproduction of parts of the excellent *Principles of Anatomy and Physiology for Physical Training Instructors in the Royal Air Force*, Third Edition, 1957. Heartfelt thanks must go also to Professor Eva Kröschlová for permission to reproduce sections from her Drama Faculty Notes entitled *Stage Movement* and *Dynamics and Swings* published by the Prague State Pedagocical Publishing House in 1988. In particular we thank her for her enthusiastic support and valuable advice.

We are also grateful to Christine Appelbee, former senior tutor in physiotherapy, who assisted us with her knowledge of anatomy and physiology, to Amanda Kimber, teacher of contemporary dance and chief examiner at SSABSA, who edited the manuscript with an understanding necessary to the specialised content of the book; to Susan Taylor, teacher of classical dance and international examiner for the Royal Academy of Dance who selflessly assisted us in the early stages of our translation; and to our illustrator Jo Williams, former dancer and mime artist, now a sculptor, who was able to grasp the essence of dance movement in her drawings.

We are indebted to Robin Cullen, Elinor Dunstan, Lynette Benjamin and Francis Williams for typing draft versions of the manuscript and to Pamela StClair-Johnson and Vassil Malandris for their help at the final stages of our project.

To those who read the manuscript and prepared testimonials in support of our work we express our most sincere appreciation. A special thank you to Jiří Kylián, artistic director of the Netherlands Dans Theater, and Meryl Tankard, choreographer, for taking the time out to show deep interest in our work, and endorsing it as a valuable tool for teachers of movement. The translators could not have successfully accomplished the work without the kind and generous help of others. We extend our gratitude to Gillian Rae Roberts, dance coordinator at the South Australian Centre for the Performing Arts; Leigh Warren, choreographer, and deep appreciation to those who have given freely of their time to provide assistance in the completion of this work.

Translators' Notes

The impetus to translate *Movement Theory* by Jarmila Kröschlová into English from the original Czech sprang from many sources. In part it stemmed from the dissatisfaction, expressed by many practitioners, with the reductionist approach favoured by contemporary writers of movement texts. Movement theory is too often presented as an analysis of the mechanics with little emphasis upon the synthesis of movement and expression.

Jarmila Kröschlová remains one of few researchers and writers about movement who has taken a holistic approach to the subject, treating movement as the language through which the body communicates the feelings of the soul. Kröschlová developed her theories by drawing upon more than fifty years experience as a dancer, choreographer and teacher. *Movement Theory* reflects her deep knowledge of the movement capabilities of the human body and displays a profound sensitivity toward form, execution and expression.

Movement Theory was written primarily as a reference text for use by teachers of movement and dance; she nevertheless recognised its broad application to mime, gymnastics, physiotherapy or any form of human activity that can benefit from knowledge and understanding of movement principles. Kröschlová develops her theory in a logically coherent fashion. She formulates the rules for correct body posture and stresses the importance of body alignment, together with conscious muscular work and relaxation, as the basis for the realisation of full movement potential free of injury. She identifies the basic movements of the various parts of the body working in the correct alignment and combines them into composite movements which are further combined into complex movements.

Throughout the book Kröschlová carefully explains the 'why' and 'how' of technically refined and expressive movement in harmony with the body, the soul and the laws of nature. To this end she provided anatomical description and illustration to assist a clear and complete understanding. In this translation the original anatomical text has been expanded and replaced with extracts taken from *Principles of Anatomy and Physiology for Physical Training Instructors in the Royal Air Force* which was selected for its clarity of expression and the excellent quality of its diagrams. In the spirit of Kröschlová we recommend that readers of this book consult the noted text to complete the study of human anatomy which forms such an essential and complementary ingredient to a full understanding of movement.

Kröschlová includes model exercises to aid teachers to grasp basic and advanced movement concepts and to serve as the basis for the creation of their own. The line and stick diagrams in the original text are not reproduced but are replaced with new illustrations which better portray the human body in movement.

Although first published more than twenty-five years ago, Kröschlová's work remains as fresh and as vital today as it did in 1975. Her work remains timeless because of the added dimension of expression that she gave to dance and movement. We commend this book to all teachers, choreographers and students of movement who strive for perfection and expression in their work.

Olga Malandris and Zora Šemberová

Preface

In my youth, at the turn of the century, there began a widespread movement of aesthetic and artistic dance education in which the ideals of classical dance were reviewed and the existence of a freer and more emotional dance expression was recognised. Classical dance ceased to be the only accessible form of stage dance art. Gradually the movement gained in popularity. Creators of new movements had already started to work abroad. The barefooted American dancer Isadora Duncan discovered a radical departure from the ballet style through her courageous art. With the help of her sister Elizabeth and her band of admirers, Isadora founded non-profit making schools of dance in which she worked with children. Elizabeth, who ran the schools, continued to develop the ideas and aims of Isadora following her untimely death.

A second pioneer was the Swiss Émile Jacques-Dalcroze, a composer and teacher of music based in Geneva. He created a faculty of rhythmic gymnastics, now known as Eurhythmics, at the Geneva Conservatorium and later founded his own school in the same city. Before the outbreak of the Great War he moved to Hellerau, near Dresden, where he was invited to teach Eurythmics in a purpose-built building which had been especially designed for him. During the war, however, he resigned from the school and returned to Geneva. The third, and most significant, pioneer in contemporary stage art was the Austro-Hungarian Rudolf von Laban. His influence on the newly-developing contemporary ballet was world wide.

The teachings of these three founders were spread throughout Europe and America by their pupils. Laban's methods, in particular, proved very popular and became well established. The three movements were well represented in Czechoslovakia. Prior to 1914, a school of Eurythmics, led by Marie Volková and Anna Dubská, was founded in Prague. After the War a school of Laban's teachings was established under the leadership of his student Milča Mayerová. A little later a school of Isadora Duncan was founded, run at first by Elizabeth Duncan and later by Jarmila Jeřábková.

I studied at both the Geneva and the Hellerau schools of

Jacques-Dalcroze. The latter was co-founded by the American, Kristina Baer-Frissel, with the Austrian, Valerie Kratina and the Hungarian Ernst Ferand, all past students of Dalcroze. Between the years 1919 to 1924 both schools adopted, as their common aim, the education of teachers of Eurythmics. Dalcroze placed his major emphasis upon rhythmic musical tuition: movement was generally limited to walking, marking time and conducting. Certain procedures were devised to allow the interpretation of the minim, dotted minim and semibreve in stepped movement. The movements corresponding to the crotchet, quaver and semiquaver were expressed by a series of steps. In addition, Swedish gymnastics classes were held at the Geneva School but were treated as extracurricular. Dalcroze's policy was not to correct students' movement.

For the second semester I transferred to the Hellerau school. Eurythmics was taught there by K. Baer-Frissel whose work, like that of Dalcroze, had a rhythmic musical basis. The movement component was taught by Valerie Kratina, and her approach was somewhat less gymnastic than that of her colleagues. Ernst Ferand taught the theory of music. I gradually became dissatisfied with all their approaches: neither of the schools provided students with any solid grounding for the methodical teaching of movement.

I commenced my own teaching activity during the last two years of my stay in Hellerau. I endeavoured to draw the attention of my students and colleagues to the rules governing movement itself according to my understanding at that time. Previously, during the War, I had studied the Gymnastics Method devised by the American Dr Bess Mensendieck under the guidance of Dr Vojáčková, one of her former students. The movement of the spine, particularly the rounded forward bend, was practised in detail. At the time I possessed a moderate understanding of the anatomical foundation of the human body, especially the spine, but I soon came to realise that the spine was not enough: I must study the working of the entire human anatomy. It was upon a fundamental understanding of the anatomy and the functioning of the human body as an integral whole that I wished to base a technique of modern dance. This would be a long term task. I reasoned that, whereas the ballet possessed a strong and reliable technique that had been perfected over centuries, the technical basis for the development of modern expressive dance was vague and not well defined. With the exception of individuals like Kreutzberg or Wigman, contemporary dancers gave an impression of being talented dilettantes. We must create a sound technical basis for modern dance education: not focused too narrowly on technique, as is classical ballet, but should offer future dancers something not present in classical technique. That was a conscious, sensitised awareness of all the components of movement expression—a feeling for form, space, rhythm and dynamics which must apply to, and be evident in, every single movement. We must demand it from the dancer and all the more from the dance teacher and choreographer. This way one captivates the whole being of the student, his/her intellect and feeling. Only an equivalent linking of these two components could satisfy our demands on modern dance expression. I took this conviction with me to Prague, to which I returned in 1924 with my eight-member dance group. The group became my experimental material.

After the Great War a large number of dancers and teachers of Eurythmics appeared in our country, thanks to the many years' activity of Eliška Bláhová from Brno. Through the Brno authorities she enforced the rule that all those who wanted to teach Eurythmics had to graduate from a teaching course. This was progressive: in Prague the authorities were giving everybody who had studied, even for a short time, permission to teach. As a protest against such ignorant bureaucracy, I introduced a two-year teaching course of gymnastics at my school, with a two-year extended study in dance.

The teaching courses and exams introduced by Bláhová, following the Dalcroze model, were aimed mainly at musical preparation for creating simple musical phrases as an accompaniment to rhythmic exercises. The perfection of movement was not important and almost coincidental. My aim was more specifically concerned with the elaboration of the movement so that rhythm and dynamics were perceptible in the quality of the movement. Strict gymnastic movement is insufficient to achieve such strong, deeply felt forms. To create perfect movement forms they must be felt with a heightened awareness of space, rhythm and dynamics and must be in harmony and compliance with the natural laws of movement. To better understand these laws I studied anatomy and the movement possibilities of the living body. At the same time I studied the fine arts of old cultures and compared the results of my findings with the live movements of my students. In many of the works of art that I examined I discovered

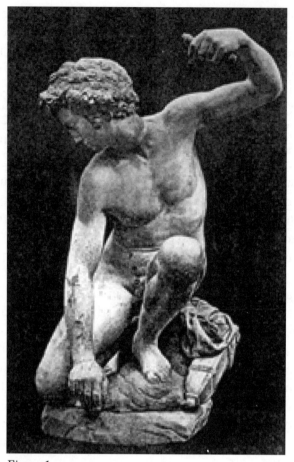

Figure 1
Michelangelo Buonarotti: The Cupid
(Victoria and Albert Museum, London)

movement intuition and strong emotional content. I realised that the
forms of movement depicted in art were in harmony with anatomical
law and, moreover, exhibited an unusual sensitivity combined with a
particular feeling for space. From my collective observations, and as
is especially evident in the art of Michelangelo, I concluded that
knowledge and awareness of muscular coordination is essential for
the achievement of movement that possesses clarity of form. I realised
the teaching of awareness of form and a feeling for space must
become an integral part of aesthetic movement tuition from the very
beginning of a student's training. I also became aware of how important is the coordination between single movements for creation of
complex ones and how this coordination relates to our feeling for

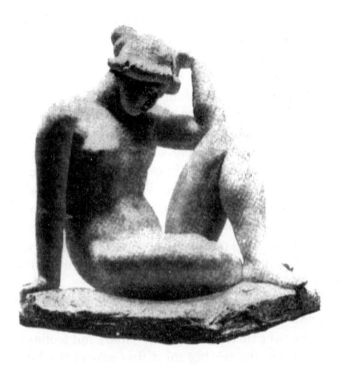

Figure 2
A. Maillol: The Sitting Woman
First half of the twentieth century. Elie Faure. History of Art: Ancient Art.
London: John Lane, the Bodley Head, 1921

rhythm. I formed the opinion that a conscious awareness of the muscles extending right to the surface of the skin was the medium
through which one perceived space as well as form, rhythm and
dynamics. I engaged upon a deep study of the potential capabilities of
the human anatomy and compared those with the actual movements
of the live body in all its weaknesses—such as imperfect muscular
control and inaccurate coordination. At the same time, I must not
overlook muscular sensation (kinaesthetic awareness) and movement
intuition. Both of these should be equally cultivated in students. My
theory of movement evolved from these foundations, combining my
pedagogical and choreographic experience accumulated during more
than fifty years of practice.

    In my theory of movement I did not exploit other existing theories,
nor did I underestimate or discount any of them. Everything that
appears in this book I have explored, sensed and tested on myself and
my students as a way of convincing myself over and over again in

practice of the essential correctness and feasibility of the theory.

This *Movement Theory* is not a text book in the usual sense, nor is it a simple collection of exercises. The exercises I present are intended to be used as models by teachers who wish to create their own. Accurate descriptions of all the basic and composite movements included in the analyses should familiarise the reader with the necessary material and its perfect execution. The only exercises that must be executed precisely and consciously are those which promote correct body posture. These exercises hold the key to perfect balance in every movement. When creating and executing their own exercises, the teacher must always check that the entire synthesis of the rules for correct body posture is maintained.

With my wishes for continued successes, I bequeath my theories of movement to my students and all future and practising teachers and choreographers.

Knowledge of the theory of movement is vital for a movement teacher who works with students in a practical manner to teach them mastery over their bodies, their minds and feelings. Before a teacher can teach, the teacher must first master the fundamentals of movement and go on to lead students to movement which is expressive and aspiring to perfection in form and spatial, rhythmic and dynamic sensation. These are the hallmarks and the qualities of movement that lead to artistry and expression not only in dance, pantomime and acting but also in sculpture and the visual arts. Proof of this can be found in the works of ancient cultures which portray perfect movement and in the works of giants of art of more recent times.

Jarmila Kröschlová

1
CORRECT ELEVATED DANCE POSTURE

The movement culture to which we aspire in the art of dance and in the all round development of young people cannot be achieved without a perfectly carried body. This fundamental and surely far-reaching knowledge should be actively pursued and taught not only by parents but especially by teachers who, if they are aware of the techniques through which correct body posture is attained, can achieve valuable results in the classroom; but who can also, if unaware, unwittingly allow considerable damage to occur.

Most of our bad posture habits are adopted in our early years. This can be easily noticed in small children after they start school. The immobility forced upon them while they bend over their desks easily tires them and causes them to stoop. Unfortunately, children require more playful movement than structured teaching can often allow.

In the early years at school the teaching of correct body posture is no less important than the teaching of the required curriculum. Primary school teachers should be given adequate grounding in the basic rules of posture so that they can teach students how to maintain a correct posture whilst they are reading and writing. No teacher should forget that they bear as . great a responsibility for the sound development of a student's physical wellbeing as their intellectual and emotional health. The lower the student's age the greater the responsibility of the teacher.

The often heard reminders by parents and teachers to children to 'Stand up straight or sit up straight!' are to no purpose if the child does not understand what he/she is doing wrong, how this is to be accomplished or of its importance. It is, therefore, vital to awaken and cultivate in children a conscious understanding that correct body posture is just as necessary a part of their whole developing personality as, say, the mastery of language.

The effort to attain, and thereafter maintain correct body posture contributes to the establishment of important features of good character. The straightening of the spine is not limited to physical correction only but leads simultaneously to the development of character traits consistent with an erect bearing. Through systematic work on correct posture the child can be led to greater self-discipline, independence and strengthened self-esteem and self-confidence. We establish the willpower and character of the student. Throughout the process it is of course necessary that the teacher serve as a good example. The teacher must adopt an erect body posture to express the balance between his/her physical and mental forces and this is the key to nobility and self-confidence. It is only in this context that these values become truly meaningful. For the teacher a controlled body posture combined with other inner qualities has an effect on bearing and demeanour in class, making the teacher more free, forthright and purposeful. The teacher's influence on the students will be lasting.

It would seem to be stating the obvious to say nobody should care so much about beautiful posture as the dancer or a movement artist. Regrettably, this is not so. An elevated posture is not only a prerequisite for technical perfection but fundamental to the aesthetics of movement. Without a correctly elevated posture the achievement of either purpose or precision of movement is impossible. Without these, the beauty of movement, which is based on that purpose and precision, is lost. Just as the singer must mould her/his voice to create a basis for correct vocal projection, so must the dancer, mime or actor acquire a balanced posture if they are to attain technical and artistic mastery over their art. Bad posture habits are the most stubborn and worst of faults to correct because they are ingrained. To correct them requires not only physical strength but great determination and sustained mental effort. It is, therefore, essential that teachers constantly strive to correct all visible faults in their students before they become entrenched, not only when standing still but during all movements on which the students work.

Elevated dance posture requires total adherence to five basic rules.

RULES FOR ELEVATED DANCE POSTURE AND CORRECT BODY POSTURE

Rule 1

Lighten and lift the pelvis by extending the front of the hip joints. Establish this by activating the abdominal and buttock muscles with the hips held in the horizontal and reducing the forward tilt of the pelvis.

Rule 2
Elongate the spine to reduce its 'S' shape curvature.

Rule 3
Carry the neck and head from the middle of the chest (thoracic spine) by first establishing their support point.

Rule 4
Establish the position of the legs by pulling the ankle, knee and hip joints up. Moderately turn out the hip joints to turn legs outward. As a result, the pelvis shifts forward to locate the body weight over the middle of the forefeet.

Rule 5
Turn out broadly spread shoulders and extend them sideways, exactly on the side of the chest. Elevate the breast bone (sternum) whilst maintaining the horizontal

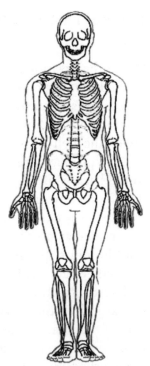

Figure 3: The Skeleton

pull sideways of the shoulders. Maintain this position when at rest or in motion.

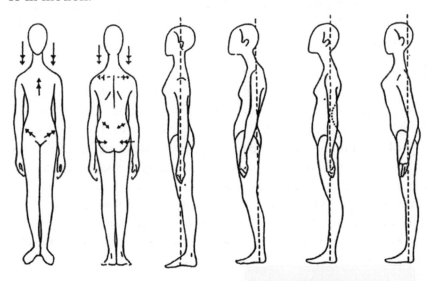

correct body alignment   incorrect body alignment

Figure 4

THE RULES IN DETAIL

Rule 1

When the position of the pelvis is correctly established, the pelvis is tilted slightly forward with the hips held in a horizontal line, the abdominal and buttock muscles work intensively. When adequately contracted, the lower segment of the straight abdominal muscle under the belly, the *rectus abdominis*, and the oblique abdominal muscles produce a pressure on the pelvis from the front of the body to the back while the contracted buttock, or gluteal muscles, produce a pressure on the pelvis from the back of the body towards the front. As a result of the kinaesthetic awareness of this complementary muscular activity, supplemented by the upward extension of the hip joints, the pelvis is tilted slightly forward, lightened and correctly established.

The contraction of the oblique abdominal muscles limits the forward tilt of the pelvis. The emphasised contraction of the lower part of the rectus abdominis avoids the contraction of the muscles in the waist and the diaphragm to leave the respiratory process undisturbed. By contracting the lower buttock muscles the thighs are rotated in the hip joints outward to allow the heads of the thigh bones, or femurs, to sink more deeply into their sockets, the *acetabulum*, supporting the pelvis. Thus the pelvis is shifted forward to place the hip joints into the body axis in a vertical plane located at the centre of the forefeet (between the third and fourth metatarsals).

Rule 2

If the pelvis is lightened and established in its basic position, the first prerequisite for an erect and elevated carriage of the spine is fulfilled by reducing its excessive lumbar lordosis. The straightening of the lumbar spine may be further enhanced by the subtle contraction of the rectus abdominus in the underbelly to draw the rib arches down. The very frequent mistake of protracting the lower rib cage, which violates the continuity of the motion of the entire trunk, may be thus avoided. Excessive neck curvature (cervical lordosis) is reduced by contracting the deep back muscles between the shoulder blades and by contracting the long neck muscles which erect the cervical spine.

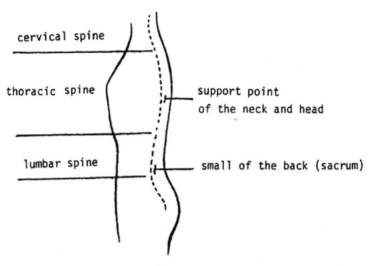

cervical spine

thoracic spine

support point
of the neck and head

lumbar spine

small of the back (sacrum)

Figure 5

Rule 3

For greater efficiency of movement of the spine, neck and head, I located the support point of the neck and head between the sixth and ninth spinous processes of the thoracic vertebrae. By drawing these processes closer together, the support point becomes established. The head is carried by the extended neck with the chin above the sternum at approximately right angles to the throat. The outer openings of the ears are located above the shoulders and the crown of the head points directly upward. When the support point

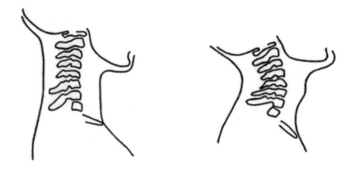

Figure 6
The process of the seventh cervical vertebra differs distinctly from the other processes. It is longer and as a result of its length it protrudes from the line of the other vertebrae.

is established, the sternum becomes moderately erect and the upper ribs arch, to allow the neck and head to be consciously moved with the upper thorax. This guided motion occurs exactly at the point of least spine mobility, coincidentally the point at which the problem of hunching the back is so often evident. A benefit of this rule is the reduction in neck lordosis and chest kyphosis.

Rule 4

The body weight is correctly placed when the legs are elongated and the hips extended upward so that the pelvis is lightened and does not sit heavily on the legs. The correct placement of body weight is achieved by a combined action: the contraction of the gluteal muscles in the buttock, which rotates the thighs outwards in the hip joints, and the slight complementary outward rotation of the shin bones together with the ankles. As the thighs are slightly turned out the pelvis is shifted forward while the outward rotation of the shin bones elevates the instep arch and causes the body weight to migrate towards the centre of the forefoot. If the shin bones are not turned out, the insteps are visibly lowered and the weight is shifted towards the big toes. (* *It is essential that the ankle joints be adequately relaxed to allow a slight forward tilt of the legs.*)

When the body weight is correctly placed, the centre of gravity can be more rapidly moved to provide greater mobility and lightness of motion. The body weight should not fall on the heel, the sides of the feet nor along the edge of the large or the small toes unless required to do so by a particular movement. By elongating the legs and hip joints we also contribute to their lightening and elevation. This rule must be adhered to in stillness and in motion.

Rule 5

To spread the shoulders wide and to carry them horizontally exactly at the sides of the chest, it is necessary to pull them along the sides of the rib cage and to moderately rotate them outward. The pulling of the shoulders sideways involves the action of the back thoracic and rhomboid muscles, which stretch the chest muscles, the *pectoralis major*.

Two separate but simultaneous actions are required to turn the shoulders out:

---

*Translator's note

1. Pull the shoulders down by contracting the lower part of the trapezius muscle while relaxing its upper part and the acromio-clavicular joints.
2. Press the shoulder blades towards the ribs, i.e. particularly their lower corners, by contracting the small chest muscles, the *pectoralis minor*, the *serratus anterior* and the upper tip of the broad back muscles, the *latissimus dorsi*. While pulling downward on the shoulders simultaneously elevate the sternum and upper ribs in the opposite direction to the shoulders. Do not pull the shoulders together.

Carrying the shoulders this way contributes to plasticity in the shape of the chest. The pattern should be adopted not only in an elevated body posture but also when moving the trunk, spine and arms and in balancing the movements of the pelvis and the legs.

THE IMPORTANCE OF THE FIVE RULES

All of the five rules are of equal importance as each is closely linked to and dependent on all the others, thus creating a unity. If any one is neglected a properly balanced body posture cannot be achieved. Each rule is inseparably dependent on the others.

Through the implementation of the five rules a greater awareness of the functional architecture of the body is acquired as its components are put into a mutually balanced position. The legs, when slightly tilted forward, carry the pelvis above the centre of the forefeet, the shoulder joints in a vertical plane above the hip joints and the openings of the ears in a vertical plane above the shoulders. When the body is positioned in this way, its central axis extends from the crown of the head, through the *sacrum*, to terminate in the middle of the slightly-turned-out feet (as seen from the profile). When standing on one foot, the axis extends from the crown of the head, through the hip joint to the centre of the foot.

Sensing of body axis

The ability to sense the existence of the body axis as a tangible reality amalgamates the separate rules into a synthesis allowing the body to be perceived as a balanced unit. A dancer interprets the architecture of his body through space, i.e. he/she perceives the vertical of the body, the horizontal of the shoulders and hips, the curves of the pelvis, chest and skull and is aware of the opposing forces which produce expressive body movement. The body sensed in this way is positioned in space ready to move.

It is possible to develop a more refined movement technique by consciously interpreting the sensations arising in the musculo-skeletal system. This perception of the position and state of movement of the body parts is known as kinaesthetic awareness. Developing this refinement depends on the following stages:

Firstly it is necessary to have kinaesthetic sense organs intact. These are the sensory receptors (nerve endings) in the skin, muscles, tendons and ligaments. These are capable of detecting and transmitting information about the changes of state in the musculo-skeletal system. These messages are conveyed along the sensory nerve fibres to the central nervous system (spinal cord and brain).

Secondly, the brain must be in a state of preparation to receive this information, i.e. a state of concentration on what is being felt. This is called a 'psychological set' of the brain which makes it ready to receive and interpret these messages from the periphery.

Thirdly, the brain formulates a response that is mediated by the motor nerves which carry messages back to the muscles concerned. In this way the brain conveys a more precise set of messages back to the musculo-skeletal system resulting in more finely differentiated and coordinated movements.

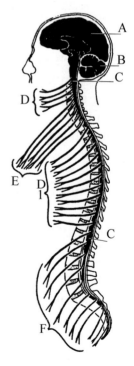

Figure 7: The central and peripheral nervous systems
A – Cerebrum ⎫
B – Cerebellum ⎬ *forming central nervous system*
C – Spinal cord ⎭
D– Peripheral nerves supplying structures on the left side of the neck.
D1– Peripheral nerves supplying structure to the left side of thorax and abdomen.
E and F – Peripheral nerves to upper and lower limbs respectively.

---

*Translator's note

I

ANATOMY: THE CENTRAL NERVOUS SYSTEM

The nervous system is the highly complex mechanism by which man reacts to his environment and coordinates his mental and bodily activities. It consists of the *brain*, protected by the skull, the *spinal cord*, protected by the vertebrae which form a special canal for it, and the *peripheral*, free running nerves which supply all parts of the body. In addition, there are small masses of nervous tissue in various parts of the body, usually near the brain or spinal cord.

The brain is the centre of appreciation, where all incoming messages, whether entering consciousness or not, are analysed and appropriate action is initiated; the spinal chord groups, transmits and relays messages to and from the brain, and the peripheral nerves transmit messages between the spinal cord and the general body tissues.

The nervous system may be compared with a complicated telephone network, and the brain with the central exchange itself. Messages are sent from all parts of the body about pressure, pain, temperature, touch and position, and from the ears, eyes, nose and mouth; they are rapidly sorted, interpreted and correlated in the brain which then relays information and instruction throughout the body.

The brain and spinal cord together are called, for convenience, the *central nervous system*. The free nerves, running from the central nervous system to all other parts of the body, make up the *peripheral nervous system*. This classification is an anatomical one.

Structure of Nervous Tissue

Nervous tissue consists essentially of nerve cells and their branches, supported by connective tissues. Nerve cells differ widely in space and size; they have a nucleus, several small branches called *dendrites* for the reception of messages, and normally one branch, the *axon* or nerve fibre, for their transmission. A nerve cell with its branches forms the basic unit of the nervous system and is called a *neurone*. Most axons, or nerve fibres, are covered by two sheaths; the outer is a thin membrane and the inner is made up of a white fatty substance. The inner membrane appears white and glistening and the masses of nerve fibres covered with it constitute the *white matter* of the nervous system. The cell body and its dendrites have no membrane and are grey. The popular phrase 'grey matter' has thus a sound anatomical basis, because the grey part of the nervous system contains the bodies of the cells where thought processes occur, but the white parts contain only the nerve fibres or mere telephone wires. The peripheral nerves are made up almost entirely of axons, and are therefore white.

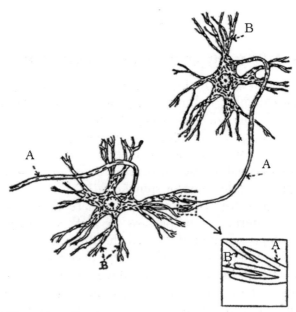

Figure 8: Two nerve cells
A – Axons
B – Dendrites
Inset – the meeting between axons and dendrites, showing the contact but anatomical separateness which is called a synapse

Function of nervous tissue

The characteristic function of nervous tissue is the carrying of nervous impulses. Nervous tissue reacts to almost any stimulus as a result of its highly developed excitability. A nervous impulse has many characteristics identical with those of a simple electric current. Electricity is commonly used to excite nervous impulses under experimental conditions but the electricity itself is not conducted through the nerve fibres; the rate of conduction of a nervous impulse in man is between 30 and 90 metres per second, according to the type of nerve fibre. This rate is many hundreds of thousands of times less than the rate of conduction of electricity.

*In a nutshell, kinaesthetic awareness occurs at the moment when the brain receives and interprets information from the kinaesthetic receptors via the sensory nerves. Without this conscious work we cannot achieve an expressive, refined and economical movement. The technique would then become mechanical.

---

*Translator's note

II

THE PROCESS OF CONCENTRATION

The process of concentration should precede each movement. It is a preparation for heightened bodily sensitivity. It could be called 'enlivened immobility', similar to a roe-deer which has stopped and discovered a scent. The roe-deer stands motionless, the head half turned against the wind which brings her near and distant scents. Her posture is light, elevated and held with minimum muscle effort. We sense her body endowed with life from inside, in perfect balance and ready to move. Such is the posture of a concentrated dancer before performance.

Let's look at the visual arts of old cultures like Greek, Egyptian, Indian, Chinese etc. Those masterpieces which portray the human body share the same quality of 'stillness enlivened from within'. All these works (like the Greek Nike, Psyche from Capua etc.) are captured in a completely balanced movement which conveys a sensitive self-awareness within the surrounding space. It is not only a matter of beauty of form but of something more substantial and deep, which enlivens matter from within.

Intuitive feeling for the source from which movement is born can also be found in some sculptors of our time, for example in the French artist Maillol (Fig.2, p. xv). From his robust female figures which are not beautiful in the sense of perfection of form and proportion, we can understand well what it means to enliven matter from within. The figures are sitting or standing, but their massive bodies are alive; they are, despite their immobility and robustness, ready to move. One must look at the beauty of the body and movement without prejudice. Each body, no matter what its proportions, has its own individual beauty as long as it is enlivened from within.

All dancers remember that rare moment when for the first time they felt light and elevated and when everything suddenly seemed easy to them. It was at the moment when they, for the first time, entered a state of balance of the body in movement and were in touch with their own inner space. They found themselves and their empowered abilities. This feeling is not permanent: it is not discovered once and for all, but must be sought and renewed again and again. The body, controlled from within and maintained in balance, glows with enlivened grace. It has, in its movement, its own individual beauty which is more captivating than the most graceful movement executed coldly, i.e. externally.

Let's look again at Maillol's figures. We see their beauty differently now that they speak to us through a new language, through that inner animation of matter which is a secret of great sculptures created by artists with intuitive understanding of the body and its movement laws.

A dancer cannot achieve a simultaneous perception of both inner and outer space without deep concentration. It is a necessary preparation before performance. This preparation requires a considerable time with the beginners. It would be unwise if the teacher rushed the student and did not allow him/her as much time as is necessary. To force students to start before they are fully concentrated, i.e. concentrated to the degree their developmental stage allows, leads to superficiality and pretence. During the course of tuition, the length of the inner preparation shortens, until finally only a few seconds are sufficient for a complete concentration. The ability to concentrate means a disciplined feeling and mind. A prepared artist must be fully present in his/her performance, i.e. fully maintaining their psycho-physical presence. Nothing at all, no irrelevant private feeling, no lost thought must weaken this concentration. The dancer must not lose inner continuity which is extremely important for movement synthesis. It is the teacher's duty to draw the students' attention to faults in concentration in the same way as other faults are criticised. The ability to concentrate is partly in-born; but it is possible and necessary to develop it to a higher intensity and greater perseverance. Concentration becomes deeper and longer through practising. The teacher knows the immense value of the ability to concentrate at will and maintain concentration. This objective should be aimed for from the start of tuition. The teacher must insist that the students execute all movements with full attentiveness so that they start movements accurately and clearly and carry them through to completion.

The students must arrive at this extremely important understanding through their own experience. The teacher must let them undertake certain tasks individually so that they can observe each other, make their own discoveries and search for their own solutions. That way, the students get used to concentrating in front of spectators, focusing on the movement and not losing even for one moment their own inner enthusiasm. Thus the teacher is able to protect them from superficiality and get them used to criticism. Criticism, which they both give and receive, refines their perception and judgement and fosters their striving for perfection. With the help of the teacher they learn about their faults and advantages in the performance of their fellow students.

Improvisation to music, which forms an important part of dance tuition, serves the same goal, namely to prolong and deepen concentration. It urges the beginner to move in harmony with music, to let the music lead and to respond through movement (even though still imperfect) to the emotional excitement awakened by music. The student will succeed all the more if he/she releases the self and surrenders, through awakened body awareness, to the melodic, rhythmic and dynamic flow of music. Right from the beginning this will encourage spontaneous response to music and gradual improvement of movement performance. The more perfectly the beginner learns to concentrate, the sooner the obstacle which prevents the perception of their own movement will disappear. The student will become aware of both personal form and expression and retain it in his/her movement memory. In this way the student will get closer to the aim of conscious dance creation.

A big danger are the so-called 'habitual movements'. We all have a reserve of movements in which we take refuge when our contact with and our immersion in music is not deep enough. When our thoughts and emotions wander outside the music we perceive it in fragments. Then the movement does not flow out of inner response to the music and is not truthful. Immersion in the task must be honest, complete and steady.

The role of the teacher also requires a high degree of concentration. The teacher must follow and observe the movements of the students through his/her own intellect and kinaesthetic awareness in order to perceive even the slightest deviations from their technical performance. The teacher must exert the same enthusiasm, as if performing the movements herself. The movement execution of her students must not be judged only by what the teacher sees but also by what he/she receives through her bodily sensations. Such symbiosis identifies deviations of technical character as well as gaps in the inner participation and concentration of the student more accurately and in more detail than eyesight and reason.

III

INNER TENSION

Explicit and deep concentration on the task evokes in a dancer's soul a certain tension which we call inner tension. This term covers everything so far discussed about inner readiness for movement before the performance: i.e. body balance, the link between inner and outer space, deep focus and readiness for movement. In summary, this preparation can be compared to the tuning of an instrument. As a musician tunes an instrument, so the dancer tunes the body, the instrument of their art; enlivens it and empowers it with the intensity of their inner tension. This preparation and its process results in a permanent state, which accompanies the performance from beginning to end in such a way that it outlasts even the closing of the last movement. Inner tension outlives a movement which is already physically brought to an end, maintaining vibration in the dancer's inner and outer space.

The excitement of the spectator also outlives the awakened artistic experience which fades away slowly. If, however, the dancer breaks creative concentration, the spectator is also disturbed. If the emotional response is broken the whole impression from the dance performance falls apart. Even the fading away of the inner tension must be in proportion. If the dancer's involvement is genuine and deep, the fading away will correspond organically to the intensity of that involvement, the inner tension.

We must not, however, mistake the inner tension for muscular tension. They are completely independent. Muscular tension changes and is governed by rhythmic-dynamic experiences and is not identical with inner tension. Inner tension accompanies and maintains a rhythmic and dynamic flow of movements; however it is unchangeable, it can disappear and renew itself again, but it either exists or not, it is superior to performance.

The movements described in the following section, ANALYSIS OF MOVEMENT, are training material for movement education; designed for workshops for future teachers who should become acquainted with the theory and practice of analysing the movement of all parts of the body. Only on the basis of this knowledge can they learn to compose exercises for movement and dance courses. (The section SYNTHESIS OF MOVEMENT illustrates a few examples.)

2
ANALYSIS OF MOVEMENT

Movement is recognised in two ways: by anatomical analysis of movement mechanics and by analysis of live movement. The difference between the two can be explained by two examples. The anatomist divides the spine into coccyx, sacrum and lumbar, thoracic and cervical vertebrae. The movement analyst considers the movement peculiarities of the spine and divides it into two parts, the upper and the lower parts. The lower part runs from the coccyx to the support point of the neck and head (a more detailed explanation is in Rule 3 of CORRECT BODY POSTURE p. 5) and the upper part from the support point to the occipital bone (the back of the head). This division of the spine from the movement point of view is justified by the fact that both parts are independent in their movement. The lower part can be demobilised and the upper part can be mobilised by itself and vice versa. However, it is possible to execute two different movements in both parts e.g. the lateral tilt of the lower part and the rotation of the upper part.

Another example: the anatomist considers the neck spine as seven vertebrae, while the movement analyst sees it as six upper-chest and seven neck vertebrae alongside of which run the long muscles of the neck. These control the neck and the head. Movement links six chest and seven neck vertebrae into the upper section of the spine which, from the movement point of view is an independent part of the spine.

To understand fully the movement mechanisms of the human body we must gain anatomical knowledge. We must be able to imagine a clear picture of the skeleton and its joint connections which have different shapes, different mobilities, and which range from firm to loose. The shape of the joints reveals their movement possibility. We must also know how the ligaments link together and establish the skeleton and to what extent they limit the movement of the joints over which they span. We also need to know, and more importantly to feel, the task of the muscle, which in response to the nervous impulses originating from an intellectual and emotional impetus, set the skeleton in motion. Individual muscles and muscle groups set in motion joints and joint units which they span. It is, therefore, important to know where the muscles originate and where they are attached, i.e. which parts of the skeleton they link. All this helps the teacher to understand the movement foundation.

The usual method of teaching anatomy in schools is detached from live movement. I consider it essential that these two subjects be tied together as closely as possible. I build my analysis on mutual interweaving of these two standpoints. The prospective teacher of movement should have regular opportunity to compare their own theoretical knowledge with the live movement of practical sessions. It is essential to have anatomical knowledge of the movement mechanics of the human body, in order to understand movement and its analysis. I recommend that all teachers read every chapter on anatomy introduced in this book and that they form a clear mental picture of the text. This visualisation is important not once but every time a teacher encounters the anatomy in a movement session. There they must test the knowledge gained against a live body and verify the results; they must learn to recognise the deviations from the norm, i.e. the ideally built human body, by deduction and by using their own developed kinaesthetic awareness, which teaches us to recognise correct and incorrect body sensations and a perfect movement line. From the very beginning the teacher must learn to recognise the body deviations and concentrate on correction. Only by mastery of these two aspects can professionalism be achieved.

A movement which is uncontrolled and technically faulty is accompanied by feelings of uneasiness, cramped strain and consequent bad body sensations. A perfectly mastered movement is accompanied by feelings of lightness, easiness; on the whole by correct body sensations. The movement teacher is expected to lead students toward gaining these sensations which in turn will enable their body to start working correctly. We achieve this by criticism: by pointing out faults in the body posture, unnecessary tension or, on the contrary, lazy work by some muscles. The more accurately the teacher identifies the fault, the sooner the student will be aware of the fault and correct it. The teacher acquires this confidence and accuracy in the evaluation of the faults only when they are able to combine anatomical knowledge with experiences of live movement awareness.

When we reflect upon movement analysis and its significance

for teaching, we arrive inevitably at a conclusion that for dance teachers as well as choreographers it is indispensable. The dance teacher and choreographer should ask themselves in what way and to what extent do the single sections of the body participate in the entire movement. The teacher should analyse the movement in detail and define the single movements of which it is composed, not resort to demonstrating the movement and asking the students to copy it. This imitation cannot satisfy the demands for dance technique and movement art because of its incidental nature, lack of accuracy and systematic work. An imitated movement is too general, too imprecise. There is also a danger that the teacher executing the movement may make mistakes which originate from different momentary conceptions or from personal physical disposition. As a consequence, the student cannot grasp the correct shape of the movement, but grasps its approximate form and with it probably also the mistakes of the teacher.

If we lack the basic knowledge of the human body, we do not know the movement abilities of all its parts and cannot analyse them in detail. We cannot work with the students systematically, and will not recognise or foresee individual problems or imperceptible variations from the norm. These problems arise either from deficiencies or discrepancies in the body structure, or from students' individual character. Bearing in mind the beauty and harmony of movement the teacher also must step in whenever that harmony is broken. This usually involves detailed work on movement itself. By correct diagnosis, and by becoming familiar with the physical and mental characteristics of the student, individual difficulties can be diminished and finally overcome without the loss of individuality. This is the result of the cooperation between the student and the teacher. It is a matter of constructive correction in mutual trust and confidence. Imitation does not lead to self-identification, to a recognition of one's own shortcomings. It does not give the student precise instruction on how to remove mistakes and does not prepare the student for conscious, creative work.

This analysis of movement has been divided into several sections, each dealing with a particular part of the body and its basic and composite movements. The chapters follow in this order: pelvis, trunk, spine, neck and head, chest, lower and upper extremities. This order differs from the anatomical sequence because it deals above all with the importance of the particular tasks each part of the body has, while coping with total body movement.

As stated before, each section is preceded by an anatomical analysis of the relevant part. In my selection I have relied upon my own teaching experience and on the discovery that it is necessary first to have the knowledge of the skeleton, the joints, ligaments and muscles in order to understand the very basis of the movement. That concerns its technical aspect. However, in the study of artistic movement we must pursue artistic aims and therefore must deal with the aspect of expression.

Artistic perfection reflects itself in a rhythmical, dynamic and spatial experience and in the experience of form. These must be a part of each artistic expressive movement. The descriptions of basic movements introduced in the analysis give data about a perfect execution; at the same time the technical aspect brings the first prerequisite to expressive movement, i.e. its precise movement form, purified from all improper 'in-between' movements, which is the result of analytical work. In regard to the rhythm and dynamics of the movement introduced in the analysis, we begin with the natural, the so-called physiological rhythm and dynamics, namely in slow tempo. The teacher wants the students to 'relish' the movement in its natural unfolding in time and strength.

In movement practice we 'transpose' the physiological rhythm and dynamics to a rhythm which can be exactly recorded in written musical values. Thus we make a step towards a dance realisation of the movement. In the analysis I introduce the *leading* and *direction* of the motion in all basic and composite movements (i.e. which body part initiates a movement). To lead a movement with one part of the body in one direction or 'in-between direction' (a direction covering any diagonal plane) is an aesthetic demand which defines even more precisely the shape of the movement (precise beginning, unfolding and ending). The *lead* of the movement awakens a spatial experience, a relationship to space. This follows the stage when students, through their work on elevated posture, became familiar with the architecture of their own bodies and began to recognise the feeling of the vertical and horizontal axes, the shape and form of the pelvis, chest and skull, i.e. to be aware of the space within their own bodies. Thus we begin to develop a relationship with the space that surrounds them, thereby including, in the simplest basic movement, an important aspect of movement expression, spatial feeling and relationship to space.

This analysis does not dispense with the necessity to classify and define movement. It deals with concepts which are uncommon or have been understood differently and need to be redefined in this context. One of these is the classification into basic, composite and complex movements which I employ in my analysis.

Basic Movement is the simplest possible movement executed by a certain part of the body in a certain joint or joint unit. It arises from given movement abilities of a joint or joint unit. The type of joint predetermines the number of basic movements that are possible. The characteristic of basic movements is that they cannot be broken up into movements that are even more simple. Such basic movement is, for example, a ventral flexing of a thigh held straight forward in the hip joint, i.e. a forward raising of the thigh. The forward movement of the thigh in the hip joint is always the same although the extent of the bending, i.e. right, obtuse or sharp angle can vary.

Composite Movement is a linkage of two or three basic movements executed simultaneously by a certain part of the body in a joint or joint unit. A new movement results which carries the characteristics of the basic movements from which it is composed. For example—if we move the thigh forward in the hip joint, simultaneously turning it out, we execute a composite movement of the thigh in the hip joint. (Not all basic movements can be joined together, for example it is impossible to link the turning out with the turning in because they contradict and negate each other. It is possible to execute them one after the other while lifting the leg forward, but the leg cannot be turned in and out at the same time.) In the descriptions I refer only to composite movements that are directionally clearly defined and that we actually use in practice.

Complex Movement is composed of basic or composite movements executed simultaneously by different parts of the body in different joints or joint units. For example, when flexing forward a turned-out leg at the hip and knee and bending the lower leg into a sharp angle with a fully stretched foot, we execute one of the complex movements of the lower limb. Through analysis we discover which parts of the lower limb participate in the movement, in what joints the movements are realised and whether they concern basic or composite movements. The example above demonstrates (a) composite movement of the thigh in the hip joint, i.e. ventral flexion in connection with external (outward) rotation, (b) a basic movement of the lower leg in the knee joint, i.e. flexion, (c) basic movement of the foot in the ankle joint, i.e. plantar flexion of the foot and (d) a basic movement of the toes in the metatarsal phalanx joints, i.e. plantar flexion of the toes.

Movements of the trunk are either rounded, which we class as basic movements of the spine, e.g. a rounded forward bend (flexion), a rounded backward bend (extension), a rounded sideways bend (lateral flexion), rotation; or concerning movement of the trunk as a whole (in its basic form) - a straight forward tilt (which is, in effect, a basic movement in the hip and ankle joints), a straight backward lean (which is, in effect, a basic movement in the knee joints); or a straight sideways shift which we subjectively perceive as a movement of the trunk in the waist but which in fact occurs in both the hip joints and spinal joints These movements will be dealt with in more detail in the next chapter.

The prospective teacher can see from the above described example the necessity for such analysis to clarify the structure of complex movements. It is on this analysis that the purity and preciseness of the movement form depends.

Explanatory Note: in my movement analysis I use certain expressions with which physical education teachers may not be familiar, e.g. the term: 'Elevated dance posture of the body, chest and head', or 'The head carried by the neck' etc. instead of the usual 'Erect body posture' or 'Straightening of the neck and head'. My reason is that I am trying to evoke in students images evoked by words. The word 'elevated' suggest lightness and space while the word 'straightened' evokes the notion of a straight line. Since it concerns the development of aesthetic perception in young human beings we must awaken and cultivate the body's sensitivity through appropriate expressions. Elevated posture is movement at rest. That is why we do not want the students to immobilise their bodies in soldier-like postures. On the contrary we try to achieve a living, lasting sensation of the body, uniting its own inner space with the space around us. I am also aware that my own way of describing the composite directional movements (e.g. forward-sideways bend-rotation etc.) may seem odd to those who do not work with these terms. Hyphens are used in my descriptions to show how composite movements are made up by a chain of single basic movements. I follow the same principle when naming the 'in-between directions', e.g. sideways-forward, sideways-downward or sideways -backward-upward etc. The hyphens are supposed to indicate at first sight that the direction e.g. sideways-forward is an oblique 'in-between direction' between two straight directions and that the movement does not pass either directly forward or directly sideways but exactly in the middle of both directions. The direction sideways-forward is the result of two straight directions, the direction sideways-backward-upward is the result of three straight directions.

The direction of movement is a very important element in dance technique and that is why I introduce it in the analysis of all basic and composite movements. When I mention a contra-direction, I mean a simultaneous feeling of two opposite directions which enhance the plasticity of the movement. The terms 'turning in' and turning out' of the limb apply to their position in relation to the middle axis of the body. The upper limb is called in movement practice an arm. I divide the arm into upper arm, forearm and hand; the lower limb is called a leg and is divided into thigh, lower leg and foot. What I call a 'hip' is the upper-lateral part of the pelvis. The so-called 'horizontal of the hips' is formed by a connecting line between the front upper processes of the hip bones; the 'horizontal of the shoulders' by a connecting line between the mid-points of the shoulder joints.

When I mention relaxation of the joints I am referring to a certain loosening of the nearest muscle fibres which support the joint capsule; it does not concern the muscles which actually move the joint while they contract and firm up. When I talk about muscle relaxation, I do not mean that the muscles must go so slack that their readiness for any movement activity disappears. There are, of course, exceptions like a passive lying down or a temporary state during the suspension in certain kinds of swings. During maximal tension, the muscles must retain a certain degree of suppleness to avoid cramped excessive tension. Even in the highest muscular activity it is necessary to achieve a sensation of general easiness which is a psycho-physical feature of movement skill.

In conclusion I must emphasise that the descriptions of the basic and composite movements in this part of the book are not exercises and that their order is not determined by any methodology but by the demands of a systematic order.

1. The Pelvis

The pelvis has been selected as the first body part, with its basic and composite movements, to be analysed here because of its important role as mediator between the upper and lower halves of the body. The pelvis, therefore, plays the most important part in body posture, whether it be in a resting position or in motion.

First of all, we must be aware of how useful a knowledge of anatomy can be in answering some of the questions which are important for movement analysis. The questions are: what is the skeletal basis of the part of the body, the movements of which are being analysed? Which joints are responsible for these movements? What are the movement possibilities of these joints? Which muscles carry out the movements that are being examined? The answers can be found in ANATOMY below.

I

ANATOMY: THE PELVIS OR PELVIC GIRDLE

The bones of the pelvic girdle consist of two hip or innominate bones, which with the sacrum, form the *pelvic girdle* (Figure 9)

In the middle portion of the outer side of each innominate bone, there is a deep socket called the *acetabulum*, which articulates with

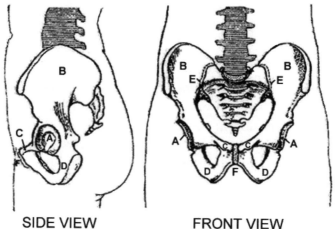

SIDE VIEW   FRONT VIEW

Figure 9: The pelvic girdle

A – Acetabulum

B – Ilium   D – Ischium

C – Pubis   E – Sacro-iliac joints

                             F – Pubic junction

the head of the thigh bone or femur. The broad flat blade of bone above the acetabulum is called the *ilium*, the arch of bone below and in front of it the *pubis*, and the part below and behind, the *ischium*; the last forms the bony prominence in the buttock.

Each innominate bone is attached to the sacrum by strong ligaments, forming the *sacro-iliac* joints. In front, the two bones of the pubis are joined together to form a slightly movable joint, thus completing the pelvic girdle. In childbirth the ligaments supporting these joints become relaxed, allowing an increase in the size of the pelvic outlet.

The main function of the pelvis is to provide a solid base through which weight can be transmitted to the lower limbs from the upper part of the body; it also provides attachment for the very powerful muscles of the legs and lower part of the back.

The Hip Joint

The hip joint is a ball and socket articulation formed by the cup-shaped cavity of the acetabulum and the head of the femur. It is surrounded by a strong capsule and very strong ligaments upon which it is largely dependent for its stability; the ligaments in front of the hip joint are the strongest in the body.

Movements of the hip joint (Figure 10) are:

(1) raising the thigh or *flexion*;
(2) bracing the thigh backward or *extension*.
(3) raising the thigh sideways away from the other leg or *abduction*.
(4) moving the thigh from a position of abduction across the other leg, called *adduction*.

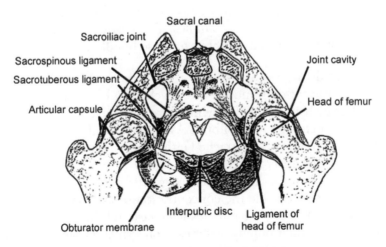

Figure 10: Frontal section of the pelvis showing both hip joints

(5) rotation of the thigh outward or *external rotation*.

(6) rotation of the thigh inward or *internal rotation*.

(7) circular movement or *circumduction*; this is a combination of the above movements.

Dislocation of the normal hip joint occurs when very considerable violence is applied. It often results from a severe impact against the knees when a person is in the sitting position, which drives the head of the femur backward over the margin of the acetabulum. It occurs in motor accidents when the knees are impacted violently against the dashboard.

THE MUSCULAR SYSTEM

The muscles of the human body constitute about 45 per cent of its total weight. There are three varieties of muscle tissue:

(1) that which produces movements of the bony skeleton, under voluntary control, called *striped* or *voluntary* muscle;

(2) that which forms the muscular coats of the intestine, bladder, arteries and many other structures; it is not under voluntary control and is known as *unstriped* or *involuntary* muscle;

(3) that which is striped but involuntary; this kind of muscle is found only in the heart and is called *cardiac* muscle.

This book is concerned with the first variety of muscle tissue only.

The structure of muscle

Voluntary muscle is made up of a large number of fibres. A muscle fibre is approximately 4 cm. long and about as thick as a human hair; under the microscope it has a characteristic transverse striping which is not present in involuntary muscle. Each fibre is enclosed in an elastic sheath and is attached to other fibres to form longitudinal strands, which are arranged in parallel bundles. The fleshy belly of a muscle is composed of an enormous number of these bundles.

Muscle tendon

The extremities of each muscle are attached to bony or other structures either by bands of strong white fibrous tissue called *tendon* or by direct attachment of muscle fibres. As a general rule, the end of the muscle nearer the trunk is attached either by its muscle fibres or by a short tendon, whereas the end further away from the trunk is more often attached by a tendon which is of greater length.

Tendons make possible the concentration of the force of powerful muscles on small areas; the muscles which extend the knee, for example, concentrate their pull by this means on a small projection of bone in front of the upper end of the tibia or shin bone. Tendons also enable muscles to act from a distance, for example, the long tendons of the muscles of the forearm which bend the fingers; the mass of muscle is thus closer to the source of its blood supply and away from the fingers whose mobility it would hinder.

The origin and insertion of muscle

The main function of voluntary muscle is to produce and control movements of the body and to maintain natural posture by acting upon the bony structure; an individual muscle is usually attached by a tendon to the bone it moves; this point of attachment is called the *insertion*; the muscle is fixed at its other end either with or without a tendon to another bone or to some other structure; this point of attachment is called the origin. Not all muscles have these simple origins and insertions on account of variations in shape, size and location.

The reverse action of muscle

The simplest mechanical form of muscle action is contraction, by which the points of origin and insertion are drawn towards each other; muscles can therefore work in a reverse way, if the bone which is usually moved is fixed; a simple example illustrates this fact; in opening a door, the door is pulled by the moving arm towards the body, but if the door is locked and the attempt to open it is continued, the hand and arm remain fixed and the body is pulled towards the door.

Lever action of muscle

Muscles are arranged in the body in such a way as to concentrate the maximum power in the minimum space; this economy of effort is mainly brought about by a system of levers and pulleys.

Muscles acting upon more than one joint

There are many instances in the body where a muscle acts upon more than one joint. A muscle can produce the same type of movement; for example, flexion in each of the joints over which it passes; or it may produce flexion in one joint and extension in another. The two different types of movement may be produced simultaneously or separately. For example, the long tendons which flex the fingers pass over several joints, producing in each one the same type of movement, namely flexion; the quadriceps muscle, however, a part of which originates from the front of the hip bone, can flex the hip and extend the knee; in walking or running, it is performing both movements; when the knee joint is held fixed, it flexes the hip; if the hip joint is fixed, it extends the knee.

Types of muscular work

It has already been mentioned that the simplest form of muscle action is contraction by which the points of origin and insertion are drawn towards each other. This type of muscle work is sometimes called *concentric*; for example, when picking up a book from a table, the muscles which flex the elbow are doing concentric work.

Static work is done when the muscles do not shorten or lengthen visibly —the book is held steady in the hand. The muscles of posture perform static work when a person is standing still.

Eccentric work is done when muscles lengthen; when the book is replaced on the table, the muscles which flex the elbow elongate as the book is lowered on to the table.

Muscles of the pelvis (Classification)

There are two muscles which lie on the posterior wall of the abdomen which act upon the lower limb. Their main action is flexion of the thigh.
  i   the *psoas**
  ii   the *iliacus*

Muscles of the buttocks (Classification)

The three muscles of the buttocks are mainly extensors and abductors of the thigh:
  i   the *gluteus maximus*;
  ii   the *gluteus medius*
  iii the *gluteus minimus*

Muscles of the pelvis (Arrangement and action)

(i)   The *psoas major* (Figure 11, p. 193) is a long muscle which is situated at the back of the abdomen; its lower portion crosses the inner surface of the upper part of the innominate bone and passes out over the rim of the pelvis into the upper part of the thigh.

Origin: from the transverse processes and bodies of the last thoracic and all the lumbar vertebrae.

Insertion: into the lesser trochanter below the neck of the femur.

Action: flexes the thigh and assists in internally rotating the femur. When the thigh is fixed it pulls the trunk forward or prevents it falling backward; it assists in maintaining the erect posture.

(ii) The *iliacus* (the muscle of the ilium. Figure 11) is a broad flat muscle lying on the inner surface of the ilium.

Origin: from the whole inner surface of the ilium.

---

*Psoas means of the loin

Insertion: into the lesser trochanter in conjunction with the tendon of the insertion of the psoas.

Action: it has a similar action to that of the psoas.

Muscles of the buttocks (Arrangement and action)

(i) The *gluteus maximus* (the largest muscle of the buttock, Figure 12, p. 191) is a very large and powerful muscle which gives the buttock its rounded appearance.

Origin: from the posterior portion of the ilium and the back of the sacrum and coccyx.

Insertion: into the posterior aspect of the upper third of the femur below the greater trochanter.

Action: extension of the hip joint; it is one of the most important of the muscles which maintain the erect posture and is also the chief muscle of forward propulsion; long distance runners always have well developed gluteal muscles.

(ii) The *gluteus medius* (Figure 13, p. 194) and (iii) *gluteus minimus* (the medium-sized and smallest muscles of the buttock): these muscles are situated underneath the gluteus maximus; the gluteus medius covers the minimus and the latter cannot therefore be seen in Figure 13.

Origins: from the outer surface of the ilium.

Insertions: into the greater trochanter of the femur.

Actions: abduction of the femur when the pelvis is the fixed point; if the femur is the fixed point, they tilt the pelvis toward their own side thus raising the opposite limb from the ground; this action occurs in walking and running. If these muscles are affected so that they cannot perform this action, the gait becomes an exaggerated waddle, like the progression of a duck; the tilting of the pelvis must then be effected by bending the whole trunk sideways from the limb which is being lifted forward.

Muscles of the abdomen

The anterior and lateral muscles of the abdominal wall consist of three pairs of broad sheet-like muscles, namely:

(i)   the *external obliques,*
(ii) the *internal obliques,*
(iii) the *transverse muscles,* and
(iv) the long pillar-like *recti abdominis* or vertical muscles of the abdomen.

The origins, insertions and actions of these eight muscles are complex, and stress is here laid upon their functions rather than their precise actions.

The oblique and transverse muscles cover the abdomen in front and on each side, lying in close contact one with another; the two recti abdominis, one on each side of the midline, extend the whole length of the front of the abdomen.

The outer layer of the abdominal musculature is formed by the two *external oblique* muscles, each of which is a broad, flat muscle extending from the lower ribs to the groin, its fibres directed obliquely downward and inward. The fleshy part of the muscle emerges into a thin but very broad, tendinous sheet called an *aponeurosis*, which transmits the pull of each muscle over a wide insertion.

Origin: from the lower eight ribs.

Insertion: by means of the aponeuroses of the two muscles which blend with one another in the midline of the body, represented by an imaginary line between the sternum and the pubic junction. Each aponeurosis is also inserted below into the *crest of the ilium** and into a strong ligament—the *inguinal ligament*—which is a condensation of the lower fibres of the aponeurosis of the external oblique, and stretches between its attachments to the crest of the ilium and the crest of the pubis**.

The middle layer of the abdomen is formed by the two *internal oblique* muscles, each lying under the corresponding external oblique muscle. Most of the fibres of the internal oblique run obliquely upward and inward. the line of pull of the muscle directly opposing that of the external oblique of the opposite side.

Origin: from the inguinal ligament, the crest of the ilium, and by a tendinous sheet from the lumbar vertebrae.

Insertion: by an aponeurosis into the aponeurosis of its fellow on the opposite side, into the crest of the pubis and the lower six ribs.

The arrangement of the aponeurosis of the internal oblique mucles is particularly interesting. The upper two thirds of each aponeurosis splits into two layers as it approaches the front of the belly and reunites again shortly before the two aponeuroses join together at the midline. The two spaces thus left between the layers of the internal oblique are filled by the two recti abdominis muscles. This arrangement adds greatly to the strength of the anterior abdominal wall. The lower third of each aponeurosis does not split but passes in one layer in front of the rectus with the aponeurosis of the inner muscle layer (see Figure 14, p. 194).

The inner layer is formed by the two *transverse* muscles (Figure 15, p. 195) which lie immediately beneath the internal oblique muscles. The fibres are directed horizontally and merge, like those of the

---

*The crest of the ilium is the uppermost margin of the innominate bone
**A ridge of bone each side of the junction of the two pubic bones in front

oblique muscles into aponeuroses, each of which joins the combined tendinous insertion in the midline

Origin: from the inguinal ligament, and the iliac crest, by tendinous bands from the lumbar vertebrae and from the lower six ribs.

Insertion: into the midline and the crest of the pubis.

The *recti abdominis.* The anterior part of the abdominal wall is supported by the two recti abdominis (Figure 14) whose fibres run in a vertical direction.

Origin: from the crest of the pubis.

Insertion: into the cartilages of the fifth, sixth and seventh ribs.

Action of oblique, transverse and recti abdominis muscles: the fibres of the three flat muscles of the abdominal wall are arranged in a crisscross fashion (Figure 15, p. 195); this arrangement not only provides strength without bulk, on the three-ply principle, but allows a considerable variety of movements.

The two powerful pillars of the recti abdominis give additional strength in front where the pressure of the abdominal contents is most concentrated. The actions of these four pairs of muscles are of a somewhat complex nature. Their first and most important function is to act as a support for the abdominal contents and indirectly as accessory muscles of respiration. They are able to accommodate themselves to varying degrees of intra-abdominal pressure. When, for example, a person who has been lying on his back, stands up, the increased pressure on the anterior abdominal wall is counteracted by these muscles; coughing, or straining as in defecation, causes a considerable increase in pressure.

The second function of the anterior and lateral abdominal muscles is to assist in maintaining erect and moving the vertebral column; the movements may be divided into:

(i)   sideways bending of the vertebral column performed by the obliques and rectus of one side assisted by the posterior abdominal and spinal muscles of the same side;

(ii) rotation of the vertebral column; this movement is carried out by the external oblique of one side acting with the internal oblique of the opposite side, in conjunction with the rotator muscles of the spine;

(iii) flexion of the vertebral column performed mainly by the recti abdominis.

The actions of the muscles of the anterior abdominal wall are not in fact separated artificially as they must be for purposes of description; it is important to remember that all muscles, particularly those in groups, act in support of one another and seldom produce a single simple movement under natural conditions of life.

Muscles of the posterior abdominal wall

The *quadratus lumborum* (the quadrilateral muscle of the lumbar region, Figure 16, p. 195): each muscle lies at the side of and parallel to the lumbar portion of the vertebral column.

Origin: from the crest of the ilium.

Insertion: into the twelfth rib and transverse processes of the first four lumbar vertebrae.

Action: the quadrati lumborum acting together draw down the last ribs and act as accessory muscles of respiration by helping to fix the origin of the diaphragm; each muscle acting alone bends the trunk to its own side. The remaining muscles of the posterior abdominal wall will be described with the muscles of the lower limb.

Muscles of the pelvis

There are four pairs of muscles forming the floor of the pelvis. The muscles of the pelvic floor will not be discussed here.*

II

THE POSITIONS OF THE PELVIS

There are four recognised positions of the pelvis, the basic position and three transitional positions. The pelvis is connected by firm joints to the sacrum and loose joints to the thigh bones (femurs). Small shifting on the femoral heads and mobility of the lumbar spine enable the pelvis to change its relation to the legs and to the thorax. In order to define the differences between the four positions we must pay attention to these changes.

The basic position of the pelvis is the established position as we recognised it in the analysis of the correct body posture. In this basic position, the pelvis forms, with the thigh bones, an obtuse angle open to the front. The pelvis is tilted slightly forward. The connecting line between the frontal tips of the iliac bones (anterior superior iliac spine) is horizontal. It is necessary to apply pressure of the abdominal muscles from the front, and of the buttock muscles from the back, till the groins elongate upward. The work of these muscles must not therefore be absent in any pelvic movement. As a result the S-shaped curvature of the spine is moderated. (Figure 17).

---

*Translator's note

The vertical 'levelled' position of the pelvis is a transitory position. It is correct with certain movements of the legs and the trunk but it must not become a permanent habit as it would limit the mobility of the spine. In the vertical position the obtuse angle between the pelvis and the thighs becomes enlarged so that both parts of the body together almost form a straight line. *The movement is led* by the coccyx which sinks from its moderately elevated position towards the thighs and points almost vertically to the ground (in the upright position of the trunk). The hips are horizontal. The spine reacts to the vertical position of the pelvis by total levelling of the lumbar lordosis so that the lumbar spine forms now, with the sacrum, an almost straight line.

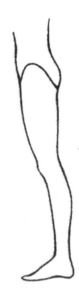

Figure 17: Basic position of the pelvis

This position is used in some squats, with legs turned out, and in some sitting positions e.g. cross-legged (Indian).

Sometimes the second position of the pelvis can also be used in the straight backward tilt of the trunk (e.g. in the kneeling position) where the pelvis is not vertical but is levelled, yet, tilted together with the trunk, backward. In the kneeling position, supported by the arms ('on all fours') the second position of the pelvis is levelled, but the position of the trunk being horizontal changes the pelvis into a horizontal position, too.

As the second position 'levels' or straightens the lumbar lordosis, it is evident that the determining factor is not the relation of the pelvis to the legs but to the lumbar spine, no matter in what position it is in relation to the ground (e.g. in the lying position on one side of the body. This position is used in some sitting positions, squats and in some movements where the trunk is tilted forward).

The levelled position of the pelvis is achieved by an increased activity of the abdominal and the buttock muscles.

The 'tucked-under' position of the pelvis is also a transitory position and it should not become a habit for the same reason as in the vertical position. The American Dr B. Mensendieck promoted the 'tucked-under' position as a corrective posture for women in the last century. The fashion of that era dictated the wearing of corsets, which emphasised and aggravated the lordosis of the spine. The habit of holding the pelvis in a permanent 'tucked-under' position, however, tempts the student to hold the thoracic spine in a slack manner. This is also harmful to the spine.

To change the basic pelvic position into the 'tucked-under' position, the pelvis changes from slightly tilted forward to moderately tilted backward. *This movement is led* by the sacrum moving backward and the coccyx changing its direction to inward (forward-down). The coccyx in this position moves towards the thighs even more. The tilting backward of the pelvis in the hip joints also causes the slight bending of the knees and the ankle joints. This position must involve the abdominal muscles more actively. The work of the abdominals is complemented by pressing the hip joints from the front and simultaneously increasing the downward pull of the lower rib cage by the straight abdominal muscles. The hips are kept in a horizontal line.

The spine reacts to this by curving its lower part, especially the lumbar section so that when seen from the side, it forms together with the pelvis a kind of a deep basin opening to the front. The curvature of the lumbar spine is performed by m. iliopsoas and its antagonist m. quadratus lumborum reacts by a maximal elongation. The perfect line of the 'tucked under' position of the pelvis demands that this antagonistic muscle activity is perceived and felt fully. (This position is used, for example, in sitting on heels and in squats with knees together.)

The tilted position of the pelvis is achieved by lifting of the coccyx and by tilting of the ilium (hip bones) forward so that the lumbar lordosis increases. Students should not achieve this position by slackening the muscles. On the contrary, the muscles should be kept active (the abdominal wall must draw the contents of the abdomen inside the abdominal cavity). This position is frequently used in Afro-American dances, jazz dance, belly dance etc.

None of these above-mentioned positions must become a habit. The second, third and fourth positions especially would result in an incorrect function of the spine and legs, and the fourth position would have a negative influence on breathing. In the cultivated movements of daily life, the first position dominates with an occa-

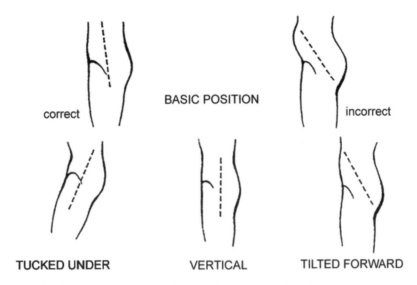

correct   BASIC POSITION   incorrect

TUCKED UNDER   VERTICAL   TILTED FORWARD

Figure 18: Basic position of the pelvis and its transitional positions

sional transition into the second and third position.

Mastery of the basic position of the pelvis and its transitory positions is a pre requisite to further technical skills. On the basis of these skills the pelvis becomes a firm and controlled centre of the moving body and it balances the harmonious beauty of its movements.

III

BASIC AND COMPOSITE MOVEMENTS OF THE PELVIS

While analysing the pelvic movements we must be aware that the pelvis cannot in reality be isolated from the neighbouring parts of the body. The movement of the pelvis necessarily affects the lumbar spine or the thighs, or both as the case may be. The structure of the body forms a whole of which the parts are connected and mutually influence each other, it is a living organism and its harmony is perfect. The centre of the body is the sacrum which is a part of the spine. The sacrum is connected, by firm sacroiliac joints, to the pelvic bones and together they form the pelvis. It is therefore obvious that when the pelvis moves, simultaneously the sacrum moves, and its movement influences the lumbar spine.

The pelvis is connected to the thigh bones via the hip joints, therefore some of its movements, such as shifting or rotating, also influence the thigh bones. We learn this through the analysis and description of these movements. By discussing basic pelvic movements I mean the ability of the pelvis to tip in the hip joint in all directions above the femoral heads and to shift, however slightly, in all directions. Furthermore we must emphasise that each movement of the pelvis is clearly defined and perceived in regard to space and shape, and from this point of view the pelvic movements are inseparable from the movement in the hip joint. Although the movements of the pelvis are impossible without the cooperation of the lumbar spine and the thighs, the division of the pelvic movements into basic and composite is an important aid to teachers and choreographers. This fact should be taken into account with the movements of the trunk, the spine and the shoulders. The least dependent are movements of the lower and upper limbs but even these cannot be completely isolated from the neighbouring parts of the body.

There are four kinds of pelvic movements:

(1) Tilting forward, sideways and backward.
(2) Shifting forward, sideways and backward.
(3) Rotation of the pelvis.
(4) Elevating one side of the pelvis while tipping the other side.

Before concentrating on the movements of the pelvis we must be aware of the architecture of the body, e.g. its vertical axis, the horizontal line of the shoulders and above all the horizontal line of the hips. This is important because while executing the pelvic movements it is easy to make a mistake by not maintaining the horizontal line of the hips or by not changing the horizontal as precisely as the movement dictates.

In all descriptions of the basic, composite and complex movements, the description of the direction and the leading of the movement plays as important a role as the preceding direction. For that reason each direction and the leading of the movement is emphasised in italics.

THE TILTING OF THE PELVIS

The tilting of the pelvis forward: the front of the hip joint is loosened, the muscles at the back extend and elongate while the pressure of the abdominal muscles and the buttock muscles on the pelvis continues. The obtuse angle which is formed by the pelvis and the extended legs can be reduced to a right angle and even an acute angle (as is the case in a full forward bend). The more the hip joints are relaxed in front, the more deeply the pelvis tilts. The body weight is kept over the forefoot. The head and upper body passively follow the movement of the pelvis so that at the completion of its movement the head and upper body hang in a relaxed manner, the crown of the head points to the ground and the relaxed arms hang from the shoulder joints downward.

The movement is led by the hips in the *direction* forward-downward.

Recovery 1: Return the pelvis into the basic position while raising the chest into the elevated posture.

Recovery 2: a gradual elevation of the trunk 'vertebra by vertebra', i.e. through a sequential spinal roll. The head is the last to return to the initial position.

The movement is led upward-backward by the hips and the sternum directed forward-upward. In the downward movement the sinking of the chest is passive while on the recovery the elevation is an active movement and therefore has its own independent lead.

The most suitable initial position for these awareness exercises is standing with the feet apart (a wide second position in ballet).

The tilting of the pelvis sideways: when tilting the pelvis to the right, it is necessary to relax, push in and bend the external side of the right hip; and to extend and elongate the external side of the left hip while maintaining the pressure of the abdominal and buttock muscles on the pelvis. The body weight shifts towards the centre of the left forefoot, the weight therefore is released from the right foot and the knee bends slightly as a result. The pelvis tilts into an obtuse angle and the right hip sinks. The more the right hip joint relaxes and pushes in, the more deeply the pelvis tilts. The upper body follows passively the movement of the pelvis so that at the completion of its movement it hangs loosely sideways towards the ground. The crown of the head is sideways right, the right arm hangs loosely from the shoulder joint sideways away from the body, the left arm in front of the body. The horizontal of the shoulders and hips changes into a slanted line at which the left shoulder and the left hip are situated higher, the right shoulder and the right hip are lower.

The movement is led by the right hip sideways-downward.

Recovery 1: return the pelvis to the basic position while raising the chest into the vertical and the shoulders and hips into a horizontal.

Leading: the left hip, the left shoulder and sternum lead sideways -upward into an upright position.

The tilting of the pelvis backward: it is necessary to relax and release at the back of the hip joints, to extend and elongate the front part while increasing the pressure of the abdominal and buttock muscles on the pelvis. Consequently, the posi-

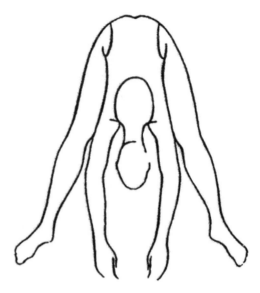

Figure 19
The pelvis is tilted forward in a standing position with the legs astride. The trunk hangs down from the hip joints.

tion of the pelvis changes from basic to 'levelled'. Then tilt the 'levelled' pelvis slightly backward. It is a small tilt in which the pelvis and the thighs form an obtuse angle opening to the back. The body weight is maintained on the centre of the front forefoot. The chest follows the movement of the pelvis passively so that at completion it hangs in a relaxed manner backward. The crown of the head points backward-downward, the relaxed arms hang down from the shoulder joints. The shoulders and hips maintain their horizontal position.

The movement is led by both hips backward-downward.

The recovery: return the pelvis into the basic position, the body is elevated simultaneously into a vertical line.

The movement is led by both hips and the sternum in the direction forward-upward.

Note: The described movements of the pelvis are introduced herein connection with movements of the spine and are not, therefore, quite pure basic movements. It is possible to practise them also in an erect standing position in such a way that the lumbar spine stays unchanged in its relation to the pelvis (with the exception of the backward tilt where the lumbar spine becomes 'levelled'). The chest always remains in the same relation to the lumbar spine so that it tilts only slightly as a unit together with the head and shoulders (it becomes 'fixed' as it were), the arms are held alongside of the trunk. Another type of 'fixing' is in the jazz dance technique when the trunk is 'fixed' in space in its original position and the pelvis moves 'by itself' (the principle of 'isolation'). All these types can be used for awareness of basic movements of the pelvis.

SHIFTING THE PELVIS

These are not independent movements but are always connected with other pelvic movements. Their execution is so important that they must be analysed separately.

The pelvic shift forward: the body is held in an elevated and upright position and while increasing the pressure of the buttock muscles, release and press slightly forward in the hip joints from the back, simultaneously stretching and extending the front part of the hip joints. It is important to maintain the pressure of the abdominal muscles on the pelvis from the front. Shift the body weight forward together with the pelvis so that when the shift is completed the pelvis is in a vertical plane above the tips of the toes with the body weight resting on them. During the movement the chest is elevated in an upright position and immobilised so that it accompanies the shift of the pelvis forward. Under the influence of the pelvic shift forward the stretched legs become tilted very slightly forward and the angle between the shin and the sole of the foot is a little more acute. The extended heels cling closely to the ground; the shoulders and hips remain in the horizontal.

The movement is led by both groins in the *direction* forward.

The recovery: return the pelvis to the basic position and the body weight to the centre of the forefoot by an increased pressure of the abdominal muscles and by a partial relaxation of the buttocks. An elevated and immobilised chest accompanies the movement of the pelvis.

The movement is led by both hips in the *direction* backward.

The shift of the pelvis sideways: when shifting the pelvis to theleft, push the right hip in without ceasing to exert pressure from the abdominal and buttock muscles on the pelvis. While the body is in an elevated and upright position, shift its weight to the little toe edge of the left foot and the big toe edge of the right foot. Both

surfaces of the soles must be held firmly to the floor. The shins tilt
slightly to the left and the lumbar spine reacts by a moderate curvature to the left. An elevated and immobilised chest accompanies
the movement of the pelvis. The shoulders and the hips remain in
the horizontal.

The movement is led by the left hip in the *direction* sideways. When
shifting the pelvis to the right the opposite procedure applies.

The recovery:gradually relax the tension of the muscles and
return to the basic position. The return is accompanied by an
increased feeling of the vertical.

The tipping of the pelvis (elevating one side of the pelvis):
while the body is in an elevated and upright position draw the left
hip of the established pelvis to the ribs. This can be achieved by
contracting the abdominal wall of the left half of the body simultaneously elongating the abdominal wall of the right half in such a
way that the right hip is pulled away from the ribs. The leg of the
drawn-up hip lightens, the heel draws away from the floor. Transfer
the body weight to the centre of the right forefoot. The chest is
immobilised in its basic elevated position. The shoulders maintain
their horizontal line but the horizontal of the hips changes into a
slanted line with the left hip raised and the right hip lowered.

The movement is led by both hips in an opposite *direction* upward
and downward.

The recovery: gradually relax the tension of the muscles and
return the pelvis to the basic position. The return is accompanied
by an increased feeling of the vertical.

The rotation of the pelvis: by an increased pressure of the
abdominal muscles on the right hip from the front and the buttock
muscles on the left hip from the back, rotate the pelvis to the right.
(The rotation to the left is vice versa). The hips are placed in a horizontal-diagonal line. The immobilised chest, neck and head are in
the meantime held in a basic, upright position. Ensure that the left
shoulder reamins frontal. The body weight rests on the centre of
the forefoot.

The movement is led by the right hip when rotating the pelvis to the
right, by the left hip when rotating to the left, in the *direction* backward. During the movement do not lose the feeling of the vertical

The recovery: return to the basic position by relaxing the abdominal and buttock muscles, retaining a strong feeling of the vertical line of the body.

Thorough detailed work on the basic pelvic movements is essential not only for the further composite movement of the pelvis but also for the movements of the trunk and the spine.

COMPOSITE MOVEMENTS

Composite movements result from a merging of two or three basic movements (which therefore must be mastered first). These must be understood as a new movement because they differ slightly in shape and direction. When merging basic movements into a new unit, firstly try to understand the specific features of each. These features are always included in the new movement.

1. Pelvic Shifts

The shift to the right forward: relax and press in the hip joints from the back (a specific feature of the pelvic shift forward). Relax and press in the left hip (a feature of the pelvic shift to the right).

Combine both movements in such a way that the forward shift is transferred more to the right half of the pelvis, press in the left hip joint and shift the pelvis in the in-between direction, right-forward. The body weight is shifted to the outer edge of the tip of the right foot and to the inner edge of the tip of the left foot. The elongated legs incline forward-right, i.e. in-between direction. The chest remains immobilised, in an elevated and upright position, the hips and the shoulders stay horizontal.

When shifting to the left-forward proceed in the opposite manner.

The movement is led by the spot between the right groin and the right hip in the in-between direction to the right-forward.

The recovery: as in both basic movements, return to the basic posture, i.e. to the feeling of the vertical line.

The shift to the right backward: combine the specific features of the basic movements so that the pressure of the abdominal muscles is increased more on the right half of the pelvis, the left hip joint is pressed in and the pelvis is shifted simultaneously backward and to the right, i.e. in-between direction right-backward. Transfer the body weight more to the heels: to the outer side of the right and to the inner side of the left. The elongated legs incline backward-right, the lumbar spine reacts by a partial levelling of the lumbar lordosis and by a moderate bend to the left. The chest remains immobilised in an upright position, the hips and the shoulders stay horizontal. They either stay facing the wall or turn as well. When shifting left-backward proceed in the opposite manner.

The movement is led by the spot between the sacrum and the right hip *in-between direction* to the right-backward.

The recovery: as in both basic movements, return to the basic posture, i.e. to the vertical.

The most frequently used composite movements are: *pelvic shifts combined with tilting of the pelvis.*

The shift forward with a backward tilt is part of the rounded backward bend of the spine as we discover its analysis.

The shift backward with a forward tilt is part of a straight-forward bend of the trunk as we discover in the analysis of the straight bends of the trunk.

The shift to the right and tilting to the left or vice versa is part of a straight shift of the trunk to the side.

The shift to the right or to the left and the tipping of the pelvis is a part of a rounded sideways bend of the spine to the left or to the right.

The shift sideways-forward or sideways-backward combined with the rotation of the pelvis is part of composite movements of the spine with torsion, for example a rounded backward bend with torsion or a rounded forward bend with torsion.

2. Rotary movements of the pelvis: circling, figures of eight

Circling: shift the pelvis along the circumference of the circle forward, forward-right, right, right-backward, backward, backward-left, left, left-forward and forward until the circle is completed or a new one starts.

The leading of the movement: each basic and composite movement is gradually completed while passing the perimeter of the circle, so the leading of the movement passes in the same way from one point on the circle to the other (as described in the above section on the individual shifts). The groins lead in the forward direction, the spot between the right groin and the right hip takes over leadership in the in-between direction forward-right, to the right etc.; so that one proceeds as mentioned before. These transitions follow from directional changes through which the pelvis passes during circling. If we can develop the feeling for the leading of the pelvis through definite points of its perimeter in all directions and between-directions, we will achieve, through movement logic, a fluent circling. The teacher must foster such bodily sensation (kinaesthetic awareness) in students; it cannot be achieved by intellectual means alone.

Perception of space while circling: the pelvis circles around the body axis and reaches the utmost limits of all the directions and between-directions through which it passes. This way, we perceive their succession and simultaneously sense the fluent path of the circling around the axis, i.e. the vertical of the body.

The movements of the figure eight situated horizontally
   – Forward and backward
   – To the right and to the left

The forward and backward figure eight of the pelvis: shift the pelvis forward-right, forward, forward-left (the forward loop); pass the centre point and continue backward right, backward, backward left (the backward loop).

The figure eight of the pelvis to the side, right and left: shift the pelvis forward-right, right, backward-right (the right loop); pass the centre point and continue forward-left, left, backward-left (the left loop).

Leading of the movements: as in circling, we arrive, through movement logic, at a fluent linking of one lead to another, along the path drawn by a figure eight.

Space awareness: in the forward and backward figure eight, perceive the path of the forward loop, the backward loop and the centre point on the body axis. The same perception occurs in the loop to the right and to the left in the sideways figure eight, with its contact point on the body axis.

Every basic movement contained in the composite movements has its own lead, for example: a pelvic shift backward combined with the rotation of the pelvis to the right. The sacrum *leads* the shift of the pelvis backward and the right hip *leads* the rotation of the pelvis to the right. The composite movement would have a lesser visual value if we did not sense the path through both leads and directions. Composite movements very often contain contra-directions, when the shifting of the pelvis backward is combined with the tilting of the pelvis forward, or the shifting of the pelvis to the left is combined with the tilting of the pelvis to the right and vice versa. The awareness of the contra-directions is even more important for the plastic beauty of the movement. Where the movement contains a rotation of the pelvis one must perceive the diagonal of the hips against the horizontal of the shoulders and the vertical of the body. The feeling of direction as well as an active leading of the movement is exceptionally important for all movements of the pelvis.

Recovery from the composite movements of the pelvis: follow the same rules as the *recovery* from the basic movements of which they are composed. Return to the basic position with an emphasised vertical line of the body by a gradual relaxation of the muscles involved. It is also possible to practise small circles and figures eight situated vertically or even tilted diagonally (in an oblique plane).

2. The Trunk

Anatomists customarily link the pelvis with the lower limbs as the 'Pelvic Girdle'. From the movement point of view, however, the pelvis is a part of the trunk and forms, together with it, one movement unit. As it is firmly bound with the sacrum, it is also connected with the movements of the spine. The trunk bends forward, sideways and backward either with a flat back, when its movement is straight and we speak about a straight forward tilt, a straight sideways shift, a straight backward lean; or it bends together with the spine and its movement is rounded. Then we speak about a rounded forward, a rounded sideways and a rounded backward bend (hyperextension) of the spine. These two types of the movement must be distinguished in the analysis clearly because they differ considerably in regard to their form.

Before the analysis of the movements of the pelvis we studied the bone structure of the pelvis and its joints connections, the ligaments and the muscles affecting its positions and movements. Now, before starting an analysis of the movements of the trunk and later on of the spine and chest, we must scrutinise closely the axial skeleton, the ribs, the breast bone (sternum) and the relevant muscles.

I

ANATOMY: THE BONY FRAMEWORK

Before describing the skeleton, it is first necessary to say a little about the nature of the material of which its various parts are composed and then to describe general types of bones, divided according to their function in the body.

Bone
Bone is a substance which provides the body with a rigid supporting framework and is especially adapted to withstand mechanical stress and strain. Two kinds of bone are found in the skeleton:
  (1) A hard, dense substance called *compact* bone; this forms the surface layer of the bone and provides the necessary rigidity. The blood supply of compact bone is maintained by numerous small vessels which pierce the surface and permeate its substance.
  (2) A soft somewhat spongy substance called cancellous bone; it forms a lattice work structure between the compact outer walls; in its interstices it contains the *marrow*.

The surface of every bone is closely covered by a strong membrane called the *periosteum*; it is richly supplied with blood vessels and acts as a medium through which the bone receives a large part of its blood supply; for this reason it plays a very important part in the repair of fractures.

Cartilage
Cartilage, commonly known as gristle, is pale, blue-white in colour and of firm but elastic consistency; though it can resist a considerable compressing force, it is of low tensile strength and can be cut quite easily with a knife. It is found in various parts of the body, for example, in the ears, nose, ribs, and in the joints where it is necessary to have rigidity and strength combined with elasticity.

Its main functions are to act as:
(1) a temporary framework for the bones and joints of children, being gradually replaced by bone as they grow.
(2) a lining to the joints between bones, increasing the accuracy of the fitting together of joint surfaces.
(3) a resilient support between bony structures to lessen the forces of shock which may be applied.

Ligament
A ligament is a collection of tough white fibres compactly fitted together to form a cord or band. Its special function is to hold bony structures together and to withstand tension; ligaments have almost no elasticity* but may become stretched under prolonged strain.

General types of bones
For the present purpose, only five types of bones need be considered; these are:
(1) the cancellous, segmental bone;
(2) the long, heavy bone;
(3) the flat, thin bone;
(4) the long, thin bone;
(5) the small, compact bone.

A typical example of the first kind of bone is one of the bones of the back, called a *vertebra*. Its main function is that of support, and it makes joints with adjacent vertebrae for movement of the vertebral column as a whole.

---

*There is a special type of ligament found between the bones of the spine which is yellow in colour and very elastic to allow spinal movement to take place.

An example of the second type, the long heavy bone, is the thigh-bone or *femur*; it is specially built to bear weight and provides a large surface at each end for strong joints.

The shoulder blade or *scapula* is an example of a flat, thin bone; its main function is to provide broad surfaces for the attachment of muscles.

A *rib* is an example of the fourth type, the long thin bone; its main function is to supply a moving framework.

The fifth type is the small compact bone which is rather like a pebble; an example is one of the bones of the wrist. Their main function is to supply the flexibility and strength necessary for the movement of the hands and feet.

THE SKELETON

The skeleton consists of the skull, the backbone, the ribs, the shoulder girdle, the bones of the upper limbs, the pelvis and the bones of the lower limbs. The anatomy of the skull does not come within the scope of this book.

The vertebral column or backbone

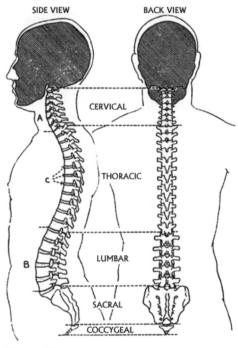

The vertebral column is divided into regions:

(1) *cervical* or neck
(2) *thoracic* or upper back
(3) *lumbar* or lower back
(4) *sacral* or base of spine
(5) *coccygeal* or tail

There are seven units, or vertebrae, in the cervical region, twelve in the thoracic, five in the lumbar; five are fused together in the sacral region to form one bone, the *sacrum*. The four small bones fused to form the *coccyx* are the remnant of the tail and serve to remind us of man's humble origin.

The vertebral column is the structure through which the weight of the upper part of the body is transmitted to

SIDE VIEW   BACK VIEW

CERVICAL

THORACIC

LUMBAR

SACRAL

COCCYGEAL

Figure 20
A – Cervical curve
B – Lumbar curve
C – Intervertebral discs

the lower limbs. There are two curves in the column which develop soon after birth, the *cervical* and *lumbar*; both curves are convex forward. The cervical curve appears when the child begins to hold up its head; the lumbar curve starts to develop when the erect position is adopted, and is at first exaggerated, giving rise to the normal hollow back and protruding abdomen of very young children but at the age of three or four, when the abdominal musculature becomes better developed, it assumes its adult shape.

The invertebral discs

A thick pad of fibrous, elastic tissue called an invertebral disc lies between one vertebra and another. These discs serve a dual purpose:
  (1) they act as shock absorbers, allowing a limited amount of movement between adjacent vertebrae;
  (2) they assist in maintaining the shape of the vertebral column, and make up about one quarter of its total length.

A typical vertebra

(Figure 21)
A typical vertebra, for example a thoracic vertebra, is composed of a body, a strong arch, four small bony processes called facets, two traverse processes and a spinous process. The body consists of a mass of cancellous bone, the upper and lower surfaces of which are flattened; the depth of the body is approximately 2.5 cm, the front and sides are rounded. The arch of bone projects backward from the body and gives protection to the spinal cord which passes between it and the body of the vertebra.

Two of the facets project upward and two project downward. These facets arise from the bases of the pillars of the arch and articulate* with the corresponding facets on the vertebrae above and below; the joints so formed allow very slight up and down and side to side movement but the aggregate of these movements in the whole vertebral column is considerable.

The transverse processes are small finger-like structures projecting outward from each side of the arch. The spinous process projects backward and downward from the top of the arch. These three

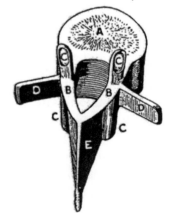

Figure 21: A typical vertebra
A – Body
B – Arch
C – Articular facet
D – Transverse process
E – Spinous process

---

*Articulate means to form a joint.

processes provide surfaces for the attachments of the muscles of the back and act as powerful levers for spinal movement.

The shape, size and structure of the vertebrae vary according to their position in the vertebral column; from the neck downward they become larger and more solid.

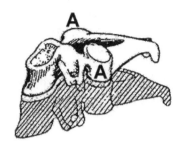

Figure 22: Cervical vertebra
A – Articular facet

The cervical vertebrae

(Figure 22)
The cervical vertebrae, with the exception of the first two, which have special characteristics and which will be described later, are smaller than either the thoracic or lumbar vertebrae, and their articular facets are shaped to allow a greater range of rotation thereby increasing the field of vision and making it nearly possible for a person to see behind.

The thoracic vertebrae

(Figure 23)
The thoracic vertebrae have small articular surfaces on the bodies and transverse processes for articulation with the ribs, which make joints with them on each side. Their spinous processes are longer than those of the other vertebrae and overlie one another closely, in this way preventing too much backward movement in the thoracic region.

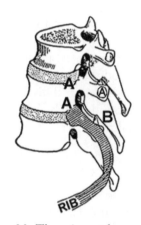

Figure 23: Thoracic vertebrae
A – Articular surface for rib
B – Spinous process

The lumbar vertebrae

(Figure 24)
The lumbar vertebrae are very much larger and stronger than

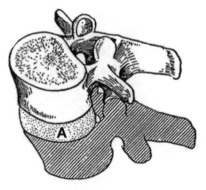

Figure 24: Lumbar vertebrae
A – Intervertabral disc

the thoracic or cervical vertebrae. For example, in the adult man, the width of the body of the fifth lumbar vertebra, the largest in the vertebral column, is about 5cm, while that of the body of the third cervical is about 13mm. The size and strength of the intervertebral discs, which lie between the vertebrae, are also increased progressively down the spine, so that they may withstand the greater weight and strain to which they are subjected.

The axis
(Figure 25)
The second cervical vertebra called the *axis* will, for the sake of convenience, be described first; it is a ring-shaped vertebra consisting of a small body, a fairly wide arch, two transverse and one spinous process for muscular attachments, and four articular facets one above and one below the base of each pillar of the arch. Its special characteristic, however, is a peg of bone which projects vertically upward from its body to articulate with the front portion of the first cervical vertebra, the *atlas*. This bony peg forms a vertical axis, as its name implies, round which the atlas and upon it, the head, can rotate in a horizontal plane.

The atlas
(Figure 25)
The *atlas*, so called because its action can be compared with that of the mythological Atlas who was thought to support the heavens upon his shoulders, is very similar in general structure to the axis, but its body

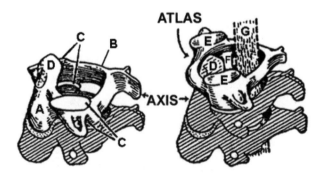

Figure 25: The axis and atlas
A – Body
B – Arch
C – Articular facet
D – Vertical peg

E – Articular facet for skull
F – Ligament
G – Spinal cord

has joined the axis to form the vertical peg. The space in its centre is divided into two parts by a strong ligament; the front part of the space is occupied by the vertical bony process of the axis and the back part by the spinal cord. The ligament holds the bony process of the axis in position and prevents it from slipping backward and injuring the cord.

The sacrum

(Figure 26)

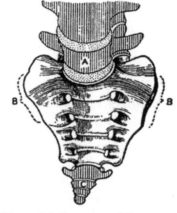

Figure 26: Sacrum and Coccyx
A – Fifth lumbar vertebra
B – Articular surface for hip bone
C – Coccyx

The five vertebrae which make up the sacrum are fused together in the shape of a concave wedge, the concavity of which faces forward. It articulates above with the fifth lumbar vertebra and, at the sides, with the inner surfaces of the two hip or *innominate* bones, thus forming the posterior part of the pelvic girdle.

The coccyx

(Figure 26)

The coccyx is continuous with the lower part of the sacrum and serves chiefly as an attachment for muscles of the pelvic floor.

II

MOVEMENT POSSIBILITIES OF THE SPINE

In terms of its movement abilities, the entire image of the spine is of primary interest to the teacher.

The spine is wedged by the sacrum in between the hip bones, and so, from the movement point of view, the sacrum is seen as the base of the spine, on which the sizeable lumbar vertebrae sit. From the lumbar section upward, the vertebrae (mainly their bodies) become gradually smaller and lower, which is significant for the mobility of the spine. The spine in motion reminds us of a stem of a plant with the head as a flower. The weakest section of the spine, the neck section, is the most mobile and the most capable of reaction. The reason for this is that it is the most articulated part of the spine, because the bodies of the neck vertebrae are lower. The differences can also be seen in size, shape and direction of the processes.

We need to pay particular attention to spinous processes. Spinous processes of the neck vertebrae are short, split on the ends into forks and point directly backward. Lumbar spinous processes have an appearance of four-angular vertical plates and they also point directly backward so that the gap between individual lumbar processes is relatively large. The spinous processes of the thoracic vertebrae are, on the other hand, long and narrow, are tilted down in a roof-like manner and the gap between individual processes is small. This fact also clarifies why the mobility of the thoracic spine in the direction ventro-thoracic (front-back) is much smaller than in the cervical and lumbar spine. The spinous processes, long and roof-like, impede above all the bending of the thoracic spine backward while its natural kyphosis, on the contrary, promotes its forward bend.

The thoracic spine has a constant tendency to stoop slightly. That is why I have created as a technical aid the term 'support point of the neck and head' and placed it in the area of the thoracic spine, between the shoulder blades. By drawing together the processes of the vertebrae we gain a firm point which helps to uplift the chest and on which the elevated neck and head are supported. It is a technical aid which proves itself in practical movement work. Without this intensified work of the spinal and neck muscles in the area between the shoulder blades, we could not achieve an elongated posture of the spine in the majority of students.

The diminished mobility of the thoracic spine is also apparent in a sideways bend, i.e. lateral flexions. The reason for this lies also in the fact that transverse processes of the thoracic spine are in a way prolonged by the ribs which cling to them. It is therefore obvious that the thoracic spine is in all directions the least mobile part of the spine and the neck spine is the most mobile.

While looking at a live human body, at its spine outlined under the skin, we realise that the seventh vertebra protrudes noticeably from the line of the neck vertebra. It differs from them, as we learnt from the anatomical analysis, by the spinous process which is longer and looks like a thickened button. Its shape resembles the spinous processes of the thoracic vertebrae. In terms of body control in movement it is an important vertebra. If we relax hold of the upper part of the chest and still lift the head, an unsightly groove between the sixth and seventh vertebrae appears. This groove becomes especially obvious during an incorrect backward bend of the neck and head where the head drops uncontrollably backward without a correct hold of the shoulders and without any back support. The front part of the neck with its protruding adam's apple and the whole neck together with the head deviate from the centre of gravity. An elevated posture of the spine in motion demands that even the seventh neck vertebra is controlled and that in the backward bend it is pushed as far as possible into line with the rest of the vertebrae, both neck and thoracic.

III

ANATOMY: THE THORAX

The bones of the thorax make up a dome-shaped structure; they are the breast bone, or *sternum*, the twelve pairs of ribs and the twelve thoracic vertebrae. Each rib is attached at the back to the body of the vertebra and the front of the transverse process. In front it is attached to the sternum by a length of cartilage called the *costal* cartilage. This cartilage gives the chest wall elasticity which makes possible the movements necessary for breathing. (Figure 27)

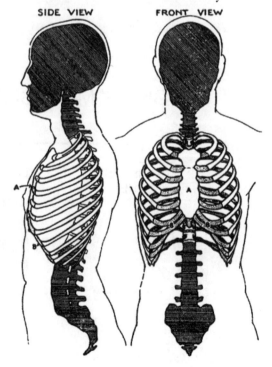

SIDE VIEW   FRONT VIEW

THE JOINTS

A knowledge of joints and their general structure, purpose and type and the direction of movement which they allow is of the greatest assistance in the understanding of muscle action. A joint, or articulation, is formed by the

Figure 27: The thorax
A – Sternum
B – Costal cartilage

meeting of two or more bones of the skeleton; it can allow free movement, slight movement or no movement at all, according to its type.

The joints of the body may be classified as follows:

(1) the *immovable* joint is a joint where the bones are united either by cartilage, for example, the cartilaginous junction between

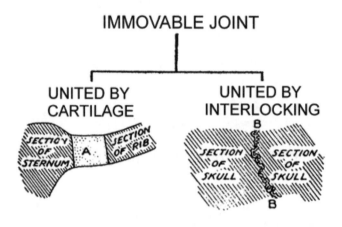

IMMOVABLE JOINT

UNITED BY CARTILAGE

UNITED BY INTERLOCKING

Figure 28: Immovable joints
A – Costal cartilage   *B – Joint between skull bones*

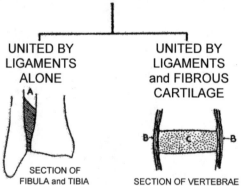

SLIGHTLY MOVABLE JOINT

UNITED BY LIGAMENTS ALONE

SECTION OF
FIBULA and TIBIA

UNITED BY LIGAMENTS and FIBROUS CARTILAGE

SECTION OF VERTEBRAE

Figure 29: Slightly movable joints
A – Ligament between lower end of tibia and fibula
B – Ligament between vertebrae
C – Cartilage

the first rib and sternum, or by a system of dovetailed edges as in the roof of the skull. (Figure 28, p. 52)

(2) the *slightly movable* joint: this consists of two bony surfaces united either by ligaments alone, such as the joint between the lower end of the tibia and fibula, or by ligaments with fibrous cartilage interposed between the bony surfaces, for example, the joints between the bodies of the vertebrae. (Figure 29)

(3) the *freely movable* joint (Figure 30): the two bone ends are covered with cartilage and connected by a fibrous capsule. The capsule is lined with smooth tissue called *synovial* membrane, which secretes a fluid to lubricate the joint, and is strengthened by ligaments, which are attached to the adjacent joint margins and whose number, strength and position depend on the particular function of the joint. A joint with a wide range of movement, such as the shoulder joint, has fewer ligaments than the hip joint which is less mobile, but which is adapted to bearing the body weight.

There are six types of freely movable joints which may be described as follows.

(i) The *gliding* joint (E): flat surfaces are in contact. Examples are the joints between the articular processes of adjacent vertebrae and between the bones of the tarsus.

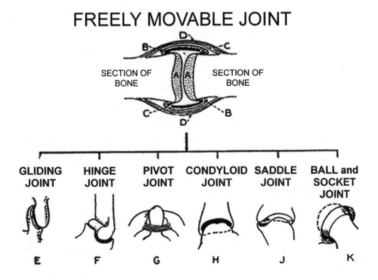

FREELY MOVABLE JOINT

SECTION OF BONE — SECTION OF BONE

| GLIDING JOINT | HINGE JOINT | PIVOT JOINT | CONDYLOID JOINT | SADDLE JOINT | BALL and SOCKET JOINT |

E   F   G   H   J   K

Figure 30: Freely movable joint
A – Cartilage
B – Capsule surrounding joint
C – Synovial membrane
D – Ligament

(ii) The *hinge* joint (F): such a joint allows movement in one plane only, at right angles to its transverse axis. Examples are the elbow, knee and ankle joints, and the joints of the fingers and toes.

(iii) The *pivot* joint (G): here a pivot-like structure, held within a fibrous ring, rotates about its long axis. Examples are the joint between the upper ends of the radius and ulna, and that between the atlas and the vertical process of the axis.

(iv) The *condyloid* joint (H): this type of joint is one in which a convex, elliptical articular surface fits into a concave articular surface. The wrist joint is an example; it allows movements in all directions, but not rotation round its central axis.

(v) The *saddle* joint (J): the surfaces of such a joint are concavo-convex and the movements permitted are like those at a condyloid joint. The carpo-metacarpal joint of the thumb is an example.

(vi) The *ball and socket* joint (K): here a spherical head fits into a cup-like cavity. Movement is permitted in any direction as well as rotation round the central axis. The hip and shoulder joints are both of the ball and socket type.

The joints of the vertebral column

The vertebral joints are:

(1) the slightly movable joints between the bodies of the vertebrae; these joints are maintained in position by two strong ligaments which run the whole length of the spine; one is attached firmly to the fronts of the vertebral bodies, and the other to the backs. Smaller ligaments bind together the adjacent surfaces of the bodies and intervertebral discs;

(2) the freely movable gliding joints between the articular surfaces projecting from the vertebral arches; each permits a gliding movement, the extent and direction of which depends upon its position in the vertebral column. The cervical and lumbar vertebrae are more freely movable than the thoracic. In addition, each thoracic vertebra has four freely movable gliding joints for the corresponding ribs.

The space between the spinous processes and arches of adjacent vertebrae is filled by a special type of very powerful ligament which is yellow in colour and, unlike the normal ligament, is very elastic; if this ligament were not elastic, forward movement of the spine would be impossible.

The movements of the vertebral column are:

(1) movement forward or *flexion*; this is the most extensive of all the movements and is most free in the lumbar region;

(2) movement backward or *extension*; this movement is most free in the cervical region;

(3) movement sideways or *lateral flexion*; this movement may take place at any part of the column, but is most free in the cervical and lumbar regions;

(4) *rotation*; this occurs to a slight extent in the cervical region, is freer in the upper region, and gradually diminishes in the lower thoracic region; it is absent in the lumbar region.

Movements in the thoracic region are limited in order to reduce interference with respiration to a minimum.

The rib joints

The head and neck of each rib form two freely movable gliding joints with the body and transverse process of the corresponding thoracic vertebrae. Each rib has its own range and variety of movement, but the movements of all are combined in breathing (see ANATOMY: THE DIAPHRAGM, p. 94.)

MUSCLES OF THE TRUNK

Muscles of the neck

(i) The *sternomastoid* (Figure 31, p. 196): each muscle passes obliquely across the side of the neck.

Origin: from the upper part of the sternum and the inner third of the clavicle.

Insertion: into the mastoid process of the skull behind the ear.

Action: contraction of the muscle of one side draws the head towards the shoulder of the same side; it also rotates the head to face towards the opposite shoulder. Both muscles acting together with the sternum as the fixed point flex the head and the cervical part of the vertebral column; but if the head is fixed by other muscular contraction, the sternomastoids are capable of acting as accessory muscles of respiration by helping to elevate the thorax.

The deformity known as *wryneck* is due to a chronically contracted sternomastoid; another condition in which the sternomastoids are affected is called *spasmodic torticollis*. Sufferers are unable to keep their heads still, either jerking them quickly or turning them in a slow and sustained fashion. It is due to a nervous disorder and other muscles of the neck and head are often affected.

(ii) The *longus colli* (long muscle of the neck, Figure 32, p. 194): each muscle is situated on the anterior surface of the vertebral column between the atlas and the third thoracic vertebra.

Origin: from the fronts of the lower cervical and upper three thoracic vertebrae.

Insertion: into the fronts of the upper cervical vertebrae.

Action: its chief action is to flex the cervical portion of the vertebral column.

(iii) The *scaleni* (scalene muscles*): there are three of these muscles on each side of the neck beneath the sternomastoids.

Origins: from the transverse processes of the cervical vertebrae.

Insertions: two into the upper surface of the body of the first rib and the third into the body of the second rib.

Actions: the scaleni bend the neck forward when acting together; when those of one side only are acting, they bend the neck to that side and turn the face toward the opposite shoulder. They can act as accessory muscles of respiration like the sternomastoid; the runner in a quarter-mile race usually finishes with his head and neck thrown well back in order to make full use of these accessory muscles of respiration.

(iv) The *splenius capitis* (the splint of the head Figure 33, p. 195): this muscle is situated over the posterior aspect of the cervical and upper four thoracic vertebrae. It takes origin from the spinous processes of cervical and thoracic vertebrae and is inserted into the mastoid process of the skull. Both muscles acting together draw the head directly backward; each splenius muscle acting separately bends the head to its own side.

(v) The *splenius cervicis* (the splint of the neck, Figure 33): arises from the spinous processes of the third to the sixth thoracic vertebrae and is inserted into the transverse processes of the upper two or three cervical vertebrae. It acts in conjunction with the splenius capitis.

Muscles of the spine

The muscles of the spine may be divided into two main groups each consisting of many muscles.

(i) the *long*, for example the large *sacrospinalis* (muscle of the sacrum and spine) on each side of the lower part of the back;

(ii) the *short*, consisting of (*a*) muscles rotating one vertebra upon another, and (*b*) muscles extending or tilting one vertebra upon another.

The long spinal muscles (Figure 34, p. 197) extend from the sacrum to the base of the skull and lie behind the angles of the ribs and the transverse processes of the vertebrae.

Origins: from the sacrum, the innominate bone, the spinous and transverse processes of the lumbar, thoracic and cervical vertebrae and the ligaments connecting these bones.

---

*Scalene means with sides of differing lengths.

Insertions: into the spinous processes of the lumbar, thoracic and cervical vertebrae, the base of the skull and the angles of the ribs; the object of this arrangement is to distribute the pull of the long spinal muscles over the widest possible area and allow movements of extension at different levels of the spine.

Actions: these muscles are mainly powerful extensors of the spine.

The *short* muscles of the spine (Figure 34) fill in the spaces between the spines of the vertebrae and their transverse processes and lie underneath the various divisions of the long muscles.

Muscles of the thorax

(i) The *intercostales* (muscles between ribs, Figure 35, p. 197): these muscles, consisting of an internal and external layer, lie between the adjacent borders of the ribs; their main action is to pull the ribs together. There are several other small muscles which assist in moving the ribs.

(ii) The *diaphragm* or midriff (Figure 36, p. 198): this is a dome-shaped muscle which separates the thoracic from the abdominal cavity. The middle portion of the dome is composed of a broad sheet of tendon, shaped like a three bladed leaf.

Origin: in front, from the lower end of the sternum and the costal cartilages of the lower six ribs on either side; behind, from the twelfth rib and the bodies and transverse processes of the upper lumbar vertebrae.

Insertion: all the fibres from these numerous origins converge to be inserted into the central tendon.

Action: the diaphragm is the principal muscle of respiration. In direct contact with the upper surface are the lungs and heart, and in contact with the lower, are the liver in the middle and on the right, and the stomach with other abdominal organs on the left.

The lower ribs become fixed in normal inspiration to enable the diaphragm to draw down the central tendon during its contraction. It moves downward without much alteration in shape, expanding the lung above it and pushing the abdominal contents downward. When the limit of downward movement is reached, which is decided by the resistance of the abdominal wall, the central tendon becomes the fixed point, being pressed hard against the abdominal contents; as a result the lower ribs move slightly forward, outward and upward thus increasing the diameter of the lower part of the chest. Normal expiration is mainly the result of the elastic recoil of the thoracic walls, helped by the contraction of the abdominal muscles which push the abdominal contents back into their previous position.

[See MUSCLES OF THE ABDOMEN Figure 14, p. 194 and Figure 15, p. 195]

IV
BASIC AND COMPOSITE MOVEMENTS OF THE TRUNK

Basic movements of the trunk

The basic movements of the trunk are:

   a straight forward (ventral) tilt

   a straight sideways (lateral) shift

   a straight backward lean

   a torsion of the trunk

In these straight movements of the trunk the spine is 'immobilised' and retains its basic elongated and elevated position with a slight S-shaped curvature. The specification 'immobilised spine' should not be taken literally. It means that the spine does not move visibly and remains in its basic position in relation to the pelvis. We should not, however, assume that the spine stiffens into a hard immobile column: in reality the movement is very lively and active. The erect spine is elastically elongated, able to react and ready to move. The upright posture, as described, is the starting position for the basic and composite movements of the trunk. The most suitable position for these exercises is standing with feet apart with moderately turned-out legs (second position in ballet). Arms to be held along-side the trunk.

A straight forward tilt (in the hip joints) starts with a composite movement of the pelvis, i.e. tilting forward with a backward shift which is executed precisely according to the description of the pelvic movements. (See the section TILTING OF PELVIS, p. 34). The abdominal muscles are elastically elongated and the 'immobilised' spine follows the pelvic tilt without bringing any change to its

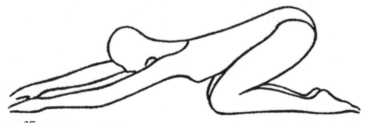

Figure 37
A straight forward tilt of the trunk in a kneeling position, executed in the hip, intervertebral and shoulder joints.

upright line. The pelvis may not always be at a right angle, but sufficiently tilted to hold the elevated sternum with the established support point of the neck and head. The depth of the tilt depends on the individual. Under the influence of the backward shift of the pelvis the angles of the thighs and shins change. The hips and the shoulders are maintained in a horizontal position.

The movement is led: the sternum leads the movement of the trunk forward; both hips lead the tilting of the pelvis forward. The coccyx leads the shift of the pelvis backward.

Direction: trunk forward.

Contra-direction: backward shift of the pelvis. The awareness of the contra-directions is important also for the technical perfection of the movement and its expressiveness.

The described execution of the straight tilt forward differs from the habitual, so-called forward tilt by: a slightly elevated thoracic spine (which is part of the elevated body posture); and the angle of the pelvic tilt which does not need to be always 90° but can be obtuse or sharp.

The straight forward tilt with an erect neck and head, and lightened chest is needed in many complex movements e.g. forward, sideways and diagonal lay-outs, a straight forward tilt of the trunk while kneeling.

A straight sideways shift (in the hip joints and in the lumbar spine): when shifting the trunk to the right, slightly tilt the pelvis to the right to an obtuse angle in relation to the legs, simultaneously shifting it to the left (see COMPOSITE MOVEMENTS OF THE PELVIS, p. 39). Start with relaxing the right hip joint and by pressing it in, then link it with an intensive elongation of the right half of the abdominal wall. The elongated trunk with its upright, elevated and immo-

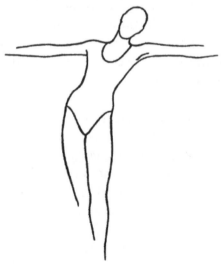

Figure 38
A straight sideways shift of the trunk in a standing position, executed in the hip, intervertebral and shoulder joints.

bilised spine follows the direction of the tilt of the pelvis, i.e. to the right. Simultaneously shift the pelvis in a contra-direction. Under the influence of the pelvic shift, the shins angle sideways-left. The hips and the shoulders must be maintained in a near horizontal line.

The movement is led: the elongated right side of the abdominal wall leads the movement of the trunk in one direction, the left extended hip in an opposite direction.

Contra-direction: pelvic shift left in opposition to the shift of the trunk to the right. The awareness of the sensation of the contra-directions is important also for the technical perfection of the movement and its expressiveness.

Straight backward lean (in the hip joints, eventually in the knee joints): start with a change of the position of the pelvis from basic to levelled (vertical) by an increased pressure of the abdominal muscles on the pelvis from the front. The lumbar lordosis almost straightens. Immobilise the whole spine including the neck and head in an upright posture. In a kneeling position the pelvis together with the trunk tilts backward from the knees. The dimensions of the movement change according to the starting position of the body. The greatest possible range for the straight backward lean is the upright sitting position (see SOME INITIAL POSITIONS OF CORRECT BEARING, p. 241). The straight backward lean always requires increased work by the abdominal and buttock muscles because the body has to maintain the pelvis in the levelled position throughout the whole movement. The degree of difficulty intensifies when executing the straight backward lean in a kneeling or standing position. In the kneeling and standing positions the lean would be quite small unless one also tilts the thighs backward together with the trunk. When standing on one foot with the free leg extended forward and its pointed toes resting lightly

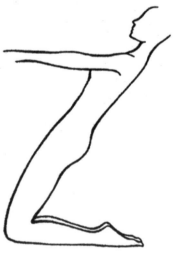

Figure 39
A straight backward lean of the trunk in a kneeling position, executed in the knee joints.

on the floor, bend the knee of the supporting leg at an obtuse angle and tilt back the thighs, pelvis and trunk. This achieves an unbroken line from the tip of the forward elongated leg to the crown of the head. The shin of the supporting bent leg tilts forward, with a sharp angle at the ankle joint. The hips and the shoulders must be maintained in a horizontal line.

The movement is led in the following manner: the crown of the head leads the movement of the trunk backward-upward, the *contra-directed movement* of the forward extended leg *is led* by the tip of the foot. In the kneeling position the *movement is led* by the crown of the head. Be aware of the contra-directory feeling in the knees.

Contra-directions: upward-backward and forward-downward.

Torsion: start with the rotation of the pelvis, the chest with the immobilised spine following the movement of the pelvis but avoiding any independent rotation of its own. The chest and the pelvis form a firm unit. In a torsion to the right, increase the pressure of the abdominal muscles on the right hip from the front and the pressure of the buttock muscles on the left hip from the back. In the case of the torsion to the left: vice versa. The hips and the shoulders move into a diagonal position in relation to the legs, which remain in their initial position of facing forward.

The movement is led: during the torsion to the right by the right hip in the *direction* right-backward, during the torsion to the left by the left hip in the *direction* left-backward.

It is necessary to maintain the exact degree and direction of the rotation because torsion is often a starting position for further movements of the trunk or spine. To experience the horizontal-diagonal of the hips and the shoulders against the frontal of the feet, while retaining the feeling of the vertical body axis against the contra-pull of the shoulders down, is necessary to spatial awareness in torsion.

The recovery is a return to the elevated posture. The spine stays immobilised even in the recovery movements. The recovery from the torsion is a consequence of gradual easing of the tension of the oblique abdominal muscles. The other recovery movements, for example from the straight backward lean to the initial position, are connected with the raising of the trunk to an upright position. The recovery of the pelvis *is led* by extended hips, the elevation of the trunk *is led* by the sternum in the direction upward.

COMPOSITE MOVEMENTS OF THE TRUNK

We combine two basic movements: a straight forward tilt with torsion, a straight sideways shift with torsion and a straight backward lean with torsion.

Straight forward tilt plus torsion to the right: rotate the trunk-with the pelvis as a whole to the right so that they form together a firm unit. Tilt the pelvis forward in 'between-direction' to the right-forward and the elongated trunk follows the movement of the pelvis, i.e. it tilts in the in-between direction to the right-forward. Simultaneously shift the pelvis to the left-backward in a movement opposite to the one of the trunk. The shins tilt to the left-backward in the direction of the pelvic shift. A straight forward tilt with torsion to the left is vice versa.

The movement of the torsion to the right *is led* by the right hip; the trunk *led by the sternum* tilts forward, in a *'between direction'* to the right-forward, the pelvic shift to the left-backward *is led* by both hips and the coccyx. The movement follows two antagonistic between-directions. In all the composite movements with torsion the hips and the shoulders have a diagonal position placed in a horizontal plane.

A straight sideways shift to the right plus torsion to the right: rotate the pelvis to the right. The trunk, with an immobilised spine, turns with the pelvis to form a firm unit. Tilt the pelvis sideways in a between-direction to the right-backward, upright trunk following the movement of the pelvis, i.e. shifting in a between-direction to the right-backward. At the same time the pelvis shifts left-forward in a contra-movement to the trunk. The shins tilt to the left-forward in the direction of the pelvic shift. A straight sideways shift to the left with torsion to the left is vice versa.

The movements are led in the following manner: the torsion to the right and the pelvic tilt *is led* by the right hip. The sideways shift of the trunk to the right-backward *is led* by the elongated abdominal wall of the right half of the trunk, the pelvic shift to the left-forward *is led* by the left groin and the left hip. The movement follows *two antagonistic between-directions.*

A straight sideways shift to the right plus torsion to the left: rotate the pelvis to the left. The trunk, with an immobilised spine, turns with the pelvis forming a firm unit. Tilt the pelvis sideways-right in a between-direction to the right-forward. The upright trunk follows the movement of the pelvis, i.e. it shifts in a between-direction to the right-forward. Simultaneously shift the pelvis to the left-backward in a movement opposite to the one of the trunk. The shins tilt to the left-backward in the direction of the pelvic shift. A straight-sideways shift to the left with torsion to the right is vice versa.

The movements are led in the following manner: the torsion to the left *is led* by the left hip, the pelvic tilt sideways-right *is led* by the right hip. The sideways shift of the trunk *is led* by the elongated abdominal wall of the right half of the trunk, the pelvic shift to the left-backward *is led* by the left hip and coccyx. The movement passes through *two antagonistic between-directions.*

A straight backward lean plus torsion to the right: rotate the pelvis to the right. The trunk, with an immobilised spine turns together with the pelvis, i.e. it forms a firm unit. Tilt the pelvis backward in a between-direction to the left-backward and the elongated trunk follows the tilt of the pelvis, i.e. leans in-between direction left-backward whilst shifting the pelvis simultaneously right-forward. The shins tilt to the right-forward in the direction of the pelvic shift. A straight backward lean with torsion to the left is vice versa.

The movements are led in the following manner: the torsion to the right *is led* by the right hip, the pelvic tilt to the back *is led* by both hips, the backward lean of the trunk by the crown of the head, the pelvic shift to the right-forward *is led* by the right hip and the right groin.

The movement passes through *two different between-directions.*

The recovery from the composite movements of the trunk is a return to the starting position. The spine remains immobilised even during the recovery movement.

The recovery of the pelvis is led by both hips, *recovery of the trunk is led* by the sternum, both in an upward direction.

CIRCULAR MOVEMENTS OF THE TRUNK
– Circling of the trunk
– Figure eights of the trunk
There are two recognised ways of circling:
– without torsion (i.e. with the hips and shoulders square to the direction faced)
– with torsion

Circling without torsion: starting with a straight forward tilt, pass into a straight sideways shift to the right, into a straight backward lean, into a straight shift to the left and into a straight forward tilt where the circle closes or a new one starts. In the transition from one basic movement into another, pass through composite movements of the trunk: a forward-sideways shift and a backward-sideways shift to the right and to the left.

The leading of the pelvis has already been described in: ROTATORY MOVEMENTS OF THE PELVIS p. 40. The circling movements of the trunk *are led* by the sternum and the crown of the head. The crown of the head circumscribes a *large circle* in space to the right or to the left, the pelvis a *small circle in the contra-direction.*

Circling of the trunk with torsion: starting with a straight forward tilt, pass into a straight forward tilt with torsion to the right, into a straight sideways shift with torsion to the right, into a straight backward lean with torsion to the right, into a pure straight backward lean, into a straight backward lean with torsion to the left, into a straight sideways shift with torsion to the left, into a straight forward tilt with torsion to the left and into a pure straight forward tilt where the circle closes or a new one starts.

The leading of the pelvis is as a basic circling of the pelvis to which one adds the *leading* of the right hip in torsion to the right and the left hip in torsion to the left. The crown of the head circumscribes a *large circle* in space to the right or to the left, the pelvis a *small circle in a contra-direction.*

Note: in a circling of the trunk and other circling movements without torsion we always stay frontal (facing forward), emphasising pure directions, i.e. forward, sideways, backward, sideways, forward. In circling with torsion we turn, under the influence of the torsion, right and left.

Figure eight forward and back without torsion: pass through a straight sideways shift to the right into a straight forward tilt, then into a straight shift to the left (the front loop), then through recovery into a straight sideways shift to the right, into a straight backward lean, into a straight sideways shift to the left (the back loop).

The lead: the movement of the pelvis *is led* gradually by the left hip, both hips, the right hip (the back loop by the pelvis), the left hip, both groins, right hip (the front loop by the pelvis). The movement of the trunk *is led* gradually by the right extended half of the abdominal wall, sternum, the left extended half of the abdominal wall (the front loop by the trunk), by the right extended half of the abdominal wall, the crown of the head, the left extended half of the abdominal wall (the back loop of the trunk).

Directions: the trunk circumscribes in space a large front and back loop, the pelvis does the same in *contra-direction* but on a smaller scale.

Figure eight forward and back with torsion: starting with a straight sideways shift with torsion to the right, gradually pass into a pure forward tilt, then gradually continue into a straight sideways shift with torsion to the left (the front loop), then through recovery from a straight sideways shift with torsion to the right into a pure straight backward lean, then into a straight sideways shift with torsion to the left (the back loop).

The lead: the movement of the pelvis *is led* gradually by the right hip, both hips, the left hip (the back loop by the pelvis), then by the right hip, both groins, the left hip (the front loop by the pelvis). The movement of the trunk *is led* gradually by the right shoulder, sternum, the left shoulder (the front loop of the trunk), then by the right shoulder, the crown of the head, the left shoulder (the back loop of the trunk).

Directions: the trunk circumscribes a large front and back loop, the pelvis does the same in *contra-direction* and on a smaller scale.

Figure eight of the trunk sideways to the right and left without torsion: pass from the straight forward tilt into a straight shift to the right, then into a straight backward lean (the right loop), then through recovery into a straight-forward tilt, into a straight shift to the left and to a straight-backward lean (the left loop).

The lead: the movement of the pelvis *is led* gradually by both hips, left hip, both groins (left loop by the pelvis), then again both hips, the right hip, both groins, (right loop by the pelvis). The movement of the trunk *is led* gradually by the sternum, the right extended half of the abdominal wall, the crown of the head (right loop by the trunk), then again the sternum, the left extended half of the abdominal wall, the crown of the head (the left loop by the trunk).

Directions: the trunk circumscribes the loop to the right and the loop to the left, the pelvis does the same in *contra-direction* but on a small scale.

Figure eight sideways to the right and left with torsion: pass from a straight-forward tilt with torsion to the right into a straight-sideways shift with torsion to the right and into a straight-backward lean in torsion (the right loop), then through recovery into a straight-forward tilt with torsion to the left, straight shift to the left in torsion and into a straight-backward lean in torsion (the left loop).

The lead: the movement of the trunk *is led* gradually by the sternum, the right extended side of the trunk, the crown of the head (the right loop), then again the sternum, the left extended side of the trunk, the crown of the head (the left loop). The movement of the pelvis *is led* gradually by the hips and groins; the torsion to the right *is led* by the right hip, the sideways shift by the left hip, the backward lean by both groins (the left hip loop by the pelvis), the torsion to the left *is led* by the left hip, the sideways shift by the right hip, the backward lean by both groins (the right loop).

Directions: the trunk circumscribes a loop to the right and a loop to the left, the pelvis does the same in *contra-direction* but on a smaller scale.

The torsion to the right or left, *led* by the appropriate hip, is followed by the chest without any independent rotation in the intervertebral joints. Despite that, both hips and shoulders are, during torsion, in a horizontal-diagonal position with regard to the vertical-frontal of the legs. The pelvis circumscribes the left loop during torsion to the right and during torsion to the left it circumscribes the right loop of the figure eight.

The technical aspect of the circular movement of the trunk is very similar to the technical aspect of the basic movements.

3. The Spine

COMMON FEATURES OF THE MOVEMENT OF THE SPINE

It is obvious from the anatomical analysis of the spine and chest and from the description of the skeleton, joints, ligaments and muscles that movement of the spine involves more than those muscles running along both sides of the spine on the dorsal and ventral sides. Some of the surface muscles of the back, muscles of the abdominal wall, hip muscles, both surface and deep chest muscles and muscles of the front area of the neck, are also involved. One can almost say that the muscles of the whole trunk take part in rounded movements of the spine.

The muscles which balance a certain movement contract and their antagonists simultaneously elongate. One controls the contraction of the muscles as well as the elongation of their antagonists through kinaesthetic awareness (muscular sensation). The spine bends in all directions and between directions. The muscles on the bending side contract actively. The sensation around the joints on that side is one of relaxation, while the opposite side elongates and the sensation around the joints is one of firmness. The ribs on the bending side move closer together, the ribs on the opposite side move apart. In the instance of the forward or sideways bend the abdominal wall on the side of the bend actively contracts and shortens, the opposite side of the abdominal wall extends and elongates. During this work it is absolutely necessary to abide by the five principles of correct body posture, otherwise the muscles will not accomplish their task to the full. This applies to all movements of the spine, basic and composite. Contraction and elongation of the muscles is active, conscious work, because it is not a matter of a passive drop of the body forward, sideways and backward which accompanies the tilting of the pelvis (see MOVEMENTS OF THE PELVIS, p. 33). It is a matter of creating balanced and harmonious arches of the spine and trunk, located precisely in space. The spine bends in basic directions, i.e. forward, sideways and backward during basic movements and in-between directions e.g. sideways-forward, and sideways-backward during composite movements.

In contrast to the straight movements of the trunk which are executed with an immobilised spine and which happen mainly in hip joints, the movements of the spine are rounded with the exception of rotation. The arc of the spine is a result of a sum of minute movements of the vertebral joints and inter-vertebral discs. The movements ripple along the length of the spine from one vertebra to another and lead into a bending of the entire spine in a certain direction or between-direction. The most important spot on the spinal arc is the sacrum. The precise and pure execution of the pelvic movement predetermines the precise and pure form of the corresponding movement of the spine.

In movement, the spine is divided into upper and lower parts. (See beginning of THE TRUNK, p. 43). Both parts can work independently. We can immobilise the lower part and bend or turn the upper part or vice versa. However, we can also move both parts simultaneously but in different ways.

In basic movements it is always a matter of compatible movement of the whole spine including the neck and head. Composite movement can be compatible movement of the whole spine but in-between directions; or it can be simultaneous but not compatible, i.e. a different movement of each or both parts of the spine.

BASIC MOVEMENTS

Anatomical terminology of basic movements of the spine:
    – forward flexion = a forward bend
    – extension =   a backward bend
    – lateral flexion = a sideways bend
    – rotation = turning
In a practical movement one uses these terms:
    – A rounded forward bend of the spine
    – A rounded backward bend of the spine
    – A rounded sideways bend of the spine
    – Rotation of the spine
My descriptions of the basic movements of the spine mainly take into consideration the bodily sensations (kinaesthetic awareness) evoked by correct and sufficient muscular work. For technical mastery it is essential to take heed from the very beginning of the leading of the movement and its spatial direction. Both elements are emphasised in the descriptions. The initial position of basic and composite movements of the spine described below is a straight posture with an erect neck and head.

Small rounded forward bend in axis: by changing the pelvic position from the basic to tucked-under, round the lower spine and

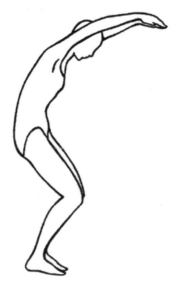

Figure 40
A small rounded forward bend in axis (started by tucking under the pelvis and rounding the spine, consequently bending the knee and ankle joints).

bend the knees (see PELVIC POSITIONS, p. 30). Control, through kinaesthetic awareness, the elongation of the posterior part of the abdominal wall and spine as far as the support point of the neck and head, while intensively contracting and shortening the front part of the abdominal wall. From the support point of the neck and head situated between sixth and seventh thoracic vertebrae, bend the upper spine forward-down. Be aware of an elongation of the neck from the support point as far as the crown of the head and, simultaneously, of a relaxation of the front of the neck. As a result, the lower spine has deviated backward from the axis, the upper spine forward. The axis of the centre of gravity runs now through the support point of the neck and head and the hip joints and above the centre of both soles of the feet, where the body weight is located. The spine is actively rounded, not slack, and forms an unbroken arch. The shoulders are maintained in their full width, do not drop them (see MOVEMENTS OF THE SHOULDERS, p. 152). The deviation of the lower spine from the axis is caused by rounding a tucked-under pelvis and by rounding the lumbar spine. The deviation of the upper spine is caused by an elongation and a rounding of the neck from the support point to the crown of the head. This results in a contra-direction of the lower spine backward-down and of the upper spine forward-down which is very important for producing the spinal arch. The established shoulders and the hips are maintained in a horizontal line.

The movement of the lower spine *is led* by both hips and the sacrum, the movement of the upper spine *is led* by the forehead.

Contra-directions are backward-down and forward-down and one must be aware of them and experience them throughout the whole movement.

Recovery: keep the pelvis in a tucked-under position. During the raising of the body, the angle of the pelvic tilt backward gradually diminishes and changes into the basic position when the erect posture is achieved.

The movement of recovery is led by the hips and the sternum. The knees straighten by the upward pull of the hips and the spine straightens by the upward pull of the sternum with a downward drawing of the shoulders in a contra-direction.

The direction of movement is *upward*.

A space awareness, above all the feeling of the body axis, is vital for the perfect form of the movement. The sensing of the body balance around the axis of the centre of gravity is characteristic of the small rounded forward bend in axis. While recovering to the upright, the leading feeling is an experience of growing, simultaneously sensing the vertical of the body as far as the crown of the head and the horizontal of the shoulders and hips. The feeling of one's own anatomical structure within space and the feeling of the spatial line of movement heightens its aesthetic quality.

Deep rounded forward bend: (a composite movement of the spine and hip joints) The vaulting of the spinal arch is similar to the one in the small forward bend in axis. It is achieved in the same manner but its depth is attained by complementing the tucked-under position of the pelvis by shifting it backward and partially tilting it forward. The tilting should be done, however, only to such an extent as the tucked-under pelvis allows. Its position should not be lost.

To add to it, relax to a larger extent all the joints of the lower limbs

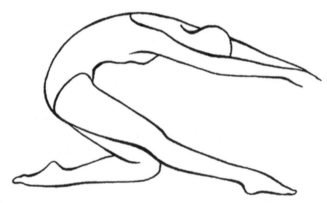

Figure 41
A deep rounded forward bend of the spine in a kneeling position on one leg, while the other leg is extended forward with toes touching the floor. This position is executed in the knee, hip, intervertebral and shoulder joints.

and bend in the hip joints, so that the arch of the upper spine points forward-down. The shoulders and the hips are kept in a horizontal.

The movement of the lower spine *is led* by both hips and the sacrum, the movement of the upper spine *is led* by the forehead.

The contra-direction is forward-down and backward-down and should be felt intensely.

Recovery is in the same manner as in the small rounded forward bend, namely by the conscious leading of the hips and the sternum in the direction upward. The significance is in the feeling of growing upward, ended by an awareness of the vertical as far as the crown of the head and accompanied by the feeling of the horizontal of the shoulders and the hips.

Small rounded backward (thoracic) bend (extension): establish the support point of the neck and the head, thus increasing the arching of the upper ribs and the sternum. Press in the seventh neck vertebra and elongate the muscles from the sternum to the chin, i.e. arch while bending the upper part of the spine backward through high release. Balance the upward-backward pull by drawing the lower ribs and the shoulders down. This way we avoid the excessive curvature of the lumbar and the cervical spine. Increase pressure of the buttock muscles on the hip joints from the back, thus shifting the pelvis and the body weight above the toes. Simultaneously, tilt the pelvis backward by an increased pressure of the abdominal muscles on the hips from the front. At the same time contract the posterior part of the abdominal wall and of the ribs, especially in the spot between the shoulder blades and below them; under pressure of the shoulder blades, the ribs ease inward. Just as in the active bend of the spine forward-down in the rounded forward bend, the active bend of the spine backward in the rounded backward bend must form a perfect, unbroken arc. This means that one must not lose the continuity of the movement in which the whole body takes part. The shoulders and the hips are maintained in a horizontal.

The movements are led in the following manner: the movement of the lower spine by the groins, the movement of the upper spine by the sternum and the crown of the head.

At the completion it is important to feel the elongation of the back of the neck in the direction of the crown of the head, i.e. not to straighten the head by drawing the chin down.

Directional feeling of the backward bend is upward-over-backward. If the direction backward outweighs or occurs before the desired height of the sternum and chin is achieved, the forming of the spinal arc is at risk.

Recovery is through an increased pressure of the abdominal muscles on the pelvis from the front and a simultaneous pressure on the ribs from the back. Return the pelvis and the spine to the initial position by elongating the back of the neck, not by moving the chin. Even here, the rule of the activity of the hips and the sternum applies during the recovery. The body weight returns to the middle of the forefeet.

The movement is led by the hips and the sternum.

Direction: upward, during which one experiences a strong feeling of a return to the vertical, and the horizontal of the hips and the shoulders.

Deep rounded backward bend — hyperextension (a composite movement of the spine and the leg joints): the forming of the spinal arc starts the same way as in the small backward bend. It is accompanied by the same body sensations which flow out of sensitively experienced muscular activity but in a more intensive and enlarged form. Increase the pelvic shift forward and the backward tilt, relax the front of the ankle joints making the angle much more acute so that the groins move in front of the toes. Retain the elongation of the front part of the body (anterior) from the ankle up to the chin. Strive to have the sternum supported by the posterior wall of the chest and the shoulder blades; the sternum must remain the highest and most emphasised spot of the arc, although not only the upper spine but the whole body tilts backward-down through high release. Through the activity of all participating muscles, one balances the

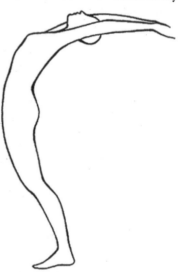

Figure 42
A deep rounded backward bend (hyperextension) of the whole spine with arms above the head, executed in the pelvis and the intervertebral and shoulder joints.

movement of the body into a perfect unbroken arc, maintaining the shoulders and the hips in a horizontal.

The movement is led by the groins, the sternum and the crown of the head in the *direction* forward-up and backward-down. The feeling of height must be attained during the whole movement as the forming of the spinal arc depends on it. The neck muscles must support the head so that the excessive bending of the neck does not interrupt the arc of the whole spine and the swelling of the front of the neck is avoided.

Recovery: first of all, raise the chest through an increased pressure of the shoulder blades on the ribs from the back and through the upward pull of the sternum. Then proceed as in the recovery from the small backward bend, i.e. increase the pressure of the abdominal muscles on the pelvis from the front, so that it returns to its basic position without interrupting the movement of the upper chest. In this way the body returns to the initial elevated posture.

The movement is led by the hips and the sternum in the direction upward. The feeling of an upward-growing leads into the feeling of the vertical of the body and the horizontal of the shoulders and the hips.

Small rounded sideways (lateral) bend: when bending the spine to the right, shift the pelvis in an opposite direction to the left and slant it simultaneously, i.e. elongate the left half of the abdominal wall and contract the right half. The left hip moves away from the ribs, the right moves towards them (see BASIC AND COMPOSITE MOVEMENTS OF THE PELVIS, p. 33). At the same time, transfer the body weight to the outer edge of the left and the inner edge of the right sole. Both elongation of the abdominal wall and the opposite contraction is transferred much further in the ribs. The ribs of the left side move away from each other while the ribs of the right side move closer to each other so that the lower and the upper ribs on this side draw together at the level of the support point of the neck and head, in this case located approximately under the armpit.

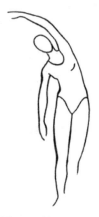

Figure 43
A small rounded sideways (lateral) bend of the whole spine executed in the pelvis and intervertebral joints.

The shoulders as well as the hips have now a slanted position, with the left shoulder higher than the right but the left hip lower than the right. Transfer the elongation of the left side of the trunk even further onto the left side of the neck as far as the area behind the ear, which is the highest spot of the small rounded lateral bend. The right side of the neck and head bend to the right, the right ear moves towards the shoulder. The chin forms a right angle with the front plane of the neck and remains above the sternum. (When adding the lifting of the arm to the movement, the fingertips are above the crown of the head.)

The movement is led in the following manner: the lateral bend to the right *is led* by the left hip, the left ear and the right temple.

Contra-directions: sideways-up (left side), sideways-down (right side). One feels distinctly the direction of the left ear upward, the left hip to the left and the contra-direction of the right temple, tilted right-downward. Even in this movement of the spine, the feeling of height must dominate. It shows above all in the elevated hold of the sternum.

Recovery: relax the extension of the left side of the body and return to the initial posture by pulling the right hip and the left shoulder down while simultaneously elevating the sternum.

The movement is led by the right hip and the left shoulder in the direction downward while the sternum *leads* in the direction upward. The return is to the vertical of the body and the horizontal of the shoulders and hips.

Deep rounded lateral bend (a composite movement of the spine and pelvis): increase the rounded lateral bend by increasing the pelvic shift in the contra-direction. Otherwise, all components of the small rounded lateral bend are retained.

Recovery: the activity of all participating muscles, above all the activity of the upper chest, increases and leads to the final balanced body posture with the emphasised vertical of the body and the horizontal of the shoulders and the hips.

Rotation of the spine: during rotation of the spine, the chest, the neck and the head rotate while the pelvis is immobilised. Stabilise the pelvis in a forward-facing position by an increased pressure of the abdominal muscles from the front on the hip opposite to the shoulder leading the rotation, i.e. the hip works in the contra-

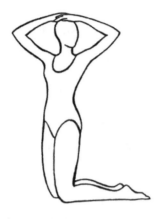

Figure 44
Variation of the rotation of the spine.

direction to the rotation of the spine. The rotation is divided into two movements: the rotation of the thorax and the rotation of the neck and the head. These can be executed separately, successively or simultaneously. During the rotation of the thorax, the shoulders move into a diagonal line above the hips, which maintain their basic horizontal position. The head, with the chin at a right angle to the front plane of the neck, does not change its basic position during the rotation of the chest and remains above the sternum. During the rotation of the neck and the head the chin deviates to the side; and in the maximum rotation it turns as far as above the shoulder. The right angle between the chin and the front plane of the neck remains unchanged. In a standing position the body weight rests on the balls of the feet.

The movement is led: during the rotation to the right the rotation of the chest *is led* by the right shoulder and by an elevated sternum. The rotation of the neck and the head to the right *is led* by the right ear. The rotation to the left is vice versa.

Direction: sideways-backward into horizontal plane. The correct hold of the shoulders with the stretched chest muscles ensures that the chest and the shoulders form one horizontal-diagonal plane. The shoulders do not move by themselves but as a result of the rotation of the thoracic spine.

Space awareness during rotation: rotate your chest, neck and the head around the body axis, i.e. in a distinctly maintained feeling of a vertical all the way up to the crown of the head. The perception of the vertical of the body, of the frontal of the hips against the diagonal of the shoulders (both in a horizontal plane) and the head is a specific space sensation of the rotation of the spine. Without this perception, the rotation will not be perfect; it will not have its full aesthetic and expressive value.

Recovery: relax the heightened tension of the abdominal muscles which immobilise the pelvis, while the chest, together with the neck and the head, returns to the basic position through a gradual relaxation of all the participating muscles.

The movement is led by the left shoulder, the sternum and the left ear (during the return from the rotation to the right); *direction* back to the initial position while the shoulders return to the horizontal and the chin above the sternum, still emphasising the vertical of the body. The relaxation during the return from the rotation must not diminish the tension necessary to maintain the elevated body posture. Only the increased muscular tension caused by the rotation gradually disappears and returns to the normal.

Let us remind ourselves that the movements of the spine need not be executed by the whole spine, but primarily by one part; either the lower part is rotated from the coccyx to the support point of the neck and head or the upper part from the support point to the skull. The rotation of the spine can be executed either in the same direction or in a contra-direction (the lower part to the right, the upper one to the left and vice versa). The rotation in the same direction can be later complemented by the rotation of the pelvis and thus enlarge the extent of turning. Strictly speaking, it is a matter of a composite movement, similar to the big forward bend, backward lean and the sideways shift.

COMPOSITE MOVEMENTS OF THE WHOLE SPINE

The composite movements of the spine result from the merging of two or three basic movements. The possibilities of merging are numerous when we consider that four basic movements have already offered so many different combinations. Moreover, the divisibility of the spine into independent lower and upper parts multiplies these possibilities. There are so many that I cannot begin to name them, let alone describe them all. Instead, I shall present some examples. Every teacher or choreographer will create further movement combinations to suit their purposes.

Refinement of form in the composite movements will only be achieved after mastering the basic movements of the spine safely and in all aspects (i.e. both technically and in terms of movement leading, as well as of its spatial orientation). This applies not only to the movement of the whole spine but also to each individual part.

Excluding rotation, the basic movements themselves show that the direction of movement of both spinal parts is not accordant but always antagonistic. For example, during the rounded forward

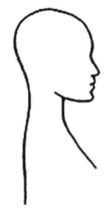
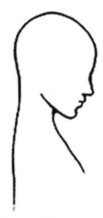
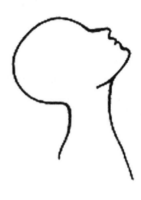

Figure 45
An erect position of the neck and head. The chin forms a right angle with the front of the neck.

Figure 46
A rounded forward bend of the neck executed in the intervertebral joints of the cervical spine. The upper chest remains elevated.

Figure 47
A rounded backward bend of the neck. The chin is in a vertical line above the middle of the sternum, the crown of the head points backwards.

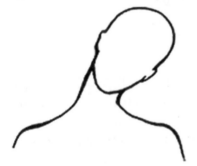
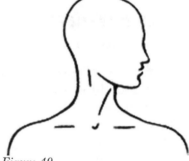

Figure 48
A rounded bend of the neck to the left and the left ear moves close to the left shoulder. The crown of the head is tilted to the left.

Figure 49
Rotation of the head and neck to the left. The chin moves left above the outer third of the clavicle while the neck remains erect.

bend the curvature of the lower part points backward-down, and the upper part forward-down. During the rounded lateral bend to the right, the lower spine curves to the left and the upper spine to the right. Also in the rounded backward bend the movement is in contra-direction, the lower part points forward, the upper part backward. It is only in rotation that the chest, head and neck move in the same direction. However, when the chest rotates in one direction and the neck and head in the opposite, it is a matter of a contra-directional rotation, i.e. of a different composite movement of the spine (see later). In such movements the directions, the leading and the technical aspect of the movement are complicated. In terms of the technique and the leading, we maintain the characteristic features of the basic movements which are contained in the composite one. That is why we need to know them well and control them effectively, i.e. practise them again and again. From the point of view of spatial orientation the composite movement has a new direction resulting from the merging of two or three basic movements. Most often, it is an in-between direction which gives the composite movement a new spatial experience.

The analysis of basic, composite and complex movements is already contained in detailed description. It is not always feasible to sketch these movements because the visual angle from which one looks at the movement does not always meet the needs of the particular movement and so partly distorts it.

A FEW EXAMPLES OF COMPOSITE MOVEMENTS OF THE SPINE

COMPLEX MOVEMENTS

To combine two basic movements:

Rounded forward-lateral bend to the right: tuck the pelvis under and round the lower spine backward-left in the direction of its shift. Transfer the body weight onto the outer edge of the left and the inner edge of the right foot. At the same time, slant the pelvis by moving the left hip away from the ribs and drawing the right hip to the ribs. The hips have left their horizontal, the left hip has lowered and the right has risen. Elongate the left side of the body as far as the ear, while contracting the right side of the ribs. The shoulders have also changed their horizontal position to a slanting one. The left shoulder is higher than the right one. The upper spine rounds forward-down and simultaneously bends to the side, so that the right ear lowers and under the influence of the forward bend is directed *in front of* the right shoulder, not *above* the right shoulder as would be the case in a pure lateral bend. The chin, however, stays above the sternum, it does not deviate from it either right or left. The rounded forward-lateral bend to the left is vice versa.

The technical aspect: see BASIC MOVEMENTS, p. 68.

Leading: the tucking under of the pelvis and the left-backward shift *is led* by the sacrum and the left hip, the slanting *is led* by the left hip. The elongation of the left side of the body *is led* by the left ear and the sternum. The bending of the spine to the right-forward-down *is led* by the forehead and the right temple.

Directions: the rounding of the lower spine and the pelvic shift occurs in an *in-between direction* backward-left, the movement of the upper spine in an *in between direction* forward-right-downward.

Rounded backward-lateral bend to the right: round the lower spine to the left-forward by shifting the pelvis to the left-forward, simultaneously transfer the body weight onto the outer edge of the left and the inner edge of the right foot, closer to the toes. At the same time, slant the pelvis and elongate to the left side of the body as far as the ear, while contracting the right side. Both the hips and the shoulders have changed their horizontal position into a slanted one, i.e. the right hip is higher, the left one lower, the shoulders are in the opposite order. The sternum and the chin rise high, the upper spine points through a high release to the right-backward-down, the lower spine to the left-forward-upward. The right ear inclines above the right shoulder. The chin forms with the front of the neck an obtuse angle opening to the front. The rounded backward-lateral bend to the left is vice versa.

The technical aspect: see BASIC MOVEMENTS, p. 68.

Leading: the rounding of the lower spine and the pelvic shift forward-left *are led* by the left groin and the left hip, the slanting by the left hip. The elongation of the left side of the body *is led* by the left ear and the sternum. The bending of the upper spine to the right-backward *is led* by the crown of the head and the right temple.

Directions: the arching of the lower spine and the pelvic shift occur in an *in-between direction* left-forward-upward, the bending of the upper spine in an *in-between direction*: right-backward-downward.

'S'-shaped lateral bend of both parts of the spine: slant the pelvis and round the lower spine to the left but instead of ending the arc of the lateral bend of the upper spine to the right *tilt the upper spine also to the left above the rounded hip*. The hips and shoulders have a slanted position: the left shoulder and the left hip move towards each other, the right shoulder and the right hip move apart. The body weight is transferred to the outer side of the left and the inner side of the right foot. Tilt the left ear to the left shoulder, with the chin above the sternum contracting the left side of the ribs, at the same time elongating the right side of the ribs and the neck to a point behind the right ear. The lateral bend of both parts of the spine to the right—vice versa. (It is a frequent movement of the Gothic Madonnas.) See Figure 122, p. 269.

The technical aspect: see BASIC MOVEMENTS, p. 68.

Leading: the movement of the lower spine *is led* by the left hip, the pelvic slant by the left hip. The movement of the upper spine *is led* by the sternum and the left temple.

Directions: the lower and upper spine have in this movement the same direction which is in contradiction with the lateral bend of the whole spine and is rather alien to our feeling.

Rounded forward bend plus rotation to the right: tuck the pelvis under and round the lower spine backward, simultaneously transfer the body weight closer to the heels. Rotate the chest to the right so that the shoulders position themselves diagonally towards the horizontal of the hips. Continuing with the rotation of the chest, neck and the head to the right, bend the head forward at the same time. The chin deviates from the sternum to the right above the centre of the right clavicle and simultaneously lowers into a sharp angle with the front of the neck. The rounded forward bend with rotation to the left is vice versa.

The technical aspect: see BASIC MOVEMENTS, p. 68.

Leading: the movement of the lower spine *is led* by both hips and sacrum, the movement of the chest *is led* by the right shoulder, the movement of the upper spine *is led* by the forehead and the right ear.

Directions: the movement of the lower spine progresses in the *straight direction* backward and the movement of chest and upper spine in an *in-between direction* to the right-forward-downward.

Rounded backward bend plus rotation to the right: arch the lower spine forward and transfer the body weight to the toes. Simultaneously, rotate the highly elevated chest to the right, so that the shoulders and the hips are horizontal but the hips are frontal while the shoulders are now located diagonally. Bend the upper spine and the head through a high release to the right-backward, so that the chin deviates from the sternum to the centre of the right cavicle. The chin forms an obtuse angle with the front of the neck opening to the right-forward. The backward bend-rotation is vice versa.

The technical aspect: see BASIC MOVEMENTS, p. 68.

Leading: the movement of the lower spine *is led* by the groin forward, the rotation of the chest *is led* by the right shoulder and the sternum, the movement of the upper spine *is led* by the sternum, the crown of the head and the right ear.

Directions: the movement of the lower spine progresses in a *straight direction* forward, the movement of the chest and the upper spine is in an *in-between* direction to the right-backward.

A combination of three basic movements:

Rounded lateral-backward bend plus rotation to the right: round the lower spine forward-left by shifting the pelvis forward-left, at the same time tilting it by pulling the left hip away from the ribs. Transfer the body weight onto the outer side of the left and the inner side of the right sole closer to the toes. Elongate the left side of the body with the sternum and the chin to the point behind the ear, while rotating the chest, neck and head to the right. The shoulders change their horizontal position into a slanting line diagonally situated, the right shoulder lowers and turns slightly to the right. Extend the upper spine together with the head through a high release backward-right, so that the chin deviates slightly to the right above the middle of the sternal part of the clavicle and the temple tilts slightly to the right shoulder. The raised chin forms with the front of the neck an obtuse angle, turned slightly to the right.

The technical aspect: see BASIC MOVEMENTS, p. 68.

Leading: the movement of the pelvis and the lower spine *is led* by the left groin and the left hip which also *leads* the slanting movement by pulling away from the ribs. The upward elongation of the left side of the body *is led* by the sternum and the left ear, the rotation of the chest *is led* by the right shoulder. The movement of the upper spine *is led* by the right ear, the right temple and the crown of the head. The entire movement passes through *contra-in-between* directions to the left-forward and to the right-backward.

When combining the lateral bend with rotation to the same side, we maintain the characteristic features of both movements except for the first feature of the lateral bend, the chin above the sternum, which must give way to the only feature of the rotation of the neck and head, i.e. the deviation of the chin from the sternum to the side because rotation of the neck and the head without this deviation cannot be done. The chin deviation in this combination is, however, smaller. The lateral bend of the neck and the head is noticeable in its second characteristic feature, i.e. the inclination of the temple to the shoulder.

Deep rounded forward-sideways bend to the left, plus rotation to the right: while kneeling on the right leg, the left leg is bent into a right angle in front of the body, with its foot resting on the ground. In this position, bend the lower spine by tucking the pelvis under, easing the left hip and shifting the pelvis to the right-back. Transfer the body weight more onto the right leg. lowering the pelvis, and stretching the leg in front. Simultaneously, elongate the right side of the body as far as the point behind the ear, bending the upper spine forward-left and rotating the chest, neck and head to the right. The shoulders change their horizontal location into a diagonal, slanting one in relation to the hips, the other slanting the opposite way. The right hip is lower than the left hip, the right shoulder and the right ear are higher than the left shoulder and the left ear. The chin deviates from the sternum above the middle of the external part of the right clavicle but owing to the forward bend it forms a sharp angle with the front of the neck.

The technical aspect: see BASIC MOVEMENTS, p. 68.

Leading: the pelvic movement *is led* by the sacrum and the right hip, the elongation of the right side of the body *is led* by the right ear and sternum, the rotation of the chest *is led* by the right shoulder and the rotation of the upper spine by the right ear. The forward-sideways bend of the upper spine *is led* by the forehead and the left temple.

Directions: the movement passes through *contra-in-between* directions to the right-back and to the left-forward, while the diagonal of the shoulders and the head merges with the *in-between direction* of the spine to the left-forward.

THE WAVES OF THE SPINE

Sagittal wave (forward-backward or frontal-thoracic): round the lower spine backward by tucking the pelvis under (see POSITIONS OF THE PELVIS, p. 30) and continue by progressively rounding as far as the upper spine. As soon as the upper spine takes over the rounding process, the lower spine starts an opposite movement, i.e. it arches forward by tilting the pelvis. The arching forward progresses towards the upper spine and, as soon as the latter takes over, the lower spine begins the backward curve anew, ie. the pelvis tucks under. Thus arises a wave composed from an alternating small rounded forward bend and a rounded backward bend, occurring simultaneously in both parts of the spine but antagonistically. The wavy movement passes through an uninterrupted succession.

The technical aspect: see BASIC MOVEMENTS, p. 68.

Leading: the rounding of the lower spine *is led* by the sacrum and the hips. The arching forward *is led* by the coccyx. The rounding of the upper spine into a forward bend *is led* by the forehead, the arching forward *is led* successively by the sternum and the crown of the head.

Directions: forward and backward. The wave progresses between the extreme end of the spine (coccyx) and the crown of the head.

Frontal wave (from side to side): bend the lower spine to the right and continue by progressively rounding the upper spine. As soon as the upper spine joins in the movement, the lower spine starts to bend to the left. The pelvis shifts from the right to the left and again to the right etc. and the upper spine follows it with a small delay. Thus arises a wave composed from an alternating rounded lateral bend to the right and left, which passes through an uninterrupted succession. In the wave starting to the left all directions are vice versa.

The technical aspect: see BASIC MOVEMENTS, p. 68.

Leading: the movement of the *lower* spine *is led* alternately by the right and the left hip, the movement of the *upper* spine *is led* alternately by the right and the left temple.

Directions: directly to the sides.

The waving movements of the spine result from its ability to transfer movement from one vertebra to the other by means of joints and inter-vertebral discs, which also greatly contribute towards the softness and fluency of the movement.

Sagittal (forward-backward) wave plus rotation of the chest: to the forward-backward wave we add a rotation of the chest alternately from right to left and left to right which is retained throughout. The shoulders change their direction into a diagonal, but the neck and head do not change, staying frontal.

The technical aspect: see BASIC MOVEMENTS, p. 68.

Leading: during curving of the lower spine the movement *is led* by the sacrum and the hips, during arching the coccyx *leads*. The rotation of the chest *is led* by the right or left shoulder. During bending of the upper spine the movement *is led* by the forehead, during arching by the sternum and the crown of the head.

Directions: forward-backward. The lower and the upper spine have the same spatial direction in this simultaneous but not identical movement.

The diagonal of the shoulders cuts through the waves in the *in-between directions* sideways-forward and sideways-backward.

COMBINATIONS OF THE ROUNDED MOVEMENTS OF THE SPINE WITH STRAIGHT MOVEMENTS OF THE TRUNK

Examples:

Straight forward bend plus rotation of the chest, neck and head: add to the straight forward tilt a rotation of the chest, neck and the head. Tilt the pelvis, shift it back and tilt the trunk forward with an 'immobilised' spine and elongated neck. At the same time, rotate the chest, the straight neck and head to the right or left, so that the shoulders and the head are positioned in a slanted line in opposition to the hips which are held horizontal. The chin moves from the sternum to the centre of the right or left clavicle.

The technical aspect: see BASIC MOVEMENTS, p. 68.

Leading: the coccyx *leads* the pelvic shift backward and both hips *lead* its forward tilt. The trunk with the elongated spine *is led* by the sternum, the rotation of the chest by the left or right shoulder, the rotation of the neck and head by the right or left ear.

Directions: straight contra-directions of the trunk forward and back cut through the directions of the shoulders and the head, which is turned into *contra-in-between* directions sideways-backward and sideways-forward.

In all movements connected with the rotation of the chest, neck and head (but not in the case of the torso), we must strictly maintain an immobilised pelvis. The pelvis easily succumbs to a rotating movement of the upper part of the body. This causes an immediate slackening of the abdominal muscles and the rotation is less effective. A conscious and sensitive adherence to the horizontal of the hips, in relation to the diagonal of the shoulders, helps to achieve a more perfect technical execution, thereby perfecting the form of this movement.

Straight sideways shift to the right plus torsion, with a small rounded backward bend (extension) and rotation of the chest, neck and head to the right: rotate the pelvis to the right. The trunk follows the movement of the pelvis, so that the hips and the shoulders are at a diagonal to the legs. The torsion to the right is thus accomplished. Shift the pelvis to the left-forward and tilt it in the direction of the diagonal to the right-backward. Simultaneously elongate the right half of the abdominal wall into a straight lateral bend and raise the sternum and chin into a backward bend. At the same time, transfer the body weight to the outer side of the left and the inner side of the right foot closer to the toes. Simultaneously, rotate the chest, the neck and the head to the right, so that the diagonal of the shoulders increases with the diagonal of the hips in torsion. The raised chin moves from the sternum above the centre of the right clavicle.

The direction of the straight lateral bend, which is in its original form pointing directly to the side, changes under the influence of the torsion and of the rotation of the chest into an *in-between* direction sideways-back. The right shoulder points almost to the back in accordance with the inclination of the neck and head, completed by their rotation.

The technical aspect: see BASIC MOVEMENTS, p. 68.

Leading: the right hip leads the torsion, the left groin and the left hip *lead* the shift of the pelvis left-forward, the elongated right half of the abdominal wall *leads* the trunk into a straight lateral-flexion, the sternum and the crown of the head *lead* the upper spine into a small rounded backward bend. The right shoulder *leads* the rotation of the chest and the right ear, the rotation of the neck and head to the right.

Directions: opposing in-between directions to the left-forward and to the right-back, with the emphasis on the backward direction.

If we want to achieve a perfect form of this and other composite movements of the spine and the trunk, we must be clearly aware of the specific features of the basic movements, in order not to neglect anything important while combining them. The leading of the movements and their direction facilitate our orientation. However, it is necessary that students develop a sense for movement logic on the basis of an instinctive awareness of movement details.

The recovery is a matter of lifting up and returning into the basic position or other initial position of the body.

The technical aspect: see *recovery*, p. 61 (trunk) and p. 69 (spine).

Leading: the lifting of the pelvis *is led* above all by both hips, the lifting of the chest and the upper spine *is led* above all by the sternum.

Direction: it is always an upward direction, returning into the vertical of the body and the horizontal of the shoulders and the hips.

While lifting the chest, *led* by the sternum in an upward direction, we must not forget the opposite direction downward of the shoulders. It is one of the five rules of a correct elevated dance posture, which must be applied in every movement.

COMPOSITE MOVEMENTS OF THE TRUNK AND SPINE

These are immensely important for a complex movement of the body and for its coordination with the movement of the lower and upper limbs. Their perfection in technique and form is considerably dependant on good work of the trunk and spine, which is a necessary prerequisite for mastering complex movements. This work is continuous: there is always something to perfect and to give it more precision.

While practising basic and composite movements of the spine, we cannot always separate lower and upper limbs from the movements of the trunk. However, initially only the simplest possible movements should be used to avoid diverting our attention from the main task. It is also desirable that the students get used to the coordination of the movements of trunk and of the limbs in complex movements. They will learn that the places where the upper and lower limbs are connected with the body, i.e. the area of the hip and shoulder joints, are especially significant for the coordination of the movements of the spine and the limbs. The work in these joints, their relaxation, elongation, bending in all directions, turning out and turning in, while the pelvis and shoulders are established, is one of the basic technical skills. All this contributes to liberating the limbs from the trunk, and on the other hand, to maintain the link of the limbs to the movements of the trunk and spine. Perfect continuity of movement, so significant for movement expression serving artistic goals, is one of the prerequisites for mastering both technique and expression.

CIRCULAR MOVEMENTS OF THE SPINE WITHOUT ROTATION AND WITH ROTATION OF THE UPPER SPINE:

Circling of the spine without rotation: start with a rounded forward bend in axis, then pass to a rounded sideways-forward bend to the right, to a pure rounded lateral bend to the right, to a rounded sideways-backward bend to the right, to a pure rounded backward bend, to a rounded backward-sideways bend to the left, to a pure rounded lateral bend to the left, to a rounded sideways-forward bend to the left and to a pure rounded forward bend by which the circle is closed or a new one started. Maintain the horizontal of the hips throughout, facing forward.

The technical aspect: see BASIC AND COMPOSITE MOVEMENTS OF THE SPINE, pp. 68, 76.

Leading of the movements of the pelvis is transferred from one point to another along its circumference (see ROTATORY MOVEMENTS OF THE PELVIS, p. 40). The *leading* of the movements of the upper spine, which starts in the rounded forward bend with the forehead, passes to the right temple, to the crown of the head, to the left temple and again to the forehead.

Directions: the pelvis circumscribes a smaller circle starting with the left-backward shift, the upper spine circumscribes a larger circle starting with a right-forward tilt, while passing through all the *primary directions* and *in-between directions*.

Circling of the spine plus rotation of the upper spine: start with a rounded bend in axis, passing into a rounded forward bend with rotation to the right (the shoulders position themselves diagonally), to the rounded lateral bend with rotation to the right, to the rounded backward bend with rotation to the right, to the pure rounded backward bend (the shoulders return to the horizontal), to the rounded backward bend with rotation to the left (again the shoulders are in a diagonal). Continuing to the rounded lateral bend with rotation to the left, to the rounded forward bend with rotation to the left and to the pure rounded forward bend (again the shoulders are in a horizontal). Thus the circle is accomplished or a new one started. The hips are kept all the time in a horizontal.

The technical aspect: see BASIC MOVEMENTS OF THE SPINE, p. 68.

Leading of the movements of the pelvis is transferred along its circumference from one point to another. The *leading* of the movements of the chest and upper spine starts in a rounded forward bend, with the forehead, then passes on to the forehead and the right shoulder, to the right temple and right shoulder, to the crown of the head and the right shoulder. In the pure backward bend the crown of the head *leads*, then the crown of the head and the left shoulder, the left temple and left shoulder, the forehead and the left shoulder and in the pure forward bend just the forehead. Thus the circle is accomplished or a new one can be started.

Directions: the pelvis circumscribes a smaller circle starting with the left-backward shift, the upper spine circumscribes a larger circle starting with a right-forward bend while passing through all the *primary directions* and *in-between directions*.

The figure eight of the spine forward and backward without rotation: facing frontally, start with a rounded forward-sideways bend to the right, pass into the pure rounded forward bend and into the rounded forward-sideways bend to the left (the front loop), continue through an upright position into the rounded backward-sideways bend to the right, to the pure rounded backward bend and to the rounded backward-sideways bend to the left (the back loop). Keep the horizontal of the shoulders and the hips facing forward. Return to the basic position.

The technical aspect: see BASIC MOVEMENTS OF THE SPINE, p. 68.

Leading: the back loop of the *pelvis* in a contra-direction to the front loop of the upper spine *is led* by the sacrum and the left hip, the sacrum, the sacrum and the right hip. The front loop of the *pelvis is led* by the left hip and the left groin, both groins, the right hip and the right groin. The front loop of the *upper spine is led* by the right temple and the forehead, the forehead only, the left temple and the forehead; its back loop *is led* by the right temple and the crown of the head, the crown of the head only, the crown of the head and the left temple.

Directions: perceive the spatial path of the movement: the front loop, the back loop, the centre point being in the body axis. The pelvic movement is perceived on a smaller scale and in the *opposite direction*.

The figure eight of the spine forward and back plus rotation of the upper spine: immediately on starting the front loop of the figure eight of the spine forward and backward, add rotation of the upper spine to the right, pass through pure rounded forward bend and complete the loop with rotation to the left. Then continue through an upright position, the back loop, while adding rotation to the right, pass through a pure rounded backward bend and complete the loop with rotation to the left. The pelvis performs both loops, on a smaller scale and in the *opposite* direction. The horizontal of the hips forward is maintained while the shoulders position themselves into a diagonal for the rotation.

Leading: to the leading which one experienced during the figure eight without rotation, add the leading of the right shoulder and the right ear wherever there is rotation of the upper spine to the right, and the leading of the left shoulder and the left ear wherever there is rotation to the left.

Directions: a forward loop, a backward loop, the centre point in the body axis; the pelvis moves on a smaller scale in the *opposite* direction. To add to this, one perceives the diagonal of the shoulders and the head during the rotation in relation to the horizontal of the hips and the vertical of the legs.

The figure eight of the spine sideways without rotation: facing frontally, start with a rounded forward-sideways bend to the right, pass to the pure rounded sideways bend to the right, then into the rounded backward-sideways bend to the right (the right loop); then through an upright position and from the rounded forward-sideways bend to the left pass into the pure rounded sideways bend to the left and to the rounded backward sideways bend to the left (the left loop).

The technical aspect: see BASIC MOVEMENTS OF THE SPINE, p. 68.

Leading: the left loop of the pelvis in contra-direction to the right loop of the upper spine *is led* gradually by the sacrum and the left hip, the left hip only, the left hip and the left groin. The right loop of the pelvis in *contra-direction* to the left loop of the upper spine *is led* by the sacrum and the right hip, the right hip only, the right hip and the right groin. The right loop of the upper spine *is led* by the forehead and the right temple, the right temple only, the right temple and the crown of the head; the left loop *is led* by the forehead and the left temple, the left temple only, and the left temple and the crown of the head.

Directions: in performing the loop to the right and the loop to the left, we are aware of the point of intersection in the body axis. The pelvis moves on a smaller scale and in the *opposite* direction.

The figure eight of the spine sideways plus rotation: it has the-same procedure as in the figure eight sideways without rotation, but at the commencement of the right loop, add concurrently a rotation to the right; and at the commencement of the left loop a rotation to the left. At the point of intersection of both loops change the direction of the rotation. Maintain the horizontal of the hips to the front.

The technical aspect: see BASIC MOVEMENTS OF THE SPINE, p. 68.

Leading: it is the same as in the figure eight sideways without rotation, but add to the leading of the right loop the right shoulder and the right ear, which *lead* the rotation throughout the right loop. To the leading of the left loop add the left shoulder and the left ear which *lead* the rotation throughout the left loop.

Directions: as well as experiencing the spatial path of the loops we perceive the diagonal of the shoulders and the head during the rotation against the horizontal of the hips.

SMALL MOVEMENTS OF THE HEAD

These concern slight movements in the cranio-vertebral joints. They are independent movements of the head between the first and second cervical vertebrae and the occipital bone. They are performed by the sub-occipital muscles (the short muscles of the neck).

The dancers from India, Cambodia and other Eastern cultures have these slight movements of the head polished to the last detail and enriched by the head shifts forward, backward and sideways. It is not common to work with head shifts in Western culture (except in mime) and they are not dealt with further.

Anatomical terminology of the slight head movements are:
– ventral flexion
– extension
– lateral flexion
– rotation
In movement practice we use the following terminology:
– pure forward tilt of the head
– pure backward tilt of the head

– pure sideways tilt of the head
– pure rotation of the head

These are slight movements of the head while the neck is immobilised. The initial position for these small movements is an upright-held chest, neck and head, with the chin above the sternum. The chin forms approximately a right angle with the front of the neck. It is important because these movements change the basic relationship of the chin towards the front plane of the neck and towards the sternum, which is their specific characteristic.

BASIC MOVEMENTS

Pure forward tilt of the head is a slight inclination of the head downward. The chin is lowered slightly and the right angle with the front plane of the neck becomes more acute; the chin, however, remains above the sternum. Elongate the short muscles at the back of the neck and the occipital bone rises slightly.

The movement *is led* by the chin in the *direction* downward.

Pure backward tilt of the head is a slight inclination of the head backward. The chin is raised a little and its right angle with the front plane of the neck changes into a slightly obtuse angle. By an active contraction of the short neck muscles, one pushes the occipital bone in slightly.

The movement *is led* by the chin in the *direction* forward-upward.

Pure sideways tilt of the head is a small inclination of the head sideways, while one side of the jaw rises slightly and the other is lowered correspondingly but the chin remains above the sternum. By active elongation of one side of the short neck muscles as far as the ear, the ear rises a little and the other is lowered correspondingly. The mastoid process (the bony point behind the ear) on the side of the inclination pushes in partly.

The movement *is led* by the ear on the side of the tilt in the *direction* down-sideways.

Pure rotation of the head is a small turn of the head to the side while the right angle of the chin with the front plane of the neck remains; the chin, however, moves from its basic position fractionally to the side above the sternal end of the clavicle. The ear on the side of the rotation turns slightly backward-sideways and the opposite ear forward-sideways, both remaining in the horizontal plane.

The movement *is led* by the ear on the side of the rotation in the *direction* sideways-back.

One controls the small movements of the head from behind by contracting the short muscles of the neck while the muscles of the front plane of the neck are relaxed.

When we retain the basic feeling of the vertical of the body and the horizontal of the shoulders and the hips, we perceive through kinaesthetic awareness the directions of the movements of the head. The head has become independent from the spine and assumes its own direction.

Recovery: release the active elongation or contraction of the short muscles of the neck and thus return the head to its initial position.

COMPOSITE MOVEMENTS

1. *Combine two basic movements:*
  – a forward tilt with a sideways bend
  – a backward tilt with a sideways bend
  – a forward tilt with a rotation
  – a sideways tilt with rotation to the same side
  – a sideways tilt with rotation to the opposite side

2. *Combine three basic movement:*
  – a forward-sideways tilt-rotation to the same side
  – a forward-sideways tilt-rotation to the opposite side
  – a backward-sideways tilt-rotation to the same side
  – a backward-sideways tilt-rotation to the opposite side

The technical aspect of the composite small movements of the head (see BASIC MOVEMENTS, p. 91.)

Maintain the technique of the basic movements from which the composite movement is composed; however where one movement affects another one must dominate, to facilitate the action without losing the integrity of the technique. For example, during the sideways tilt-rotation, the technique of both movements is mutually affected. Here the typical feature of the rotation of the head dominates, i.e. the deviation of the chin away from the sternum. The chin moves above the sternal end of the clavicle which is originally required in the pure rotation of the head. The lateral tilt is then expressed by its further typical characteristic, i.e. the lowering of the ear and the jaw on the same side. The techniques of the backward and the sideways tilt also affect each other. The problem is solved if you push in one side of the mastoid process by contracting the short neck muscles, as is required by the lateral tilt. Try to elongate the chin, at least partially, in the backward tilt.

Leading of the movement: adhere as much as possible to the leading of all the basic movements from which the composite movement is composed.

Directions: the composite movements pass through *in-between* directions, e.g. the forward-sideways tilt with rotation has the following directions: forward-sideways-down; the backward-sideways tilt with rotation has the following *directions*: upward-sideways-backward etc.

The *leading* of the pure movements of the head differs slightly from the leading movements of the head and neck together. For example, in the forward tilt, the lowering of the forehead is so small that we cannot perceive it as leading. Rather, we are aware of the position of the chin and the change of its angle to the front of the neck; that is why the leading is transferred to the chin.

II

RESPIRATORY MOVEMENTS OF THE CHEST

The most important movement of the chest is its ability to expand and contract the ribs. In this way, the whole thorax expands and narrows. This ability is applied in the first place during breathing but it is also, as we have learned, a complementary activity with the movements of the spine. For example, in the rounded backward bend, the ribs on the front of the chest move more apart and the ribs at the back move closer together. In the rounded forward bend it is vice versa*. (In a rounded sideways bend, the ribs on one side move closer to each other, and on the other side they move apart.) The movements of the ribs are mainly affected by the muscles between them (intercostal muscles). The external layer expands the ribs and the internal one draws them closer together. Closely connected with these intercostal muscles are the muscles of the abdominal wall and of the back. (See the description of the bone structure of the trunk and the spine and their muscles, p. 51.)

The activity of the diaphragm makes a major contribution to the respiratory movements of the chest. Its movements influence

---

* Translator's note: See Figures 35, 36, pp.194, 195.

the enlargement and the reduction of the chest cavity during inhalation (inspiration) and exhalation (expiration). The ribs expand the chest cavity by moving apart, lifting and opening in all directions. The chest cavity reduces with the ribs drawing closer and simultaneously lowering. During inhalation, the diaphragm enlarges the chest cavity by sinking into the abdominal cavity and pushing down its contents. During exhalation, on the contrary, it arches back into the chest cavity, helping to expel the used air from the lungs. Its movement is automatic, but it can be made more effective by the complementary movement of the ribs. It is possible to control and direct the movements of the ribs independently from respiration. That is why practising the movements of the ribs is important not only with regard to the overall mobility of the chest, but also for increasing the breathing capacity. Closely connected with this is an improvement in the heart activity, blood circulation and the activity of the organs situated in the abdominal cavity.

Normal respiration may, for the purpose of description, be divided into quiet and deep respiration; there is no essential difference between them.

III

ANATOMY: THE DIAPHRAGM

Quiet Respiration
(Figures 50 and 51, p. 198)

Quiet respiration is performed by the diaphragm, the intercostal muscles and the abdominal muscles. At the beginning of inspiration the diaphragm begins to move down taking its fixed point from the lower margins of the ribs (Figure 50) and in so doing draws air into the lungs through the bronchial tubes, and at the same time pushes the abdominal contents before it until the resistance of the abdominal muscles prevents further downward movement; the level reached by the diaphragm depends upon the force of its contraction and the tone of the muscles of the abdominal wall. When this level is reached, the central tendon of the diaphragm becomes the fixed point for its action (Figure 51) and, working in conjunction with the intercostal muscles, it lifts the lower ribs which in turn push forward and raise the sternum and upper ribs. The movement of the diaphragm in Figures 50 & 51 has been exaggerated, the actual range in quiet respiration being about 19 mm with very little alteration of diaphragmatic shape.

The abdominal muscles adjust their tone in relation to the pressure within the abdominal cavity; they are therefore in a state of greater tone at the end of inspiration than at the beginning.

Expiration is effected by the elastic recoil of the thoracic walls assisted by the action of the abdominal muscles which push back the displaced viscera and pull down the sternum.

Deep Respiration

The mechanism of deep inspiration is the same as that of quiet inspiration with additional muscular help to produce an increased expansion of the thorax. The head, neck and upper part of the trunk are established or flexed forward to enable the sternomastoid and scalene muscles to act on the sternum and upper ribs; the shoulder girdle is braced back so that the pectoral muscles can raise the ribs sideways; the trapezii help indirectly to expand the thorax by taking the weight of the shoulder girdle off the chest wall. The latissimi dorsi and quadrati lumborum fix the lower ribs, enabling the diaphragm to make stronger and more extensive movements. During forced expiration, all the muscles of the abdominal wall contract strongly.

The influence of the correct body posture on respiration is substantial. Only through adhering to all five rules of the elevated body posture are all parts of the body balanced in such a way that they fulfil the conditions for a fully ensured function of respiration. Caving-in of the chest, slackening of the abdominal wall, an undesirable tension caused by lifting of the shoulders and an uncontrolled caving-in of the neck vertebrae so that the front of the neck swells and the 'adam's apple' protrudes excessively forward. All create obstacles to a free air-flow during respiration.

This explains why it is necessary to emphasise that work on correct, elevated body posture for regulating respiration is the most important factor for students at all levels of development. Respiration and movement are closely connected. Both activities depend on each other to such an extent that incorrect and insufficient respiration spoils movement and uncontrolled, deformed movement spoils respiration. By holding the body incorrectly, one destroys the harmony of both movement and respiration.

The process of breathing comprises two activities: exhalation and inhalation. Sufficient exhalation is a condition for a sufficient inhalation. That, of course, does not mean that one expels all air from the lungs so forcefully that the fluent rhythm of respiration is brought to a standstill. When starting on breathing exercises, begin with exhalation. In the first stage of work on movement, the teacher guides the students not to hold their breath back in the moment of exertion, but on the contrary to exhale. One starts work on breath control by becoming aware of the body sensations connected with correct breathing.

Correct exhalation: while lying down on the back and feeling the body axis correctly, we concentrate our attention on the intercostal spaces between the ribs. Through body awareness we are conscious of closing up the intercostal spaces and simultaneously expelling the air through the nose or mouth. The relaxed exhalation finishes with a calm pause before inhaling again.

Correct inhalation: after a brief rest, inhale with a closed mouth. Through body awareness we control the chest expansion sideways, backward and upward, while the ribs move apart and rise sideways and backward. The sternum and the upper ribs arch forward-upward while the sacrum, the hips and the lumbar spine move fractionally towards the floor. The arches of the lower ribs must not protrude forward. The abdominal wall is elongated during a correct inhalation. It must not be 'sucked in'! The inhalation finishes with a pause before a new exhalation or it softly changes into exhalation.

The whole breathing process can theoretically be divided into three stages: abdominal, costal (rib) and sternal (upper) chest breathing. These three stages link up and during the correct breathing process they merge and counterbalance each other, harmonically bound in one rhythmic breathing stream.

Faults during breathing: we often observe that through the influence of a certain incorrect body posture, a habit is formed by which one of the above mentioned stages of breathing dominates at the expense of the others. A certain small deformity of the chest is developed at the same time. Thus, during predominantly abdominal breathing where the costal and the upper chest breathing is neglected, the upper part of the chest is rather flat and underdeveloped.

On the other hand, the habit of predominantly costal breathing develops the *lower part* of the chest at the expense of its upper part. The waist becomes wide and firm, i.e. the side and back part of the abdominal wall firms up and its front part becomes slack as a result of an insufficient arching of the upper chest. This part of the chest is usually flat and under-developed as it is during predominantly abdominal breathing. The habit of mainly upper chest breathing causes an over-developed arching of the upper chest to the detriment of the lower part. The waist is usually narrow, the back abdominal wall is sunken, the ribs protrude excessively forward. In addition, the accompanying habit of pulling up the shoulders often develops so that the neck becomes 'shorter'. The breath tends to be superficial, too fast and the desirable relaxation of the intercostal muscles during exhalation often does not eventuate.

I do not claim that these types of breathing are always so clean-cut, but the signs of a particular type can be found in the body posture and the shape of the chest and these reveal faulty breathing habits. These facts demonstrate that our first task is to develop a correct body posture in students. We cannot arrive at a perfect mastery of movement if there is no simultaneous control over the respiratory involvement in it. The key to both lies in the pursuit of a perfectly balanced body posture.

In the course of general tuition teachers must take notice of how the students breathe and should see to it that their respiration adjusts to the rhythm and dynamics of the movement. Above all, the teacher should guide the students not to hold their breath, but to let it flow freely together with the rhythmic and dynamic feeling, later also with the spatial one. Respiration helps in the coordination of movement. It aids the accurate start and length of individual movements and the duration of the pause before the build-up to the peak of the movement. One works on respiration mainly by a controlled awareness. Respiration is connected with the function of inner tension and the union of these two factors enlivens movement within.

4. The Lower Limbs

The movements of the lower limbs are clearly connected with the movements of the pelvis. Here I recommend a renewed study of the description of its bone structure, joints and muscles.

I

ANATOMY: THE LEGS

The bones of the leg

(Figure 52, p. 199)

The skeleton of the leg consists of:

(1) the thigh bone or *femur*;
(2) the knee cap or *patella*;
(3) the shin bone or *tibia*;
(4) the *fibula* which is a long thin bone lying along the outer side of the tibia.

The femur

The femur has a head, a neck, a shaft and a large lower extremity; it is the longest bone in the body. The head is spherical and articulates with the acetabulum. The neck is about 33mm in length, rounded and very strong; it joins the shaft of the femur at an angle of 125 degrees. The shaft has a slight forward convexity. A large bony prominence called the *greater trochanter*, projects from its upper extremity, and on the inner side of the shaft just below its neck, there is a small blunt spur of bone, the *lesser trochanter*. Certain important hip muscles are attached to these trochanters.

The shaft of the femur is directed slightly inward, forming an angle of about 170 degrees with the shaft of the tibia, when the body is in the upright position and the feet are together. The lower end of the shaft of the femur widens out to form two large articular surfaces called *condyles*, the inner condyle being slightly lower than the outer. These two condyles articulate with the upper end of the tibia to form the knee joint.

The patella

The patella is situated in front of the knee joint in the tendon of the muscles which extend the knee. It is roughly circular in outline and about 32mm in diameter and 12mm thick; it has an inner and an outer surface; the inner surface articulates with the condyles of the femur. Its function is to improve leverage by its pulley-like action as it glides in the groove between the smooth surfaces of the condyles. If the outer side of the groove is abnormally flat or if the angle between the shafts of the femur and tibia is considerably less than 170 degrees, the patella may dislocate to the outer side of the joint.

The tibia

The tibia is so named on account of its likeness to the Roman flute; it has an upper and lower extremity and a shaft. The upper extremity provides a broad horizontal plateau which has an inner and an outer articular surface for the corresponding condyles of the femur. The shaft is straight and tapers slightly towards its lower end; it is triangular in cross-section. The lower extremity has a downward projection, the *internal malleolus*, on its inner side. The end of the shaft and the inner aspect of the internal malleolus forms the inner aspect of the ankle joint.

The fibula

The fibula is a long, thin bone which has a head, shaft and lower extremity. Its head articulates with the outer side of the upper end of the tibia and its lower extremity is fixed by strong ligaments to the outer side of the lower end of the same bone. Its lower end, called the *external malleolus*, forms part of the ankle joint. The fibula does not transmit any weight, its main function being to supply a framework for muscle attachment and help to protect certain important blood vessels.

The bones of the foot

(Figure 53, p. 199)

The skeleton of the foot is made up of:
  (1) the seven bones of the main part of the foot which together make up the *tarsus*;
  (2) the five bones of the fore-foot called *metatarsals*;
  (3) the bones of the toes or *phalanges*.

The tarsus

The two largest bones of the tarsus are the ankle bones or *talus*, and the heel bone or *calcaneus*, sometimes called *os calcis*. The upper surface of the talus articulates with the lower end of the tibia and fibula forming the ankle joint. The rounded surface on the front of the talus articulates with the *navicular* bone which in turn articulates with the three small *cuneiform* bones. The under surface of the talus makes three small joints with the upper surface of the calcaneus; the calcaneus, in addition to its articulation with the talus above it, forms a joint with the *cuboid* bone at its anterior extremity.

The metatarsals and phalanges
The metatarsals are similar in shape to the corresponding bones of the hand, but they are of greater size and strength. The proximal ends of the inner three metatarsals articulate with the three cuneiform bones and the proximal ends of the outer two with the cuboid bone. The phalanges are generally shorter and thicker than those of the hand. There are two phalanges in the big toe and three in each of the remaining toes.

The arches of the foot
(Figure 54, p. 200)
Very great strains are imposed upon the feet, particularly during strenuous exercise. The foot is able to meet these strains because of the strength and flexibility of its structure. It is constructed in the form of arches which are held together by ligaments and supported by muscles. The arches are:
  (1) longitudinal, extending from the heel to the toes;
  (2) a series of transverse arches across the foot.

The longitudinal arch
The longitudinal arch consists of an inner and an outer portion which rest on a common pillar behind, namely the calcaneus. The inner part of the longitudinal arch is formed by the calcaneus, the talus, the navicular, the three cuneiform bones and the inner three metatarsals with their phalanges. The outer portion is formed by the calcaneus, the cuboid bone, the outer two metatarsals and the corresponding phalanges. The inner portion of the arch, the instep, is high, only touching the ground at the calcaneus behind and at the distal end of the first metatarsal in front; the distal end of the first metatarsal is called the ball of the foot. The outer portion of the arch is low and rests on the ground. The talus is the keystone of the arch and receives the body weight which it transmits through the pillars of the arch to the ground.

The longitudinal arch is supported chiefly by the long muscles of the leg and the short muscles of the foot; it is strengthened also by ligaments. If it becomes flattened owing to muscular weakness, the foot is deprived of its normal spring and a shuffling, flat-footed gait develops.

The transverse arches

The tarsal and metatarsal bones are arranged with a slight convex, transverse curve on the upper surface of the foot and a slight concave, transverse curve on the sole of the foot. This arrangement forms a series of arches from one side of the foot to the other, extending from the distal ends of the metatarsals in front to the navicular and cuboid bones behind. The transverse arches are supported by small muscles of the foot and by ligaments.

The knee joint

(Figure 55)

The knee joint is made up of the two condyles of the femur and the upper end of the tibia; it is a hinge joint. Two crescent-shaped pieces of cartilage are attached to the upper end of the tibia; the purpose of these cartilages is to provide a smooth and accurately fitting articulation between the surfaces of the condyles and the upper end of the tibia. The knee joint has a loose capsule supported by a strong ligament on

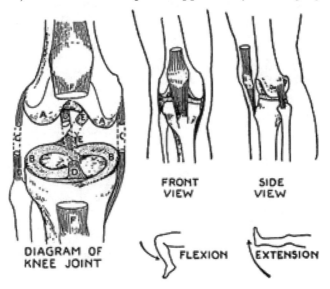

FRONT VIEW   SIDE VIEW

DIAGRAM OF KNEE JOINT   FLEXION   EXTENSION

Figure 55: The knee joint
A – Condyle of femur
B – Cartilage
C – Internal and external ligaments
D – Anterior cruciate ligament
E – Posterior cruciate ligament
F – Quadriceps tendon

both sides. There are also two strong ligaments called *cruciate* ligaments, which arise from the tibia and are attached between the condyles of the femur; these ligaments are directed diagonally across the middle of the joint, in such a way that they do not interfere with joint movement, but prevent the femur slipping forward or backward on the tibia. The front of the knee joint is supported by the very strong combined tendon of the muscle which extends the knee, called the *quadriceps*. The patella, which is fixed within this tendon, articulates with the groove between the two condyles.

The knee joint appears to be one of the least secure joints, because the leverage imposed upon it by the two longest bones in the body is very great, the joint surfaces are not close fitting and the movement allowed is considerable; nevertheless this joint is very strong owing to the support of the powerful ligaments and muscles around it. Dislocation only occurs as a result of extreme violence.

The condition of 'water on the knee', or *synovitis*, is caused by an excessive secretion of synovial fluid as a result of disease or injury to the joint. Synovitis can occur within any joint which has a synovial membrane, that is to say within any freely movable type of joint. It is seen more commonly in the knee than elsewhere because this joint is not only very exposed to minor strains and injuries, but it also has a relatively large and superficial synovial membrane which makes the detection of fluid a simple matter.

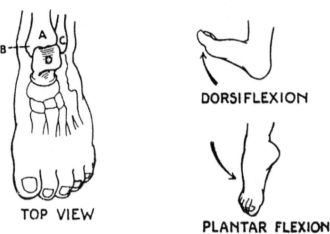

Figure 56: The anatomy and movements of the ankle joint
A – Lower end of tibia
B – Internal malleolus
C – Lower end of fibula (external malleolus)
D – Upper articular surface of talus

The cartilages in the knee are often damaged; they may then interfere with the normal working of the joint. Injury to a cartilage may be caused by a violent twisting movement of the body when one foot is firmly fixed on the ground with the knee bent; if, for example, the individual has all their weight upon the right foot with the knee bent and they twist suddenly in an anti-clockwise direction, they may injure their inner cartilage; if they twist in a clockwise direction the outer cartilage may be damaged.

Immediately after a cartilage has been injured the knee joint may remain locked; in such a case any would-be helpers should resist the temptation to unlock the joint, and call for medical assistance. It is a great help to the doctor in forming an exact diagnosis if they see the joint in the locked position.

The ankle joint
(Figure 56)
The ankle joint is formed by the lower end of the tibia with its malleolus, the lower end of the fibula, and the upper articular surface of the talus. It is a hinge joint and its capsule is supported by strong ligaments on both sides with smaller ligaments at the front and back. The ligaments at the side are sometimes ruptured when the ankle is twisted, but quite often the ligaments remain intact, tearing off a piece of bone from the lower end of the fibula or from the internal malleolus.

Movements of the ankle joint are:
(1) raising the foot upward towards the knee or *dorsiflexion*;
(2) bending the foot downward away from the knee or *plantar flexion*.

The joints between the talus and calcaneus and between the talus and navicular
(Figure 57, p. 200)
These are strongly constructed gliding joints; they are important in so far as they permit turning of the sole of the foot to face inward and outward called *inversion* and *eversion* respectively. The range of eversion is very small. These joints also permit a limited movement of the forefoot inward, *pronation* or *internal rotation*, and outward, *supination* or *external rotation*. It is important to understand that no inversion, eversion or rotation can occur at the ankle joint; movements are purely dorsiflexion and plantar flexion.*

---

*Editor's Note: Although in plantar flexion there is some rotary instability due to the shape of the mortise of the ankle joint.

COMPARISON OF FUNCTION OF THE UPPER AND LOWER LIMBS

The functions and movements of the upper limb differ widely from those of the lower limb, although there is much similarity of anatomical structure between the limbs themselves. The reason for this can be explained on a purely mechanical basis.

Muscles of the thigh

These may be classified as shown below.

The *anterior* group, mainly muscles which extend the knee:

(i) the *quadriceps*, which has four large divisions with separate origins and a combined insertion. The action is mainly extension of the knee. It is by far the most important muscle in this group;

(ii) the *sartorius*, which crosses the quadriceps;

(iii) the *tensor fascia lata*, which is of some importance as a muscle of posture.

The last two muscles are not extensors of the knee, but are included in this group for convenience of description.

The *posterior* group, muscles which flex the knee and extend the hip:

(i) the *biceps femoris*;

(ii) the *semimembranosus* and *semitendinosus*.

The *internal* group of three muscles which adduct the thigh on the pelvis: the *adductores longus, magnus* and *brevis*.

Muscles of the leg

The muscles of the leg may also be divided into three main groups.

The *anterior* group, which is concerned mainly with the extension of the five toes and dorsiflexion of the foot.

(i) the *long extensors* of the *toes*;

(ii) the *anterior tibial muscle*.

The *posterior* group containing flexors of the toes and plantar flexors of the ankle:

(i) the *long flexors* of the *toes*;

(ii) the *posterior tibial* muscle;

(iii) the *gastrocnemius* and the *soleus*.

The *lateral* group containing muscles whose main function is eversion: the *peroneus longus* and *peroneus brevis*.

Muscles of the foot

There are four layers of small muscles in the foot and though their function is extremely important, their general anatomical arrangement will not be set out in detail.

ARRANGEMENT AND ACTION

Muscles of the thigh

Anterior group

(i) The *quadriceps* (the four-headed muscle. Figure 58, p. 199) is a very large and powerful muscle occupying most of the front of the thigh; it has four divisions or *heads*, an inner (medial), an outer (lateral), an intermediate and a fourth head, called the rectus femoris (the straight muscle of the thigh). In Figure 58, the intermediate head cannot be seen as it is overlapped by the lateral head. The fibres of all four muscles converge towards the patella.

Origin: the medial (inner), lateral (outer) and intermediate heads arise from the front and sides of the shaft of the femur; the rectus femoris arises from the a6nterior portion of the ilium.

Insertion: all four heads converge into a single tendon which after enveloping the patella is inserted into a bony prominence on the front of the upper end of the tibia.

Action: extension of the leg upon the thigh: the rectus femoris assists in flexion of the thigh at the hip joint. The quadriceps is a most important muscle of posture.

It may be noticed in Figure 58 that the fleshy part of the medial head of the quadriceps extends almost to the level of the knee joint and that its fibres are directed downward and outward. The reason for this arrangement is that the pull of the other three heads of the quadriceps is approximately along the line of the femur (BA in Figure 59, p. 201). If the outward component of this pull were not counteracted in some way, the patella would dislocate outward; the medial head, however, pulls on the patella along the line BC and the resultant force of the whole muscle group is directed along the line BR, thus keeping the patella in the correct line of movement.

The medial head of the quadriceps is mainly responsible for moving the knee through the last 20 or 30 degrees of extension and when full extension has been reached it keeps the knee braced back. For this reason, when injuries of the knee which limit extension have occurred, the medial head is usually the first part of the quadriceps to become wasted; its strength, therefore, is an index of the degree of recovery of the injury to the knee.

In cases where one or more ligaments of the knee have been completely ruptured, it is absolutely essential to maintain the power of the quadriceps and particularly of the medial head by appropriate exercises; if this is done conscientiously the instability of the joint may be largely overcome. There are many men with ruptured cruciate ligaments who can still play vigorous football and indulge in other strenuous forms of sport, because they have been properly instructed in maintaining a powerful quadriceps, which can control any laxity of the knee joint almost as efficiently as the ligaments themselves.

(ii)   The *sartorius** (Figure 58G, p. 201) is the longest voluntary muscle in the body; it is narrow and rather like a strap.

Origin: from the front of the ilium.

Insertion: into the inner aspect of the upper end of the tibia,

Action: it flexes the thigh and the leg; it also rotates the thigh outward and abducts it.

(iii)   The *tensor fascia latae* (Figure 58H) is the muscle which tightens the broad tendinous sheet or *fascia* on the outer side of the thigh. It arises from the anterior portion of the crest of the ilium and is inserted into the fascia on the outer side of the leg.

Action: it tightens the fascia and, continuing this action, abducts the thigh. In the erect posture it steadies the pelvis on the thigh and the thigh on the leg

Posterior Group

(i)   The *biceps femoris* (the two-headed muscle of the thigh. Figure 60, p. 201) occupies the outer portion of the back of the thigh.

Origin: the long head from the ischium* and the short head from the upper part of the back of the femur.

Insertion: into the upper end of the fibula by a tendon, commonly known as a hamstring.

Action: this muscle is a very powerful flexor of the knee joint. With the legs fixed, each muscle draws the trunk backward as in rising from a stooping position; it plays an important part in maintaining the erect posture.

(ii)   the *semimembranosus* and *semitendinosus* (Figure 60) are situated on the inner side of the back of the thigh.

Origins: from the ischium.

Insertions: into the inner aspects of the upper end of the tibia by strong tendons; these are the inner hamstrings.

Actions: like that of the biceps femoris.

---

*This muscle is known as the tailor's muscle, so called because it brings the lower limb into the crossed leg sitting position.

Medial Group

The *adductor longus, adductor magnus* and *adductor brevis* (the long, the large and the short adductors. Figure 61, p. 199). These three muscles lie one upon the other at the inner side of the thigh; together they form a thick sheet, the shape of a half-haddock.

Origins: from the pubis* and ischium.

Insertions: into the posterior aspect of the shaft of the femur; the adductor magnus extends above and below the insertions of the other two muscles.

Actions: adduction of the thigh on the pelvis. They also assist in flexion of the thigh. The fibres of the adductor magnus which arise from the ischium extend the thigh on the pelvis.

The adductor muscles are used more than any other muscle group in riding, the sides of the saddle being grasped between the knees by their contraction.

Muscles of the leg

Anterior group

(i) The *long extensors of the toes* consist of two muscles (Figure 62, p. 202), one of which extends the big toe and the other the four lesser toes.

Origins: mainly from the anterior surface of the shaft of the fibula.

Insertions: each muscle becomes tendinous just above the ankle; the tendons pass in front of the ankle joint and across the foot, one being inserted into the last phalanx of the big toe, and the other splitting into four divisions, which are inserted into the last two phalanges of the corresponding toes. As the tendons cross the ankle joint, they are held in position by fibrous ligaments, and to prevent friction against these ligaments, the tendons are enclosed in special tendon sheaths which contain a lubricating fluid.

Actions: extension of the toes; both muscles also assist in dorsiflexing the foot.

(ii) The *anterior tibial* muscle lies mainly over the tibia; it can be felt lying along the sharp edge of that bone.

Origin: from the shaft of the tibia.

Insertion: its tendon passes over the front of the ankle joint to be inserted into the first cuneiform and first metatarsal bones on the inner border of the foot.

---

*The *pubis* is that part of the innominate bone below and in front of the acetabulum (the socket for the head of the femur); the *ischium* is that part below and behind the acetabulum.

Action: dorsiflexion of the foot; it is also a strong invertor of the foot and supports the inner border of the longitudinal arch.

Posterior group

(i)   The *long flexors of the toes*: these two muscles lie on the posterior surfaces of the tibia and fibula.

Origins: from the posterior surfaces of the tibia and fibula.

Insertion: the tendons pass round the inner side of the ankle and under the foot; one tendon is inserted into the distal (last) phalanx of the big toe, the other splits into four divisions which are inserted into the last phalanges of the corresponding toes.

Actions: in addition to flexing the toes they assist in plantar flexion of the foot.

(ii)   The p*osterior tibial* muscle is an important muscle situated between the tibia and fibula at the back of the leg.

Origin: from the posterior surfaces of the tibia and fibula.

Insertion: its tendon passes with the long flexor tendons round the inner side of the ankle joint and is inserted into every bone of the tarsus, except the talus, and into the bases of the middle three metatarsals.

Action: its chief action is plantar flexion, but it is also a strong invertor of the foot. By means of its broad insertion it acts as the main support of the inner side of the longitudinal arch of the foot.

(iii)   The *gastrocnemius* (the belly-shaped muscle of the leg. Figure 63, p. 202) and the *soleus* (the muscle shaped like the sole fish. Figure 63) together form the calf muscles. The soleus covers the long flexor and posterior tibial muscles and is itself almost covered by the gastrocnemius.

Origins: the gastrocnemius arises by two separate attachments, one to each of the condyles of the femur; the soleus arises from the posterior surfaces of the upper ends of the tibia and fibula.

Insertions: the tendons of the two muscles blend into one to form the well known Achilles tendon which is inserted into the back of the calcaneus. The Achilles tendon is the strongest and thickest in the body. This fact must have been well known to Thetis, the mother of Achilles, when she gripped him by this tendon to dip him in the waters of the Styx.

Actions: mainly plantar flexion; this is usually performed with the foot as fixed point, thus raising the body on the toes; the gastrocnemius, by reason of its attachment above the knee joint, assists in flexing the knee joint.

These two muscles provide the normal spring to the gait; they are the chief jumping muscles.

External group

The *peroneus longus* and *peroneus brevis* (the long and short muscles of the fibula); both muscles are situated on the outer side of the leg.

Origins: from the outer side of the fibula.

Insertions: the tendon of the peroneus longus crosses the lateral side of the ankle then underneath the longitudinal arch of the foot to be inserted into the base of the first metatarsal and into the adjoining cuneiform bone. Thus with the tendon of the posterior tibial muscle it forms a sling which supports the crown of the longitudinal arch. The peroneus brevis is inserted into the base of the fifth metatarsal.

Actions: The *peroneus longus* acts as elevator of the foot.

Muscles of the foot

The four layers of small muscles in the foot are covered by a very strong and broad tendinous sheet which acts as the tie-beam to the arch of the foot. The muscles, with very few exceptions, run parallel to the longitudinal arch, because their main function is to pull on its two pillars and thus prevent it flattening.

The arch of the foot is primarily maintained by muscular support and secondarily by ligaments. As mentioned above, the peroneus longus and posterior tibial muscle support the crown of the arch by a sling-like arrangement; the small muscles maintain the pillars in their correct position. The ligaments give additional support, but soon become stretched if they are subjected to prolonged strains. A flat foot, that is one in which the longitudinal arch has flattened, need not necessarily give rise to pain; the presence of pain depends on the state of the small muscles. Most ballet dancers have flat feet, but very strong foot muscles and supple joints of the tarsus. This type of flat foot is not accompanied by any disability or pain; but the flat foot in which the muscles are weak usually has stiff tarsal joints and the condition becomes painful because the muscles are too weak to do their normal share of work. The whole body weight is then thrown on the ligaments and if the condition persists the ligaments become slightly inflamed, painful adhesions* start to form around them and the foot becomes gradually stiffer. This results in postural defects and difficulty in walking, because the foot is no longer sufficiently flexible to make delicate adjustments of balance.

*An adhesion is scar tissue which forms as a result of the healing of some local inflammation; scar tissue contracts as it heals, binding together the surrounding structures, and may thus cause pain.

The muscles which support the arches of the foot are the anterior tibial, the posterior tibial, the long flexors of the toes, the peroneus longus and the small muscles of the foot (Figure 64, p. 202).

Corrective exercises should be given upon the following lines:

(1) Instruction in walking with the feet parallel to one another; also walking on the outer borders of the feet to strengthen the invertors (the anterior and posterior tibial muscles).

(2) Heel and toe walking; the toes should be made to grip the ground.

(3) To strengthen the supporting muscles of the transverse arches encourages slight external rotation of both shin bones by standing with toes gripping the floor while flattening them thereby lifting the arches.

II

BASIC AND COMPOSITE MOVEMENTS OF THE LOWER LIMBS

The lower limb is divided into the thigh, the lower leg and the foot. The foot is divided, for movement purposes, into the heel, the arch of the foot, the instep, toes and the sole. The front of the foot including the toes is also called the 'forefoot'.

The movements of the lower limbs are classified into the movements of the thigh in the hip joint, movements of the lower leg in the knee joint, movements of the foot in the ankle joint and movements of the toes in the metatarsals and the phalanges. The movements of the individual toes will not be given any attention in this text. The movements of the lower limbs, as they are carried out in dance practice, are mainly complex movements because all parts of the lower limbs participate in them. They can be separated from each other. Analysis enables us to discover which sections of the lower limbs take part in the complex movement and to examine whether or not these movements are basic or composite.

The knowledge of the cooperation of all the joints of the lower limbs in any complex movement and the knowledge of all its movement abilities is important for a teacher as well as a choreographer. They have to be able to analyse any complex movement. To gain the necessary analytical perception it is essential to study separately the individual parts of the lower limbs with their basic and composite movements. This is despite the fact that in practice one always deals with complex activity and only very rarely with an isolated basic or composite movement.

Before starting the movement analysis of the lower limbs, we must recognise how important the unifying awareness of the body axis is in movement practice. In movements of the lower limbs, standing on both feet constantly alternates with standing on one foot either with stretched or bent legs. During this action the first priority is a conscious awareness of the axis of the centre of gravity which is only possible by maintaining the five rules of the correct body posture (see section: CORRECT ELEVATED DANCE POSTURE, p. 1). The foot should be firm and the instep flexible.

We learn how to achieve this through detailed analysis. The analysis reveals the details of the movement but its synthesis is only achieved on the basis of a conscious awareness of the axis of the centre of gravity. The students must learn to perceive the axis through body awareness, which is the basis for achieving harmony and efficiency in each movement and the participation of the entire body in it.

To revise:
The axis of the centre of gravity while standing on both feet passes through the crown of the head, promontory of the sacrum and the centre of the joined feet.

The axis of the centre of gravity while standing on one foot runs through the crown of the head, the hip joint and the knee of the weight bearing leg and the centre of the sole.

Standing on one foot is more difficult because the support base is more narrow and the body balance demands that none of its parts deviate from the axis of the centre of gravity. It is usually the hip and the inside or outside ankle of the standing foot which deviate. Such a stance is unbalanced and therefore unsteady.

We differentiate movements of the non-weight bearing leg and movements of the weight bearing leg. The movement abilities of the participating joints are the same, but as far as diversity of form, the non-weight bearing leg has many more possibilities. It can combine basic and composite movements of its parts in various ways gaining a rich variety of shapes and having a bigger span of movements in space.

HIP JOINT

MOVEMENT POSSIBILITIES OF THE HIP JOINT

In the anatomical terminology they are:
- Flexion and extension   = moving thighs forward and moving thighs backward.
- Abduction and adduction = moving away from the centre of the body and moving towards the centre of the body.

- External rotation
- Internal rotation

Movement practice uses the following terms for directional movements:
- a forward lifting (raising)
- a backward extension or lifting
- a sideways lifting (raising)
- turning out
- turning in

These movements take advantage of the possibilities of flexion, extension and rotation in the hip joint.

Common characteristics of the thigh movements in the hip joint: in the analysis we concentrate on the movements of the hip joint (for exercises promoting awareness of the movement of hip joints it is best to choose a lying down position).

We can move the thigh in the hip joint in all directions and between-directions (diagonally). In general, when moving a joint in a particular direction, some parts of the structure on the side of the particular joint become slack while those on the opposite side become taut. For example, when raising the leg forward in the direction of the movement, the capsule and the ligaments adjacent to the front of the hip joint become slack while those on the opposite side become taut. The bigger the release on the side of the direction of the movement, the bigger the range of movement achieved. The visual effect of these movements is completed by a consciously guided work of the antagonists (extensors) through their elongation which must flow together with the spatial perception of the movements. For example, in the raising of the leg forward, the muscles of the front of the thigh and hip contract while on the back they elongate. When we emphasise the elongation of the antagonists during the simultaneous maximal slackening of the front of the hip joint, we increase the range of the movement and at the same time reinforce a spatial feeling of the thigh and the entire lower limb elongating in the forward direction. The movement will therefore be more expressive. This applies not only to the movements of the thigh of the stretched leg, but also to the movements of the thigh of the bent leg.

This is equally valid when raising the leg to the side, lifting it backward and executing composite movements in the hip joint, as we shall see later. This rule also concerns the rotatory movements of the thigh in the hip joint. The side of the outward or inward rotation must become slack to the maximum while those on the opposite side become taut. This way we increase the rotatory range in the hip joint as long as we can keep the pelvis firm and immobilised. *Leading* in the case of thigh movements is as important as in movements of the pelvis, trunk and spine. The thigh movements in the hip joint of the non-weight-bearing leg may be performed with a bent knee and the movement *is then led* by the knee as well as with a fully extended leg. In the latter case, the movement *is led* by the tip of the toes and then it is not only a matter of the movement of the thigh in the hip joint, but also of the movement of the foot in the ankle joint. If the plasticity of the movement is to be convincing, we must perceive, simultaneously, and with the same intensity, the leading of all single movements, as well as feeling the direction of the movement.

The basic position of the hip joint, from which the thigh movements should originate, is in practice one of extension. This is also a part of the elevated dance posture. We ensure the extension of the hip joint by maintaining the basic alignment of the established pelvis (see POSITIONS OF THE PELVIS, p. 30) controlled by the abdominal and buttock muscles. The buttock and abdominal muscles keep the pelvis firm and immobilised so that the hips do not deviate from the axis of the centre of gravity. While working on the basic movements of the thigh in the hip joint, we maintain a parallel or a slightly turned-out position of the lower limb. In common practice, however, we usually turn out the leg a little more, in order to join two basic movements in the hip joint—a forward leg-raising and an outward rotation. In this case the movements are composite.

MOVEMENTS OF THE NON-WEIGHT-BEARING LOWER LIMB

Basic Movements

Forward raising: ensure that the centre of gravity is over the supporting leg. When raising the leg forward, in the direction of the movement, the capsule and the ligaments adjacent to the front of the hip joint become slack while those on the opposite side become taut. Transfer the elongation of the back of the hip to the muscles on the back of the thigh and by contracting the muscles on the front of the thigh and hip, lift the leg forward. (See example under COMMON CHARACTERISTICS OF THE THIGH MOVEMENTS IN THE HIP JOINT, p. 112.) In opposition to the lifting leg, press with abdominal muscles on the pelvis on the side of the lifting leg. This way we avoid inward hip rotation following the movement of the thigh. The forward raising of the leg forms a right angle with the trunk at the same time keeping the hips and the shoulders in the horizontal plane.

The movement is led by the tip of the toe of the straight leg or by the knee of the bent leg.

The direction: straight forward.

To achieve a pure and technically perfect movement form, it is absolutely essential to perceive and be aware of the horizontal position of the hips. This applies to all basic and composite movements of the leg in the hip joint.

Backward lifting (extension) of the non-weight-bearing lower limb: ensure that the centre of gravity is over the supporting leg. (The leg we are lifting is held in a parallel position.) During lifting backward the capsule and the ligaments adjacent to the back of the hip joint become slack and those on the front become taut. Transfer the elongation onto the muscles of the front of the thigh and by contracting the muscles on the back of the hip and thigh, raise the leg backward. In opposition to the lifting leg press with buttock muscles on the hip and do not allow the hip to rotate. The hip follows the movement of the thigh. The long back muscles must work strongly to hold the spine upright, as well as the buttock and the lower abdominal muscles of the supporting leg in order to stabilise the pelvis and thus prevent it from tilting forward and the lumbar spine from excessive arching (hyperlordosis). The backward lifting of the leg forms an obtuse angle with the trunk. The hips should be kept in the horizontal.

The movement is led by the tip of the extended leg.

Direction of the movement: straight back-down.

To elevate the lower limb higher, one must add rotation of the leg outward in the hip joint.

Lifting the lower limb sideways: ensure that the centre of gravity is over the supporting leg. The leg is lifted in parallel position i.e. the toes and the knee caps are pointing forward. In the direction of the sideways lifting, the capsule and the ligaments adjacent to the outer side of the hip joint become slack while those on the opposite side become taut. Transfer the elongation onto the muscles of the inner thigh and contract those on the outer side of the thigh and hip while raising the leg sideways. To keep the hip level on the side of the lifting leg, the muscles of the supporting hip and the lateral abdominal muscles on that side must develop pressure on the pelvis to stabilise it in the horizontally level position. The lifted leg should be powerfully elongated to the side in opposition to the action of the pelvic muscles; simultaneously, a stretch should be felt in the muscles of the inner thigh which limits or completely avoids hitching of the same hip. Substantial work by the trunk muscles keeps the trunk in an upright position. The shoulders, together with the hips, are kept in a horizontal. The sideways raising of the leg forms an obtuse angle with the trunk.

The movement is led by the tip of the toe, or the knee in the case of a bent leg.

Direction: straight sideways.

A parallel held leg has a smaller movement range than a turned-out leg (as in ballet). In the forward, backward and sideways lifting of the leg the same rules apply whether the tip of the foot touches the floor or the leg is raised.

Recovery: the leg returns to its initial position by contracting the muscles of the inner thigh. This is not a passive movement, the thigh does not drop, but actively joins to the thigh of the supporting leg, over which the centre of gravity is constantly maintained.

The movement is led by the heel of the lowering extended leg in the direction downward.

Turning out of the thigh: it has several degrees, moderate-medium-maximum. Transfer the body weight onto one leg while letting the other leg hang down freely. The outward rotation of the leg is preceded by a maximal elongation of the hip joint which we perceive as moving the thigh away from the pelvis so that the hip joint is burdened as little as possible. While rotating the free leg outward, the capsule and the ligaments adjacent to the postero-lateral side of the hip joint become slack while those on the opposite side become taut. Keep an established pelvis and an intact axis of the centre of gravity over the supporting leg. The heel of the rotated leg moves in an inward direction, the toe outward-sideways, the hips and the shoulders are in a horizontal.

The movement is led by the outer part of the thigh in *the direction* backward.

Turning in of the thigh: it has two degrees, moderate and maximum. During the maximal rotation inward, elongate the outer side of the hip joint in order to achieve a maximal slackening (release) in its antero-medial side. At the same time keep an established pelvis, the hips and the shoulders horizontal and an intact centre of gravity over the supporting leg. The heel of the turned-in leg points sideways-outward, the toes inward.

The movement is led by the inner thigh in the *direction* inward.

Recovery: it is a return to the initial position – standing with feet together. Besides feeling the downward direction in the leg we also feel the vertical of the body and the horizontal of the hips and of the shoulders, particularly at the completion of the movement.

The basic movements of the thigh in the hip joint, the forward, backward and sideways lifting of the extended leg and their joining, *are led by primary directions*: forward and down, backward and down, sideways and down. They can be executed at various ranges, i.e. in obtuse, right and acute angles to the trunk.

When executing these basic movements, in-between directions or in connection with an outward or inward rotation, we create composite movements. The outward or inward rotation have a significant influence on these movements. Their range is greater when the thigh is turned out and the leg is bent. When the leg is parallel and lifted backward, the thigh achieves only an obtuse angle in relation to the trunk, whether the leg is stretched or bent. When we want to lift the leg higher to the back, we must complement the movement of the leg with the movement of the pelvis, i.e. by its tilting forward. This easily leads to a frequent fault, an excessive arching of the lumbar spine (i.e. hyperextension).

COMPOSITE MOVEMENTS OF THE THIGH

We combine two basic movements: the forward, backward or sideways lifting of the leg + an outward or inward rotation.

The forward-sideways raising: lift the leg between two primary directions sideways-forward. The right leg is right-forward-diagonal.

The forward raising diagonally crossed: lift the leg forward in-between directions crossed over in front. The right leg is diagonally forward over left (adduction crosswise).

The backward-sideways raising: lift the leg between two primary directions sideways-backward. The right leg is right-backward-diagonal.

The backward raising diagonally crossed: lift the leg behind between-directions crossing over back. The right leg is diagonally backward over left (abduction crosswise).

The technical aspect: simultaneously elongate the antagonist muscles used in those basic movements which are contained in the composite movements, i.e. in the forward-crosswise lift we elongate the muscles of the back and outer side of the thigh; in the forward-sideways lift the muscles of the back and inner side of the thigh. In the backward-crosswise lift we elongate the front and the outer side of the thigh, in the backward-sideways lift the front and the inner side of the thigh. When the leg is turned out or in, we must feel relaxation of the side of the hip joint in the direction of the outward or inward rotation.

Directions: most composite movements pass through *in-between-directions* (i.e. diagonally). For example, the forward-crosswise lift passes through *in-between-direction* forward-sideways-inward and the forward-sideways lift through *in-between-direction* forward-sideways-outward. The back crosswise lift passes through the *in-between-direction* backward-sideways-inward and the back-sideways lift through the *in-between direction* backward-sideways-outward.

The leading of the movements is the same as the leading of the basic movements. Using the extended lower limb, the pointed toes lead. For a bent leg, the knee or the heel leads.

Directional features of the outward or inward rotating extended lower limb are the same in all directional movements of the leg, with the exception of the sideways lift. A safe way to determine if the pointed elongated leg is correctly turned out or turned in is to identify the direction of the heel and the tip of the toe.

When the leg is turned out, the heel points sideways-inward and the tip of the toe is more or less sideways-outward, depending on the degree of rotation. This also applies to the forward and the backward sliding, starting from a stance with legs together (*battement tendu*).

When the leg is extended to the side, the direction of the heel and the tip of the toe is different. When the leg is turned out to the maximum, the heel points forward, otherwise forward-down. When the leg is turned in to the maximum, the heel points backward, otherwise backward-down depending on the degree of the outward or inward rotation of the leg in the hip joint.

In the movements with a bent leg, it is the whole shin that takes over the direction of the heel and the tip of the toe. This element is important for the plasticity of the complex movements of the legs which will be mentioned again at an appropriate place.

Circular movements of the thigh

Due to the position of the hip joint and its spherical shape, and also due to the shape of the head of the femur which is an approximate hemisphere (moving in the deep concave socket of the joint or *acetabulum* which is located in the middle portion of the outer side of the pelvic bone or *ilium*), we can move the thigh in all directions and between-directions. To a certain extent it also enables us to execute circular movements along the perimeter of the socket within the limits of the ligaments and the function of the joint capsule.

A large raised arc of the extended non-weight-bearing lower limb: start with a turned-out leg, elongated to the tip of the toes by crossing diagonally (adduction) in front. Pass through a maximal forward lifting, a forward-sideways lifting, pure sideways raising, backward-sideways lift at which point the arc starts to descend and the turning out is cancelled, the leg passes through a backward lift until it finishes the whole arc in the position of the backward-crosswise extension. The leg passes through basic and composite movements during which the antagonist muscles must be kept elongated as has already been described.

The technical aspect is the same as the technique of the execution of the individual basic and composite movements at their highest points.

The movement is led by pointed toes or the extended heel.

Directions: all the directions and between-directions alternate here from the forward-crosswise stretch to the backward-crosswise stretch along the perimeter of the furthest possible extension. The whole movement should be accompanied by the perception of the shaping of a large arc.

CIRCULAR MOVEMENTS OF THE EXTENDED LOWER LIMB

We can locate them differently in space.

The frontal circular movement: the highest point of the upper curve is at the moment of the highest elevation of the leg and the lowest point of the lower curve is at the level of the ankle of the support leg = low forward lifting;

- Forward-sideways: facing diagonally.
- Sideways: facing to the side.

The directions backward-sideways and backward are much less suitable for these circles. The circles are executed with the extended working leg held either parallel (pointing forward to the front) or rotated out or in the hip joint. During the circle, it is best to change the outward rotation of the leg into the inward rotation: for example, the circles facing to the side. When circling, the frontal part of the circle is executed with the leg turned out and the back part with the leg turned in.

The technical aspect: see BASIC AND COMPOSITE MOVEMENTS OF THE LOWER LIMBS, p. 110.

Leading: extended tip of the toe or heel.

Directions: as in the large rounded arc (the same principle).

Small circles of the extended lower limb: these concern minimal circling of the extended leg freely hanging from the hip, close to the support leg, and the foot flexed at the ankle. Circle with a minimal muscular effort. It is a more advanced exercise for loosening the hip joint. We can also connect circling with directional movements, i.e. in primary directions as well as *between-directions*. In this case they are fully active movements. They start low and gradually move higher (thus creating a spiral) along the path of the primary direction or the *between-direction*. For example, during the gradual lifting and circling of the extended leg forward.

The technical aspect: we combine the technique of circling with the technique of the directional movement.

The movement is led by the extended tip of the toe or the heel in a primary direction or a *between-direction* which is simultaneously combined with the direction of the circling to the right or to the left.

FIGURES EIGHT OF THE EXTENDED FREE LOWER LIMB

– vertically located.

– horizontally located.

These can be executed with a leg in an elongated parallel position or a turned-out leg. It can be made more complex by adding a rotation alternately out and in, in the hip joint during the figure eight. In this latter composite movement, the direction of the leg rotation always changes near the extreme points of the loops in the vertical figure eight, that is, at the uppermost and the lowest point in the horizontal figure eight, facing to the front. (And at the furthest right and left points.)

The vertical figure eight frontally located has an upper and lower loop. Its movement is ascending and descending following the line of some of the directional movements of the leg with the point of intersection between the upper and lower loop (approximately at knee level). The best way to execute it is firstly with the leg in a constant, slightly turned-out position. (This applies also to the horizontal figure eight.) Other options include the following example. Initial position: the lower limb is extended forward with the tip of the toe touching the floor, and rotated outward. While ascending, start to turn the leg and draw the inner section of the lower loop in the direction sideways-inward (adduction) until reaching the point of intersection. Continue to draw the outer section of the upper loop in the direction sideways-outward while turning the leg out (abduction) until passing its peak. Then, while descending, gradually rotate the leg inward and reaching the point of intersection continue to draw the outer section of the lower loop in the direction sideways-outward, which is completed by the leg returning to the initial position.

The horizontal figure eight consists of two loops (left and right) described in the air, e.g. by the right leg. The initial position is as in the vertical figure eight, but with the foot raised above the ankle level of the weight bearing leg. *Left loop* - move the right leg left-downward, crossing in front of the left leg ('adduction'). Continue upward and return by descending to the point of intersection. *Right loop* - move the right leg downward-right ('abduction'), continue upward and return by descending to the point of intersection.*

The technical aspect: see BASIC MOVEMENTS OF THE LOWER LIMBS, p. 110.

The movements are led by an extended tip of the toe or the heel.

Directions: of the vertical figure eight are characterised by an ascent and descent along a vertical path. The horizontal figure eight is characterised by a horizontal path and we execute it at different heights, the ankle height, the knee and the hip height.

Circular movements of the extended working leg can be led not only by an extended toe but also by an extended heel. This is unusual but beneficial. It increases the sensitivity of the sole and results in a stronger extension of the whole leg. In the movements of a slightly extended leg we combine the feeling of the directions and the path of the movements. The feeling of the directions helps us to:

– lead from the source of the movement (in this case from the hip).

– always reach the furthermost limits of the directions and between-directions thereby broadening the perimeter of the circular movement.

Both the technical and artistic aspects of the movements gain tremendously from this.

The movements of the thigh in the hip joint of the weight-bearing lower limb: these are a self-evident part of the complex movements of the leg. In complex, i.e. integrated movements, all parts of the leg: thigh, shin, sole and all three joints: hip, knee and ankle always take part. Now let us examine only the thigh movements of the weight-bearing leg. In a weight-bearing straight leg the thigh movements (i.e. positioning and angling at the hip joint) do not differ essentially from the same movements of the non-weight-bearing leg. The thigh of the weight-bearing leg angles to various degrees forward, backward, sideways and in-between-directions, e.g. in different lay-outs, lunges or kneeling positions etc. The span of these

---

*Translator's note: 'adduction' may be combined with a gradual turning in and abduction with a gradual turning out.

positions can reach the right angle in relation to the trunk, e.g. in the 'splits'. We can execute them straight, turned-out and turned-in, but not all can be carried out to the same degree.

It is slightly different in the case of the thigh movement with a weighted, bent leg. They can be directed forward or sideways, but they cannot be directed backward. Only in the case of a maximal outward rotation of the hip joint can the thigh point sideways-backward. In all movements of the weight-bearing bent leg the direction of the knee and of the lengthwise axis of the sole must be congruent. The thigh (respectively knee) must never roll sideways-inward past the big toe. It is one of the frequent faults in the movements of the bent weight-bearing leg, e.g. in lunges, demi-plié and grand plié. If these movements are correctly executed, the alignment of the thighs, shins and feet must be seen to be accurate. That is the reason why the teachers should take care that the students—as long as they are not capable of a large range of outward rotation in the hip joints—do not turn the feet out beyond the capability of the hip joint (see BASIC MOVEMENTS AND COMPOSITE MOVEMENTS OF THE FOOT, p. 128).

The technical aspect of the movements of the thigh of the weight-bearing and bent leg is similar to the directional movements of the non-weight-bearing leg; however, it requires more intensive work of all participating muscles and their antagonists. We must also pay particular attention to the establishment of our pelvis so that it does not deviate from the correct axis and alignment. It is also important to maintain the hips in a *horizontal line* and not disturb it by elevating or lowering one hip. We change the frontal horizontal line into a diagonal one when executing a forward lunge with torsion of the trunk (see BASIC AND COMPOSITE MOVEMENTS OF THE TRUNK, p. 58). In this case the frontal horizontal of the shoulders changes into a diagonal with the legs; and the directions of both hips and the shoulders must be absolutely precise and clear. To achieve complete technical mastery of movements (i.e. positioning and angling) with a bent weight-bearing leg, we must also control the line of the shins in the knee and ankle joints. This point will be analysed in the next chapter.

Leading: the movements of the bent weight-bearing leg *are led* by the knee in *straight directions* forward and sideways and *in-between directions* forward-crosswise, forward-sideways, and (rarely) sideways-backward while maintaining the horizontal of the hips.

KNEE JOINT

Basic movements of the leg at the knee joint are flexion-extension (anatomical terminology) or bending stretching (in movement practice).

The movements of the lower part of the leg are almost always a part of a complex movement of the lower limb. This means that we combine them with basic and composite movements of the thigh in the hip joint and with the movements of the foot in the ankle joint. Bending the knee joint is possible only in one direction, and we classify it into three degrees: a right, obtuse and sharp angle. We can execute the basic movements of the lower leg, i.e. bending and stretching, while standing on one foot, lying on the abdomen or lying on the side. During these movements the thigh is still.

Backward flexion of the non-weight-bearing lower leg: while standing in a balanced posture on one foot (e.g. left), we bend the right lower leg from the knee backward towards the thigh, forming a right angle at the knee, while the sole of the foot is relaxed. The thigh and the knee of the free leg should be held in a parallel position to the thigh and the knee of the stationary leg. The flexion of the lower leg is performed by the back thigh muscles of the working leg. The anterior thigh muscles, serving as antagonists, elongate moderately.

Leading: as the sole of the foot is passive, this movement is not led into space. However, in practice we combine the movement of the lower leg with a plantar flexion (bending-down), or a dorsiflexion (bending-backward) of the foot (see further text). In that case the movement *is led* by an extended tip of the toe or the heel; the muscles of the lower leg and foot also participate.

Direction: directly backward

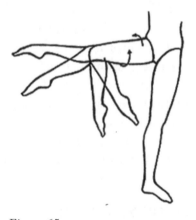

Figure 65
Standing on one leg. The free lower limb, turned out and lifted sideways, is bent in the knee. The thigh and the lower leg form either right, obtuse or acute angles. The axis of this position runs through the hip joint, knee joint and the middle of the foot.

An obtuse angle, backward flexion of the non-weight-bearing lower leg, is executed in the same way as the right angle flexion, but with a lesser effort of the back thigh muscles. The anterior thigh muscles, being antagonists, elongate slightly (in cooperation with the foot as in the right angle flexion).

A sharp angle backward flexion of the non-weight-bearing lower leg is the same as the right and obtuse angle flexion but with maximum contraction of the back thigh muscles. The anterior thigh muscles, being antagonists, elongate to their maximum (in cooperation with the foot as in the right and obtuse angle flexion).

Direction: backward-upward.

The recovery: the lower leg returns to the initial position (straight legs together) through the same path. When the lower leg and foot work cooperatively, both the lower leg and the foot are active. The movement is completed by transferring the body weight onto both feet and by elongating the whole body in elevated posture. Take care not to hyper-extend the knees!

Leading: The movement is actively led by the sole of the foot in the completion of the movement.

Direction: downward with a distinct final awareness of the vertical of the body and the horizontal of the hips and of the shoulders.

The lower leg extension in the knee joint always links the whole leg into a straight line with the thigh and subordinates the lower leg to the movement of the thigh in the hip joint. The lower leg is immobilised when the foot is fixed in a plantar or dorsiflexion. Foot and lower leg are moved like a long lever by the movements in the hip joint. In the case of an independent movement of the lower leg with plantar or dorsiflexion of the foot, the sole is also fixed and throws the work onto the lower leg at the knee joint.

COMPOSITE MOVEMENTS OF THE NON-WEIGHT-BEARING LOWER LEG IN THE KNEE JOINT

In view of the fact that the rotatory movements of the lower leg in the knee joint are not possible with a stretched leg and are always connected with a bent knee, they are classified among the composite movements of the knee joint.

1. OUTWARD AND INWARD ROTATION OF THE LOWER LEG IN THE KNEE JOINT OF THE NON-WEIGHT BEARING LEG

The best way to execute rotatory movements is with a relaxed knee and the lower leg hanging vertically towards the ground. To achieve this position one must hold the thigh forward or sideways.

Outward rotation: lift the thigh forward or sideways into a right angle and simultaneously relax the knee joint and the lower leg muscles. The lower leg hangs in a relaxed manner and at a right angle to the thigh. In this relaxed position turn out the lower leg by using the thigh muscles, mainly the lateral hamstring. You may also combine the outward rotation with active dorsi- or plantar flexion.
  Leading: the heel leads in the direction inward.

Inward rotation: as already described, the lower leg hangs vertically and at right angles to the thigh, while we rotate the lower leg inward by using muscles the thigh, mainly the medial hamstring.
  Leading: if the foot is active with dorsi- or plantar flexion, the heel *leads in the direction* sideways-outward. If the foot is relaxed, the inward rotation of the lower leg has no directional leading in space.

2. CIRCULAR MOVEMENTS
  – Ellipse
  – Circle
  – Figure eight

Ellipse of the lower leg: the thigh is raised in front and the lower leg hangs vertically and at right angles to the thigh, but with active plantar or dorsiflexion of the foot. Turn in the lower leg in the knee joint, simultaneously extending it to an obtuse angle and moving forward gradually. Then turn out to a sharp angle and move back. The elongated ellipse is so formed. The movement is also executed vice versa. The corresponding movement of inward and outward rotation in the hip joint increases the range of the lower leg movement.
  Leading: by a tip of the toe or by the heel *in the direction* forward with a deflection sideways-outward, then backward with a deflection sideways-inward, or vice versa.

Circle of the lower leg: when the path of the bending and extending is shortened, a small circle is formed with the lower leg.

The movement is led by an extended tip of the toe or by the heel.

Direction: the perimeter of a small circle starting sideways-inward or sideways-outward.

The figure eight with the thigh raised forward: starting position: the thigh is raised in front at a right angle to the trunk and the lower leg hangs vertically towards the floor. The weight-bearing leg is extended. The lower leg gradually extends while describing the front loop and gradually bends in the knee to a sharp angle, describing the back loop or vice versa. By turning the lower leg in and gradually out (front loop) and by turning out and gradually out (back loop), the figure eight is completed.

The movement is led by an extended tip of the toe or an extended heel, as far forward and backward as possible.

The figure eight with the thigh raised sideways: starting position: the thigh is elevated sideways and turned out to the maximum, the knee is bent into a 90 degree angle so that the thigh is horizontal.

The lower leg describes first the inner loop in the direction inward-backward-forward, through the point of intersection, and continues the outer loop by moving outward-backward-forward. The figure eight can also be executed with a gradual turning in and turning out of the lower leg.

The movement is led either by an extended tip of the toe or an extended heel.

Direction: the path of a horizontal figure eight with an inner and outer loop. Rotatory movements increase sensitivity and mobility of the leg. They are used in Spanish dances and the can-can.

The figures eight performed this way are located in space slightly aslant (they are neither horizontal nor vertical).

COMPOSITE MOVEMENTS OF THE LOWER LEG IN THE ANKLE JOINT

The lower leg can tilt at the ankle in all directions and in-between directions. It can tilt forward or backward in movements of the whole body or the leg only. When angling the lower leg or the whole leg, it is necessary to establish the ankle joint and to actively elevate the instep while flexing the foot. These movements are usu-

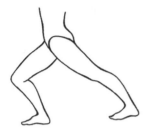 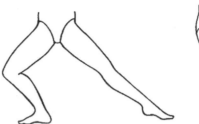 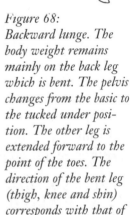

Figure 66
A forward lunge in the basic position. The front lower limb is bent and the hip and knee stretch behind the body. The weight of the body rests mainly on the front leg. The thigh, bent knee and tilted shin, lie on a vertical plane directly above the foot.

Figure 67
Sideways lunge. The body weight remains mainly on the turned-out leg which is bent in all three main joints (hip, knee and ankle). The other leg is turned out and extended in the opposite direction. The pelvis changes to a vertical levelled position with the hips held in the horizontal. The knee of the bent limb points sideways and lies on a vertical plane directly above the foot.

Figure 68:
Backward lunge. The body weight remains mainly on the back leg which is bent. The pelvis changes from the basic to the tucked under position. The other leg is extended forward to the point of the toes. The direction of the bent leg (thigh, knee and shin) corresponds with that of its foot.

Diagrams 66, 67, 68 are complex movements involving all joints of the lower limbs. The extent of the bending in the joints depends on the depth of the lunges.

ally combined with an outward or inward rotation of the hip joint and to a lesser degree of the knee joint. These positions into right, obtuse and acute angles are classified as composite movements.

During their execution, the foot of the weight-bearing leg must be firmly established with a correctly placed body weight. At the same time, the weight shifts from the exact middle of the forefoot closer to the toes or to the heel towards the outward or the inward edge of the foot. The ankles, however, must not roll to the sides but must maintain a firm position. If the placement of the body weight is inaccurate and unstable, and if the shin is not actively turned slightly in or out in the ankle joint, the balance of the posture is unstable whether or not the leg is extended or bent.

Example 1: When standing on 3/4 pointe, complement the plantar flexion of the foot by a slight outward rotation of the shin bones, together with the ankle joint and simultaneously supinate the foot (i.e. slightly lift the inner edge of the foot). In this way we establish the foot and the ankle joint in a vertical position of the instep towards the floor. Consciously transfer the body weight to the big and second toes.

The turning out is led by the outer ankle *in the direction* backward.

Example 2: In a standing position with a turned-in leg (extended or bent), it is necessary to turn the whole leg in the hip joint.

The turning in is led by the inner ankle *in the direction* backward.

The rotation in these movements is slight.

Tilting of the shin of the bent leg is always a part of complex movements of the lower limb. These can be theoretically divided into single movements:

– movements of the thigh in the hip joint
– movements of the lower leg in the knee and ankle joints
– position of a fixed foot

BASIC AND COMPOSITE MOVEMENTS OF THE FOOT OF THE NON-WEIGHT-BEARING-LEG IN THE ANKLE JOINT

BASIC MOVEMENTS

According to anatomical terminology:
- Plantar flexion = bending downward
- Dorsiflexion = raising upward
- Abduction = drawing away from the central axis of the body (lateral direction)
- Adduction = drawing towards the central axis of the body (medial direction)
- Pronation = lifting of the outer edge of the foot
- Supination = lifting of the inner edge of the foot

In practice we use the following terminology:
- bending of the foot downward
- raising the foot upward
- twisting sideways-out
- twisting sideways-in
- inward rolling or pronation
- outward rolling or supination

Basic position of the foot of the non-weight-bearing leg: this is a position from which we start and to which we always return. The relaxed foot hangs from a loose ankle joint. The foot forms with the lower leg an obtuse angle with the opening to the front, it is partially pointed downward. This is the initial position for all active movements of the foot of the non-weight-bearing leg, but it is possible to use other positions as well.

Bending the foot downward (plantar flexion) can be done in two ways:
- by pointing toes downward
- by drawing the heel to the calf

In the first case the instep is arched and its shaping passes into the toes which point downward. The front of the ankle joint is stretched and taut, the back is bent and relaxed. The instep almost forms a straight line with the lower leg. In the second case the instep is also arched but not as much, the front of the ankle joint elongates passively but the toes remain in their basic position, relaxed. The heel is active and forms a sharp angle with the lower leg.

The movement is led in the first case by pointed toes *in the direction downward*; *the movement is led* in the second case by the heel in the *direction upward*.

The first variation is used in movements when the tip of the toes draws straight, rounded and curved lines in space etc. The second variation is used in all natural movements of skipping, jumping and in any case which requires elastic rebound and a soft landing in order to complement the activity of the instep.

Raising the foot upward (dorsiflexion) can also be done in two ways:
- by flexing an extended flat foot, loosening the front of the ankle joint and drawing the instep to the shin.
- by extending the back of the heel, loosening the front of the ankle joint and flexing the foot with toes as relaxed as possible.

Movement in the first case *is led* by the toes of the stretched flat foot, in the *direction* upward, the *movement* in the second case *is led* by the heel in the *direction* downward.

The first case is used in circular movements of the lower leg and the whole leg with an stretched flat foot and in part of the circular movements of the foot and in all instances where the toes of the stretched flat foot lead the movement in space.

The second case, combined with the drawing of the heel to the calf in plantar flexion, is a part of natural movement in a bouncy walk, running, skipping and jumping. It is in everything that requires activating the heel and extending the instep with soft flexible toes in order to melt into the floor and elastically rebound.

If the feet are held stiffly, the heels and insteps are not used with mobility and elasticity. If the knees are allowed to slacken in walking, running and jumping, the movement is stilted and clumsy and rebound is difficult.

Abduction of the forefoot: in the basic position of the foot relax the ankle and on the same side contract the muscles under the ankle towards the heel.

The movement is led by the outer edge of the foot *in the direction sideways-out.* It is a movement which exercises the sensitivity and mobility of the foot, but it can also be used in standing positions with a leg turned out to its maximum in the hip and at the ankle. The foot in these positions is in maximum abduction, i.e. it moves outward. The abduction of the foot, however, must never exceed the degree of the turning out in the hip and at the ankle. When the weight-bearing leg is bent, the thigh, the lower leg and therefore also the knee must point exactly above the third metatarsal or toe (see previous chapter). Neither the inner nor the outer ankle must deviate from the axis of the lower leg. The larger the abduction of the foot the larger must be the turning out of the thigh in the hip joint and the lower leg at the ankle, in order to achieve a balanced posture.

Adduction of the forefoot: in the basic position of the foot, relax the inner edge of the ankle joint and contract the muscles under the inner ankle towards the heel.

The movement is led by the inner edge of the foot in the *direction sideways-in.*

The span of the adduction is smaller than the span of the abduction. In both cases, the inner edge of the foot applies pressure on the knuckle of the big toe.

Rolling in or lifting of the outer edge of the foot (pronation): in the basic position of the foot, contract the muscles under the outer ankle and along the whole outer edge of the foot, which we lift by this contraction.

The movement is led by the outer edge of the foot in *the direction upward.*

Rolling out or lifting of the inner edge of the foot (supination): in the basic position of the foot, contract the muscles under the inner ankle and along the whole inner edge of the foot, which we lift by this contraction. Simultaneously, apply pressure on the knuckle of the little toe.

The movement is led by the inner edge of the foot in the *direction upward*.

Both movements serve to cultivate sensitivity and mobility and occur in circular movements of the foot.

COMPOSITE MOVEMENTS

We combine two basic movements:

Abduction of the forefoot plus raising upward (dorsiflexion): technical aspects and specific characteristics of both basic movements are combined.

The movement is led by an extended tip of the toe in the *directions upward-sideways-out*.

Abduction plus bending downward (plantar flexion) is hardly feasible.

Adduction plus bending downward (plantar flexion): technical aspects and specific characteristics of both basic movements are combined.

The movement is led by an extended tip of the toe in the *direction downward-sideways-in*.

Adduction plus dorsiflexion is not feasible.

Abduction plus pronation (eversion) is easier to achieve in dorsiflexion (see Dorsiflexion, below). The technical aspects and specific characteristics of both basic movements are combined.

The movement is led by the outer edge of the foot in the *direction upward* and the tip of the toe in the *direction sideways-out*.

Abduction plus supination is not feasible.

Adduction plus supination (inversion) is easier to achieve in plantar flexion (see Bending downward, below).

The technical aspects and specific characteristics of both basic movements are combined.

The movement is led by the inner edge of the foot in the *direction upward* and the tip of the toe in the *direction sideways-in.*

Adduction plus pronation is not feasible.

The noted composite movements are a part of the circular movements with pronation and supination. *They can also be led* by the heel in the opposite direction on a smaller scale. *We combine three basic movements:*

Dorsiflexion plus abduction plus pronation (which is minimal): the technical aspects and specific characteristics of the three basic movements are combined.

The movement is led by an extended tip of the toe in the *direction upward-sideways-out.*

Bending downward (plantar flexion) plus adduction plus supination: the technical aspects and specific characteristics of the three basic movements are combined.

The movement is led by an extended tip of the toe in the *direction downward-sideways-in.*

These two movements are also a part of the circular movements of the foot, namely circling with pronation and supination.

CIRCULAR MOVEMENTS OF THE FOOT OF THE NON-WEIGHT BEARING LEG

– Circling
– The vertical Figure eight
– The horizontal Figure eight

Circling of the foot—there are two variations.

– In the first variation, basic and composite movements without pronation and supination alternate.
– In the second variation pronation and supination are added.

Circling without pronation and supination: raise the foot (dorsiflexion), pass to angling sideways-out (abduction of forefoot), point down (plantar flexion), pass to angling sideways-in (adduction of forefoot etc.)

Circling with pronation and supination: the foot is raised up to dorsiflexion, passes to abduction of forefoot with pronation, continues to plantar flexion and passes to adduction of forefoot with supination.

The movement is led by an extended tip of the toe in all *directions* and *between-directions* along the perimeter of the circling.

Circling without pronation and supination can also be led by the heel, but in the opposite direction. We use in this case the second variation of raising and pointing down of the foot (see description in DOWNWARD BENDING AND RAISING OF THE FOOT, pp. 129). Circling of the first variation *is led* only by an extended tip of the toe and in the second by the heel.

Vertical figure eight of the foot occurs between the maximum raising and the maximum pointing, i.e. between the dorsi- and plantar flexion of the foot: adduction, dorsiflexion, abduction = upper loop, through the point of intersection; adduction, plantar flexion, abduction = lower loop.

Horizontal figure eight of the foot occurs between the maximum abduction and adduction of the foot, i.e. between angling sideways-out and angling sideways-in: dorsiflexion, abduction, plantar flexion = outer loop; dorsiflexion, adduction, plantar flexion = inner loop.

The movements are led by an extended tip of the toe through *directions and between-directions* along the path of the figure eight.

Both figures eight can also be executed with added pronation in the upper loop and supination in the lower loop of the vertical Figure eight, and with added pronation in the outer and supination in the inner loop of the horizontal figure eight. The figures eight without pronation and supination can also be led by the heel in the opposite direction.

BASIC AND COMPOSITE MOVEMENTS OF THE FOOT OF THE WEIGHT-BEARING LEG

The foot of the weight-bearing leg is immobilised, fixed and in a definite position. *The position of the fixed foot in the basic standing position is a moderate dorsiflexion combined with moderate abduction.*

The technique of expressive dance essentially took over the five positions of the classical ballet technique, but reduced the angle formed by both feet from 180 degrees to 160 degrees at the most. It limited the size of the angle because a 180-degree angle interferes with the principles of correct body posture. Usually, the pelvis tilts excessively forward and therefore the lumbar lordosis increases too. There is also a danger here that the inability to turn out the whole leg sufficiently is compensated by an excessive abduction of the feet. Consequently, the body weight cannot remain on the middle line of the lengthwise axis of the foot, but deviates to its inner edge (rolling). At the same time, the inner ankle protrudes sideways.

The angle of 60 degrees serves here as a basis; however, angles ranging from 90 degrees of inward up to 160 degrees of outward rotation of both feet are used.

DANCE POSITIONS

- 1st position = basic position (natural position)
- 2nd position = open position with legs astride
- 3rd position = closed moderately crossed position
- 4th position = open fully crossed position
- 5th position = closed fully crossed position

- In the 1st position: the heels are close together.
- In the 2nd position: the heels are in a horizontal line, approximately 40cm apart.
- In the 3rd position: the heel of one foot touches the instep arch of the other foot.
- In the 4th position: the heel is approximately the length of one foot in front of the tip of the other foot.
- In the 5th position: the heel of one foot touches the tip of the other foot.

It is necessary to make sure that the range of the turn out is equal in both feet (see diagram IV POSITIONS OF THE FEET in the Diagrams Supplement, p. 322)

All the above mentioned dance positions can be done:
- with parallel feet
- with legs turned out to the maximum

The weight can be supported either on the whole feet, or only on the big toe and the heads of the first and second metatarsals.

All these variations can also be executed with bent knees involving ankle joints (Figures 66, 67, 68, p. 127).

POSITIONS ON THE DEMI-POINTE

When one rises to a position on high demi-pointe the movement of the weight-bearing foot changes from dorsiflexion to maximal plantar flexion of the foot. The body weight rests in these positions on the two phalanges of the big toe and on the heads of the first and second metatarsals. The heel pulls actively towards the calf.

The legs in all the above-mentioned positions are extended to their maximum with the whole leg turned out in the hip and established ankle. In all positions of the whole foot, the feet are secured to the floor. In the described positions on the demi-pointe the heels in all positions must be kept in the direction sideways-in. The most suitable angle of the feet is 90 degrees.

THE PARALLEL STANDING POSITION

In this position the thighs do not turn out, the patellae and the axes of the feet point forward and the feet are in a moderate dorsiflexion without abduction. These positions are also used in the technique of the expressive dance; however, they are not basic positions. Very subtle turning out in the hip joint and at the ankle correspond with the straight hold of the parallel feet pointing directly forward. The feet are in a partial dorsi flexion without abduction.

BASIC AND COMPOSITE MOVEMENTS OF THE TOES IN METATARSAL - PHALANGEAL JOINTS

Anatomical terminology:
   – Plantar flexion = bending down
   – Dorsiflexion   = bending upward
   – Extension   = stretching
   – Abduction   = moving away from the second toe
   – Adduction   = pulling towards the centre

In movement practice we use the following terminology:
   – Tilting down of the toes
   – Raising of the toes
   – Stretching of the toes (elongating)
   – Spreading toes sideways-out
   – Spreading toes sideways-inward

These movements in the joints link the metatarsals with the first phalanges of the toes and the phalanges of the toes between one another. The big toe has two phalanges and the rest of the toes have three each.

The toes have a certain basic position from which their movement originates and to which they return again. The basic position of the double phalanged big toe is an extension in the metatarsals joint and in the inter-phalangeal joint, i.e. the big toe is extended. The basic position of the rest of the toes is a moderate dorsiflexion of the first phalanges (i.e. moderately lifted) and a plantar flexion of the second and third phalanges (i.e. they are tilted down). When the foot bears the body weight, then the third phalanges rest on the floor and are extended. When the tip of the toe of the non-weight-bearing foot is pointed, all the toes including the big toe are elongated and maximally tilted down, thus extending the instep arch (e.g. dance on pointe in ballet).

The above-mentioned basic possibilities of the movements are natural for all the toes but in practice they are executed only as a collective movement. The toes are not usually able to move separately and independently of the others. They execute all the described basic movements together. Together they bend, stretch, rise, tilt down, pull away from each other and pull together again. Under the influence of civilisation and urban lifestyle they have lost the ability of independent movement. However, theoretically, their ability for such independent movement does exist. There are cases where necessity has forced some individuals to develop the ability of the toes to such a degree that they could substitute for the fingers, e.g. mastering a musical instrument, drawing, painting, sewing etc.

In dance technique we strive for a heightened sensitivity of the sole and the toes, but always only in their common function. We use the sole and the toes for rebounding in walking, running, skipping and jumping and above all, we use their ability for dynamic changes from relaxation, through normal activity, up to a rebound, which represents the height in dynamics. As long as we work with bare feet, we are able to develop a sensitive landing of the sole, clinging to the floor and gradually detaching from it. To achieve this, however, we need natural ground where the soil is undulating and uneven. In indoor dance studios we cannot arrive at such a genuine sensitivity.

So far it has been considered sufficient for dancers, their teachers and choreographers to have a developed sensitivity of the foot as a whole and its division into the tip of the toe, heel, instep, the sole, the ankles and the outer and inner edges of the sole. The dancer should be aware of the tip of the foot even in the detailed sensation of the toes. Through kinaesthetic awareness the movements of both the lower leg and the foot in the ankle joint should be distinguished and the sensitivity of elongation or relaxation of the instep arc perceived. The dancer should also be able to concentrate muscle sense on the outer edge of the sole and on the outer and inner ankle. Then the sensitivity of the soles of the dancer's feet will be considered as sufficient for the task defined by the dance technique, i.e. to serve as a firm and sensitive support for the dancing body. We know, however, from Eastern dance cultures, that Indian, Cambodian and other dancers achieve such eloquence of feet, soles and toes that it can compete with the eloquence of arms and hands.

5. The Upper Limbs

Let us first turn our attention to the anatomical analysis:

I

ANATOMY: THE SHOULDER GIRDLE AND UPPER LIMBS

The upper limbs

The bones of the upper limbs consist of the two collar bones or *clavicles* and the two shoulder blades or *scapulae*, which form the shoulder girdle (Figure 69), and the bones of the arms and hands (Figure 70, p.140).

The shoulder girdle

(Figure 69)

The shoulder girdle is a structure that provides a strong, mobile base by which each of the upper limbs is attached to the trunk. It is not adapted for weight bearing like the pelvic girdle, but for the performances of complex movements.

The *clavicle* is about 150mm long and is attached at its inner end to the sternum by a joint which allows a fairly free range of move-

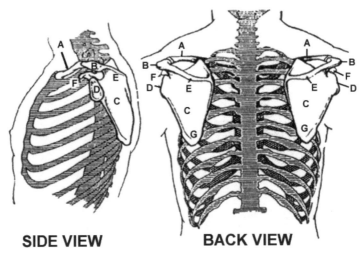

SIDE VIEW   **BACK VIEW**

Diagram 69: The shoulder girdle

A – Clavicle   *D – Glenoid fossa*   *G – Inferior angle of scapula*

B – Acromion   *E – Spine of scapula*

C – Scapula   *F – Coracoid process*

ment. Its outer end articulates with the inner aspect of the *acromion* which is described below. The clavicle acts as a prop to maintain the scapula and upper limb at the correct distance from the chest wall. Fractures of this bone, due to a fall on the outstretched arm, are very common; fortunately they usually unite rapidly and without residual disability.

The *scapula* is a flat, triangular bone which, in the position of rest, covers an area on the back of the chest extending from the second to the seventh rib. At its outer angle there is an oval surface, facing outward and about 25mm in diameter, with which the head of the humerus articulates; this is the *glenoid fossa*. Across the back of the triangular portion of the scapula runs a prominent ridge of bone, called the *spine* of the scapula which extends outward and overhangs the shoulder joint; this overhanging part is called the *acromion*.

The scapula, by its broad flat surface and wide muscle attachments, maintains a very strong purchase on the chest wall, so providing a firm basis upon which movements of the upper limb can take place.

For additional information see the sections THE TRUNK, p. 43., THE THORAX, p. 51. and THE JOINTS, p. 51.

The bones of the arm and hand
(Figure 70)
The skeleton of the arm and hand consists of:
   (1) the bone of the upper arm or *humerus*;
   (2) the bones of the forearm, the *radius* and *ulna*;
   (3) the eight small bones of the wrist forming the *carpus*;
   (4) the nineteen bones of the fingers called *metacarpals* and *phalanges*;

The humerus
The humerus is a long bone and consists of a head, a neck, a shaft and a lower extremity. The head, which is the shape of a half-sphere, articulates with the glenoid fossa of the scapula to form the shoulder joint; the lower end articulates with the *radius* and *ulna* bones to make the elbow joint.

The radius
The radius is a long thin bone consisting of a head, neck, shaft and lower extremity. The head is shaped like a thick disc, and its upper surface has a shallow depression which articulates with the outer part of the lower extremity of the humerus; the sides of this disc articulate with the upper portion of the ulna. The shaft of the radius is slightly curved; it lies on the outer side of the ulna when the palm faces forward, and across the ulna when the palm faces backward. Its lower end helps to form the wrist joint and also articulates with the lower end of the ulna.

The ulna

The ulna consists of an upper extremity, a shaft and a lower extremity. The upper extremity has a crescent-shaped notch which articulates with the inner and posterior portion of the lower end of the humerus. The tip of the upper extremity is a beak-shaped process of bone called the *olecranon*. When the arm is extended, this process fits into a depression at the back of the lower end of the humerus, locking the elbow joint and preventing further extension. The ulna articulates with the radius at its upper and lower ends. Its lower extremity also forms part of the wrist joint.

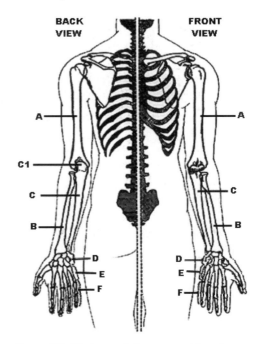

BACK VIEW   FRONT VIEW

Figure 70: Skeleton of the arm and hand
A – Humerus   *D – Carpus*
B – Radius   *E – Metacarpals*
C – Ulna   *F – Phalanges*
C1 – Olecranon

The carpus

The carpus consists of eight small pebble-like bones closely fitted together in two rows, four bones in each row; it provides a flexible yet firm basis upon which the muscles of the forearm and hand can exert themselves. The upper end of the carpus has a smoothly rounded surface which articulates with the lower end of the radius and ulna to form the wrist joint. The lower end of the carpus articulates with the upper extremities of the metacarpals.

The metacarpals and phalanges

The metacarpals are five in number; they each have a straight shaft and an upper and lower articular surface. The first metacarpal forms the bony support of the base of the thumb; the remaining four provide a framework for the palm of the hand; the lower ends of these bones articulate with the upper ends of the first row of phalanges to form the knuckle joints. The phalanges are the bones of the fingers and thumb; there are three phalanges in each finger and two in the thumb.

See Joints in the section THE TRUNK, p. 43.

Joints of the shoulder girdle

The joint between the sternum and clavicle is a freely movable gliding joint; it is the only point at which the shoulder girdle articulates with the trunk. This joint permits movement of the clavicle in all directions. The outer end of the clavicle forms the *acromioclavicular* joint with the acromion process of the scapula; this is a freely movable joint and permits gliding movements.

Both the above joints are subjected to considerable strains and are therefore supported by strong ligaments.

The shoulder joint

The shoulder joint is of the ball-and-socket type formed by the hemispherical head of the humerus and the shallow glenoid fossa of the scapula. Structurally it is a weak joint and for such strength as it does possess, it is dependent more upon the muscles which surround it than on the ligaments. The articular cavity, or *glenoid fossa*, which receives the head of the humerus is deepened by the attachment of a ring of fibrous cartilage round its rim. The whole joint is enveloped in a capsule and is strengthened by certain ligaments above and in front; seven important muscles give their support mainly to the upper

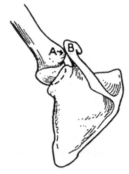

Figure 71: Amount of abduction possible without external rotation of the arm A – Greater tuberosity impinging on acromion

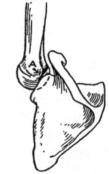

Figure 72: Amount of abduction possible with external rotation of the arm A – Greater tuberosity facing backward, allowing movement of abduction to continue

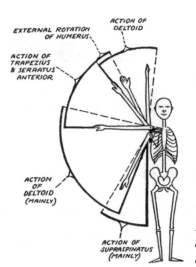

EXTERNAL ROTATION OF HUMERUS

ACTION OF DELTOID

ACTION OF TRAPEZIUS & SERRATUS ANTERIOR

ACTION OF DELTOID (MAINLY)

ACTION OF SUPRASPINATUS (MAINLY)

Figure 73: The approximate range of action of the muscles which perform abduction in the shoulder

part of the joint capsule. The lower aspect of the capsule is thus the least protected part, so when a dislocation of the shoulder occurs, it is usually through this lower and weaker part of the capsule.

The movements of the upper limb can be described as follows.

(1) Movements of the shoulder girdle;
    (i) forward or *protraction*;
    (ii) bracing the shoulders backward or *retraction*;
    (iii) shrugging the shoulders or *elevation*;
    (iv) downward movement of the shoulders or *depression*;
    (v) forward rotation;
    (vi) backward rotation.
(2) Movements of the shoulder joint:
    (i) forward elevation of the upper arm or *flexion*;
    (ii) backward swinging of the upper arm or *extension*;
    (iii) sideways movement of the upper arm away from the body or *abduction*;
    (iv) movement of the upper arm from the abducted position towards the body and across the chest towards the opposite shoulder; this is called *adduction*.
    (v) outward rotation of the upper arm or *external rotation*;
    (vi) the reverse movement, called *internal rotation*;
    (vii) circular movement or *circumduction*; this can combine all the above movements.

The elbow joint
(Figure 74)
The elbow joint is of the hinge type and is formed by the articulation of the lower end of the humerus, the upper extremity of the ulna and the head of the radius*. The elbow joint is strengthened by two strong ligaments on each side and by powerful muscles in front and behind.

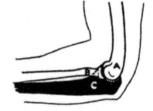

Figure 74: Left elbow joint
A – Lower end of humerus
B – Upper end of radius
C – Upper end of ulna

    The movements at the elbow joint are:
(1) bending the elbow or *flexion*;
(2) straightening the elbow or *extension*.

The joints between the radius and ulna
(Figure 75)
The upper and lower articulation between the radius and the ulna are

*The head of the radius increases the stability of this hinge joint, but is not absolutely essential to its function. When fractured, it is often removed and the functional result is usually very good.

both pivot joints; in the upper joint the neck of the radius rotates within a ring-shaped ligament, and in the lower joint the end of the radius revolves round the ulna.

The movements in which the radius and ulna take part are

(1) turning the palm of the hand downward towards the ground or *pronation*; after this movement the radius lies across the ulna;

(2) turning the palm upward or *supination*; this is the reverse movement; after full supination the radius lies to the outer side of and parallel to the ulna.

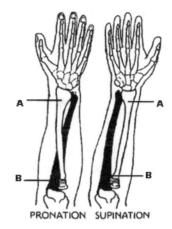

Figure 75: *The joint between the radius and the ulna (right forearm)*
A – Radius
B – Ulna

The wrist joint

The wrist joint is a condyloid articulation formed by the lower end of the radius, a disc of cartilage attached to the lower extremity of the ulna, and the upper aspect of the carpus. It is strengthened by ligaments on both sides and at the back and front of the joint.

The movements permitted at the wrist joint are:

(1) forward bending or *flexion*;

(2) backward bending or *extension*;

(3) sideways movement; when the ulnar border of the hand is moved in such a way that it decreases the angle between itself and the ulna, the movement is called *ulnar deviation*; the opposite movement, i.e. moving the radial border of the hand, is called *radial deviation*.

(4) circular movement, or *circumduction*, is a combination of all the above movements.

Any force which may be transmitted through the wrist joint is first taken by the lower end of the radius; it is in this part of the bone that a fracture so commonly occurs as the result of a fall.

Figure 76:
Movements of the wrist

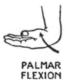

PALMAR
FLEXION

DORSI-
FLEXION

ULNAR
DEVIATION

RADIAL
DEVIATION

MUSCLES OF THE UPPER LIMB CLASSIFICATION

Muscles connecting the vertebrae to the upper limb
(Figure 77, p. 202; 78, p. 203)
They lie on the posterior aspect of the thorax and are mainly concerned with movements of the shoulder girdle, with the exception of one muscle which moves the upper arm.
- (i)   the *trapezius*;
- (ii) the *latissimus dorsi*;
- (iii) the *rhomboideus major and minor*;
- (iv) the *levator scapulae*;

Muscles connecting the walls of the thorax to the upper limb
These three muscles are situated at the sides and front of the thorax, their main function is to draw the whole of the upper limb forward and inward and to rotate the scapula:
- (i)   the *pectoralis major*;
- (ii) the *pectoralis minor*;
- (iii) the *serratus anterior*.

Muscles of the shoulder girdle
(Figure 79, p. 203)
These consist of one large muscle which covers the shoulder joint and five smaller muscles which pass from the scapula to the neck of the humerus. The function of these muscles is to move the arm and to control its movements at the shoulder joint:
- (i)   the *deltoid*;
- (ii) the *supraspinatus*;
- (iii) the *infraspinatus* and *teres minor*;
- (iv) the *teres major*;
- (v)   the *subscapularis*.

Muscles of the upper arm
The *anterior* group whose most important function is flexion of the elbow joint:
- (i)   the *biceps brachialis*;
- (ii) the *brachialis*;
- (iii) the *coracobrachialis*.

The *posterior* muscle whose main function is extension of the elbow joint is the *triceps*.

Muscles of the forearm

It is necessary to know the actions rather than the names of the muscles of the forearm, and they will therefore be classified according to function. They consist of:

(i) flexors of the wrist, fingers and thumb;
(ii) extensors of the wrist, fingers and thumb;
(iii) rotators of the forearm.

Muscles of the hand

(i) the short, superficial muscles of the thumb and little finger;
(ii) the deep muscles of the hand.

ARRANGEMENT AND ACTION

Muscles connecting the vertebrae to the upper limb

(i) The *trapezius** (Figure 80A, p. 203): each muscle is broad, flat and triangular in shape; it lies immediately under the skin of the back. All its fibres converge toward the upper part of the shoulder.

Origin: from the back of the skull, the elastic ligament between the cervical spines, and the spinous processes of the seventh cervical and all the thoracic vertebrae.

Insertion: into the outer border of the clavicle, the acromion, and the spine of the scapula.

Action: the trapezius can elevate, depress or brace the shoulder backward. When the shoulders are fixed the trapezii, acting together, can draw the head backward; acting singly, the muscle can bend the head sideways; it has a very important part to play in controlling the elevation of the arm above shoulder level.

(ii) The *latissimus dorsi* (the broadest muscle of the back, Figure 80B, p. 203): this is a large triangular muscle which covers the lumbar and lower half of the thoracic region; its fibres are directed upward and outward and converge toward the armpit.

Origin: from the crest of the ilium, the sacrum, the spinous processes of the lumbar and lower six thoracic vertebrae, the lower four ribs and sometimes from the inferior angle of the scapula.

Insertion: by a single tendon into the medial and anterior surface of the humerus about 50mm below the head; as may be seen in Figure 80, the muscle twists on itself at C so that the upper fibres are inserted below the lower fibres.

Action: its main action is to bring the arm from an abducted position to the side of the body; in its reverse action, it pulls the body up

---

*It is called trapezius because the two muscles together roughly form a trapezium, a four-sided figure with no two sides parallel.

to the arm; it is also an extensor of the upper arm. The latissimus dorsi assists, by its attachment to the lower four ribs, in fixing the origin of the diaphragm when the latter is called upon to contract more power-fully than usual, as, for example, during coughing, sneezing, and straining in defecation. The upper part of this muscle passes across the lower third of the scapula and helps to maintain the close proximity of this bone to the chest wall, when pushing movements are performed.

(iii) The *rhomboideus major and minor* (the large and small rhomboid shaped muscles, Figure 81, p. 203): these two muscles lie between the scapula and the upper part of the vertebral column.

Origins: the major, from the spinous processes of the second to the fifth thoracic vertebrae, and the minor, from the spinous processes of the seventh cervical and first thoracic vertebrae.

Insertions: into the inner or vertebral border of the scapula.

Actions: the two muscles have a similar action in drawing the lower angle of the scapula upward and inward, thus depressing the point of the shoulder.

(iv) The *levator scapulae* (the elevating muscle of the scapula, Figure 81): this muscle lies underneath the trapezius; its fibres are directed upward and inward towards the base of the skull.

Origin: form the transverse processes of the first four cervical vertebrae.

Insertion: into the upper and inner border of the scapula.

Action: this muscle helps to elevate the scapula when the cervical part of the vertebral column remains fixed; when the shoulder is fixed, each muscle bends the head and neck to its own side.

Muscles connecting the walls of the thorax to the upper limb

(i) The *pectoralis major* (the large muscle of the chest, Figure 82, p. 204): this is a broad, thick triangular muscle which stretches across the front of the chest from the sternum to the armpit.

Origin: the upper portion of this muscle arises from the inner third of the clavicle, and the lower portion from the sternum and the carti-lages of the upper six ribs.

Insertion: the fibres all converge to be inserted into the humerus immediately in front of the insertion of the latissimus dorsi; those fibres arising from the sternum and costal cartilages twist upon them-selves before they reach their insertion, so that the upper fibres of the sternal portion of this muscle are inserted below the lower fibres.

Action: the chief action is adduction but the muscle also produces internal rotation and flexion of the upper arm. The upper or clavicular portion of the muscle completes the movement of adduction initiated by the lower or sternal portion. Briefly, all movements of adduction or internal rotation are performed mainly by the sternal portion of the pectoralis major. Flexion or forward elevation of the upper arm is performed by the clavicular portion of the pectoralis major.

The latissimus dorsi and the pectoralis major are the most important climbing muscles of the upper limb.

(ii) the *pectoralis minor* (the small muscle of the chest): this small triangular muscle lies underneath the outer part of the pectoralis major.

Origin: from the outer surfaces of the third, fourth and fifth ribs.

Insertion: into the coracoid process of the scapula.

Action: it assists in drawing the scapula forward round the chest wall; it also depresses the point of the shoulder.

(iii) The *serratus anterior** (Figure 83, p. 204): this muscle covers most of the side of the chest wall and its posterior portion lies underneath the scapula.

Origin: by fleshy slips from the upper eight ribs.

Insertion: along the under surface of the medial or vertebral border of the scapula. The strongest part of the muscle is inserted into the inferior angle of the scapula where it can exert its greatest pull at the point of maximum leverage.

Action: the serratus anterior is the chief pushing and punching muscle; it draws the scapula forward round the chest wall and plays a most important part in abduction of the arm. The arm is moved through the first 90 or 100 degrees of abduction by the deltoid and the smaller muscles of the shoulder, while the shoulder girdle remains fixed by the action of the serratus and the trapezius on the scapula. Abduction from approximately the horizontal position to 45 degrees above it, is performed by the serratus anterior and trapezius which rotate the scapula while the shoulder joint remains fixed by the deltoid. When this position is reached, further rotation of the scapula does not occur and the deltoid cannot pull the arm up to the vertical position because the highest point of the humerus is impinging upon the acromion. The humerus must therefore be externally rotated and the limb can then be brought into the vertical position by further movement at the shoulder joint by the action mainly of the anterior fibres of the deltoid.

Muscles of the shoulder

(i) The *deltoid**: this thick triangular muscle covers the shoulder joint. From the point of view of function, its fibres may be divided roughly into anterior, middle, and posterior fibres.

---

*This muscle is so called because its origin from the ribs is serrated or notched like the teeth of a saw. (There is also a small muscle, the serratus posterior, which will not be described.)

Origin: from the outer third of the clavicle, the acromion, and the spine of the scapula.

Insertion: the fibres converge into a single tendon which is inserted into the lateral surface of the humerus about halfway down its shaft.

Action: the chief action is abduction of the arm from the side to approximately the horizontal position; it acts most strongly between the range of 15 to 90 degrees of abduction; this action is performed mainly by its middle fibres. The anterior fibres draw the upper arm forward (flexion) and bring it into the vertical position above the head; the posterior fibres draw the upper arm backward (extension).

(ii) The *supraspinatus* (the muscle above the spine of the scapula): this muscle lies in the groove above the spine of the scapula and its tendon crosses the tip of the shoulder joint.

Origin: from the posterior surface of the upper part of the scapula. (Supraspinous fossa).

Insertion: into the highest point on the neck of the humerus.**

Action: it plays the chief part in moving the arm through the first 10 or 15 degrees of abduction.

(iii) The *infraspinatus* (the muscle below the spine of the scapula and the *teres minor* (the small rounded muscle): these two muscles are situated below the spine of the scapula and their tendons pass behind the shoulder joint.

Origins: from below the spine of the scapula. (Infraspinous fossa).

Insertions: into the neck of the humerus, the insertion of the infraspinatus being immediately above that of the teres minor and below that of the supraspinatus.

Actions: both muscles rotate the upper arm externally and assist in adduction (drawing the arm to the side).

(iv) The *teres major* (the large rounded muscle): this thick, somewhat rounded muscle, crosses from the inferior angle of the scapula, behind the armpit, to the upper part of the humerus in front.

Origin: from the inferior angle of the scapula.

Insertion: into the medial and anterior surface of the humerus about 25mm below the head.

Action: the muscle rotates the upper arm internally and draws it inward and backward.

(v) The *subscapularis* (the muscle lying under the scapula): this muscle is situated on the anterior surface of the body of the scapula, between that bone and the ribs.

---

*It is called deltoid because it has the triangular shape of the Greek capital *delta*, represented by an equilateral triangle.
**This point is called the *greater tuberosity*.

Origin: from the flat anterior surface of the scapula.

Insertion: into the front of the neck of the humerus.

Action: it is chiefly an internal rotator of the arm, but when the arm is raised it helps to adduct the arm to the side. The tendons of all the smaller muscles of the shoulder joint are closely blended with the joint capsule and thus form a very strong tendinous cuff which envelops the top and sides of the head of the humerus contributing to the stability of the joint. During abduction of the shoulder, these muscles contract and hold the head of the humerus firmly in apposition to the glenoid fossa and thus counteract the natural tendency of the head of the humerus to ride upward over the joint margin. As soon as the head of the humerus is held down firmly, the movement of abduction by the supraspinatus can be started.

Muscles of the upper arm
Anterior group

    (i)   The *biceps brachialis* (the two-headed muscle of the arm): this muscle lies along the front of the forearm.

Origin: by two tendons or heads; one called the *long* head arises from a point just above the glenoid fossa, the other, the *short* head from the coracoid process of the scapula.

Insertion: into the medial aspect of the radius about 18mm below its head.

Action: it is primarily a supinator of the forearm and secondarily a flexor of the elbow joint.

The tendon of the long head of the biceps acts as an accessory ligament of the shoulder joint and is closely blended into the joint capsule.

    (ii) The *brachialis* (the muscle of the arm, Figure 84, p. 204): this muscle lies over the lower end of the humerus and the front of the elbow joint.

Origin: from the front of the lower half of the humerus.

Insertion: into the upper end of the ulna about 12mm below the elbow joint.

Action: it is the chief flexor muscle of the elbow joint.

    (iii) The *coracobrachialis* (the arm muscle attached to the coracoid process, Figure 84): this is a small, straight muscle situated on the medial side of the upper arm.

Origin: from the coracoid process.

Insertion: into the medial side of the humerus about midway down its shaft.

Action: this muscle is a weak adductor and flexor of the upper arm.

Posterior muscle

The *triceps* (the three-headed muscle): this muscle covers the whole of the back of the humerus.

Origin: by three separate origins or *heads*: the *long* head arises from immediately below the glenoid fossa, and the other two heads, a *lateral* and a *medial*, from the middle of the posterior aspect of the humerus. They blend into one tendon.

Insertion: into the olecranon process of the ulna.

Action: extension of the elbow; it also assists in adduction of the upper arm.

Muscles of the forearm

(i)   *The Flexor Group*

The long flexors of the fingers and thumb: these muscles lie mainly on the medial side of the front of the forearm. They are more powerful than the opposing extensor muscles because they are the chief muscles of gripping; the extensors are seldom called upon to do work against active resistance, their chief function being to open the fist and extend the fingers. The long muscles of the fingers perform the strong, coarser movements of the fingers whereas the short muscles in the hand, which will be mentioned later, perform the movements of precision.

Origins: from the bony prominence or condyle on the medial side of the lower end of the humerus, and from the fronts of the shafts of the radius and ulna.

Insertions: into the last two phalanges of the fingers and thumb.

Actions: flexion of the fingers and thumb: they assist in flexion of the wrist.

Flexors of the wrist (Figure 85, p. 204): there are two muscles whose main function is flexion of the wrist. They arise from the inner condyle of the lower end of the humerus and from the ulna and are inserted into the carpus and the bases of the metacarpals.

Actions: flexion of the wrist when acting together.

(ii)   *The Extensor Group*

The long extensors of the fingers and thumb: the extensor group is situated on the lateral side and the back of the forearm.

Origins: from the bony prominence or condyle on the lateral side of the lower end of the humerus, and from the posterior aspects of the shafts of the radius and ulna.

Insertions: into the last two phalanges of the fingers and thumb.

Actions: extension of the fingers and thumb; they assist in extension of the wrist.

Extensors of the wrist: there are three; they arise mainly from the outer condyle of the lower end of the humerus and are inserted into the bases of the metacarpals on the back of the hand, one on the ulnar and the others on the radial border.

Actions: acting together they dorsiflex or extend the wrist; acting separately they produce either radial or ulnar deviation.

(iii) *The rotators of the forearm.*

(*a*) The *pronator teres* and *pronator quadratus*;

(*b*) The *brachioradialis* and *short supinator*.

The *pronator teres* (the rounded muscle of pronation): this muscle lies among the flexor group.

Origin: from the common flexor origin on the lower end of the humerus and from the upper end of the ulna.

Insertion: into the outer aspect of the middle of the shaft of the radius.

Action: its chief action is pronation, which it performs by rolling the lower part of the radius round the ulna. Its subsidiary action is flexion of the elbow joint.

The *pronator quadratus* (the rectangular muscle of pronation): this muscle arises from the lower end of the ulna and is inserted into the lower end of the radius; it acts as a pronator only.

The *brachioradialis* is a flexor of the elbow though it is situated in the extensor group.

Origin: from the outer part of the lower end of the humerus.

Insertion: into the outer aspect of the lower end of the radius.

Action: it is a flexor of the elbow and acts most strongly when the forearm is in the position midway between full supination and full pronation.

The *short supinator* is a small but important muscle situated between the upper ends of the radius and ulna.

Origin: from the outer side of the elbow joint and the outer aspect of the upper end of the ulna.

Insertion: into the outer surface of the upper third of the radius.

Action: it assists the biceps in performing supination of the forearm. Supination is an extremely important component of complex movement of the wrist.

The small muscles of the hand

(Figure 86)

These are (i) the *superficial* muscles at the base of the thumb and little finger, and (ii) the *deep* muscles between the metacarpal bones and between the tendons of the hand. The muscles of the thumb are among the most important in the whole of the upper limb; they bring the thumb into apposition with any one of the four fingers and thus make precise grasping movements possible. Both groups of muscles arise from the bones and ligaments of the carpus and are inserted into the phalanges of the thumb and little finger. The thumb muscles have four separate actions:

(1) they draw the thumb across the palm of the hand to oppose the other fingers; this movement is *opposition*;

(2) they move it directly away from the palm of the hand in a plane at right angles to its surface; this movement is *abduction*;

(3) they press the adjacent margins of the thumb and index finger together; this movement is called *adduction*;

(4) they flex the joints of the thumb.

The deep muscles of the hand are the four *lumbrical* muscles, named for their likeness to earthworms, and the seven *interosseous* muscles which lie between the metacarpals. The action of the interossei is to straighten the interphalangeal joints, bend the metacarpo-phalangeal joints and to spread the fingers and to draw them together.

II

BASIC AND COMPOSITE MOVEMENTS OF THE SHOULDERS

The shoulder girdle, commonly called the shoulders, represents with the arm one unit for a movement teacher, the parts of which are mutually dependent on each other. The anatomical analysis has clarified for us the skeletal basis of the shoulders and their joint connections. The main link of the shoulder girdle and arms with the chest (thorax) is, however, a muscular connection, which is of great importance for the movement of the shoulders. Its advantage is a high mobility and adaptability of the shoulders but it also represents a considerable danger. The shoulders succumb to an incorrect posture of the chest, spine, neck and head and also to an uncontrolled movement of the arms. It is not easy to establish and maintain the shoulders in the correct basic position; and yet the movement of the entire upper part of the chest, including the arms, depends on this if we want to achieve a controlled movement which is perfect in form.

The shoulders have a mediator's role between the trunk and the arms. The movement teacher must always be aware of it. This can happen only when the muscles which connect the chest with the arms, and especially posterior thoracic muscles, are perfectly controlled and trained, so that their sensitivity towards this role is developed. For a movement teacher this means having a knowledge of the functioning of appropriate muscles, a keen perception and a body sensitivity for this muscle region.

The hold of the shoulders is usually faulty, either limp or cramped. This fact is unfortunately often overlooked by movement teachers who lack the appropriate knowledge. They do not give attention to the shoulder posture and its movement, despite its great importance. There are even some movement teachers who insist on the old army style of shoulder posture with the shoulder blades pushed together and neck squeezed in between.

A more detailed explanation of the fifth rule of the elevated dance posture on page 3 defines the basic alignment of established shoulders. To develop this posture, it is necessary to keep active the muscular connections both between the shoulders and the chest and between the shoulders and the arms. It is an important task for a movement teacher to develop and maintain a harmonious interaction of all the muscles which participate in the movement of the shoulders and arms. Arm movements without active participation of the back and the chest are cut off from the whole: they lack expansion, fluidity and strength and are, in a way restricted.

The anatomical terminology of the movements of the shoulder girdle refers primarily to the movements of the shoulder blades:

- fixation of the shoulder blade   = establishing the shoulder blade
- elevation of the shoulder blade   = raising of the shoulder blade
- depression of the shoulder blade = lowering of the shoulder blade
- protraction of the shoulder blade = pulling forward of the shoulder blade
- retraction of the shoulder blade = pulling backward of the shoulder blade
- adduction of the shoulder blade = pulling the shoulder blade towards the spine
- outward rotation of the lower angle of the shoulder blade

In movement practice we talk about:
- establishment of the shoulders
- elevation of the shoulders

- pulling downward of the shoulders
- pulling sideways of the shoulders
- pulling forward of the shoulders
- pulling backward of the shoulders
- pressing the shoulder blades towards the ribs

BASIC MOVEMENTS

The initial position of all basic and composite movements of shoulders and arms is an upright posture of the chest with established shoulders.

Establishment of shoulders = basic position of shoulders: relax the upper part of the trapezius and acromioclavicular joints. Through a proportionate activity of the lower trapezius and the muscles under the clavicle, pull shoulders down and draw the clavicles towards the ribs. Feel as if you are expanding the large chest muscles (pectoralis major) which mark off the armpits in the front and contract the large back muscles (lattissimus dorsi), particularly that part which marks off the armpits at the back. By using these and the serratus anterior, press the shoulder blades, especially their lower angles, towards the ribs. With this complex and proportionate activity, not maximal, establish the shoulders and keep them exactly on the sides of the chest. The tension of the above-mentioned muscles corresponds to the relaxed, elevated posture of the whole body. This certain tension is necessary to maintain the horizontal of the shoulders, in contrast to the vertical of the trunk. The neck, together with the head, is free, able to move in a relaxed and elevated manner, without any unnecessary and harmful tension of the upper part of the trapezius and the front neck muscles. This is the basic posture of the shoulders from which we execute basic and composite movements.

Upward pull of the shoulders: raise the shoulders by activating the 'lifter' muscle of the shoulder blades (levator scapulae) and try not to narrow the shoulders, i.e. exclude as much as possible the upper trapezius in this movement. We must not lift the shoulders haphazardly upward, but raise them in the basic position. Above all, we must not lose the feeling of the width and the horizontal of the shoulders.

The movement is led by the points of the shoulders (acromions) in the *direction* sideways-upward.

Downward pull of the shoulders: pull the shoulders by increased contraction of the lower part of the trapezius and the sub-clavicular muscles down towards the ribs while simultaneously raising the sternum in the opposite direction.

The movement is led by the lower angles of the shoulder blades and the acromial section of the clavicles in the *direction* downward.

Sideways pull of the shoulders: while the pectoralis major is stretched, be aware of the horizontal of the shoulders in contrast to the vertical of the trunk (be conscious of each shoulder separately and then both together).

The movement is led by the acromions in the *direction* sideways.

Forward pull of the shoulders: pull the widely-spread shoulders by increased contraction of the pectoralis major forward without slackening the chest.

The movement is led by the front part of the acromions in the *direction* forward.

Backward pull of the shoulders: using the lower part of the trapezius, pull the shoulders backward without narrowing them.

The movement is led by the back part of the acromions in the *direction* backward.

Pressing the shoulder blades to the ribs: by increasing the contraction of the muscles which border the back part of the armpits and contracting the serratus anterior, press the shoulder blades to the ribs and draw away from the spine.

The movement is led by the lower angles of the shoulder blades in the *direction* sideways-forward.

Forward tilt of the shoulders: by increased elongation of the muscles of the back of the armpits, while contracting the pectoralis major tilt the shoulders forward-down without narrowing them.

The movement is led by the front part of the acromion in the *direction* forward.

The recovery from the basic movements of the shoulders is a return to the basic shoulder posture by the relaxing of the maximal tension of the involved muscles.

COMPOSITE MOVEMENTS, ROTATING MOVEMENTS

These movements are best executed with arms lifted to the side.

Turning the shoulders in consists of three basic movements:
- sideways pull of the shoulders
- downward pull of the shoulders
- forward tilting of the shoulders

The pectoralis muscles are stretched to the sides, the upper part of the trapezius is relaxed and the sub-clavicular muscles contracted. The lower angles of the shoulder blades withdraw slightly from the ribs and the acromions turn forward-down.

The movements are led by the acromions in the *direction* forward-down.

Turning the shoulders out consists of four basic movements:
- downward pull of the shoulders
- sideways pull of the shoulders
- backward tilting of the shoulders
- pressing of the shoulder blades to the ribs.

The arching of the upper part of the chest increases under the influence of this composite movement, the ribs of the posterior part of the chest draw closer to each other where the support point of the neck and head is situated and the neck and head raise themselves considerably. The activity of all used muscles must be maximal.

The movement is led by the acromions in the *direction* backward-down.

The rounded backward bend (extension) of the neck and head and all the rounded backward bends of the whole spine must start by turning out the shoulders. The quality of each complex movement with a rounded backward bend depends on this particular composite movement.

Recovery from the composite movements of the shoulders: relax the increased tension of all muscles used until the normal level of tension is reached and return the shoulders to their initial basic position.

CIRCULAR MOVEMENTS OF THE SHOULDERS:
- circling
- circling in the opposite direction
- vertical figure eight
- vertical figure eight in the opposite direction

Circling the shoulders: gradually link, one after another, the upward pull of the shoulders, backward pull of the shoulders, downward pull of the shoulders and forward pull of the shoulders. In the transition from one movement to the other we pass through appropriate composite movements, upward, upward-backward, backward, backward-down, down, down-forward, forward. In the opposite direction it is vice versa.

The movement is led gradually by those parts which have led in the basic movements. They are bound together along the perimeter of circling. All *directions* and *in-between directions* alternate.

Circling the shoulders in opposite directions: there are two kinds:
1. Both shoulders rise together, then one shoulder moves back and the other forward, they move together downward and finally each shoulder completes its circle.
2. One shoulder starts upward, the other one downward, then one moves forward and other backward and so they continue in their circling. The opposite direction is vice versa.

The movement is led gradually by these parts which have led in the basic movements, but now each shoulder moves differently. All *directions* and *between-directions* alternate along the perimeter of the circling.

Vertical figure eight of the shoulders: the shoulder moves forward, upward and backward (top loop), then forward, downward and back (lower loop) This is done individually, or both shoulders together.

Leading: as in circling, but along the path of the figure eight.

Vertical figure eight in opposite directions: one shoulder executes the upper loop while the other one executes the lower loop.

Leading: as in circling, but along the path of the figure eight.

Similarly, we can also move the shoulders in a horizontal figure eight, forward and backward.

III

BASIC AND COMPOSITE MOVEMENTS OF THE ARMS

Just as the majority of the leg movements are a total of basic and composite movements of the parts of the leg, so the arm movements are mostly complex movements in which all individual parts of the arm participate. Through movement analysis we explore what kind of movements are executed in a complex movement by the upper arm in the shoulder joint, the forearm in the elbow joint, the hand in the wrist joint, etc. We also discover the movement possibilities of these joints.

Anatomical terminology of movement possibilities of the arm in the shoulder joint:

- flexion   = bending (moving arm forward)
- extension   = stretching (moving arm backward)
- abduction   = moving away
- adduction   = moving towards
- inward rotation   = turning in
- outward rotation   = turning out

In movement practice we use terms which indicate the direction of basic movements (as has already occurred with leg movements in the hip joint). In basic movements the arm moves in the shoulder joint in different basic directions (forward, sideways, backward, upward, downward):

- raising arms forward
- raising arms sideways
- raising arms backward
- raising arms upward
- turning in
- turning out

With incorrect carriage of the chest and shoulders, the movements of the arms are also faulty. We must connect the basic posture of established shoulders with an elevated hold of the chest and with the basic position of the arms. Thus we gain a perfect starting position of all arm movements in the shoulder joints, including turning out and turning in.

Basic position of the arm: the arm hangs freely along the body from established shoulders. It is slightly turned in at the shoulder joint so that the elbows are away from the body and point sideways-outward. Also the forearm is slightly turned in by its own weight so that the palm of the hand faces the body and the thumb points forward-inward. As the elbow is slightly bent the arm forms a moderately rounded line. The arm position is often faulty, as a consequence not only of an incorrect chest and shoulder posture, but also of an excessive tension of the forearm and hand muscles. As a result of such tension the arms do not hang from the shoulders in a relaxed manner but bend the elbows or press them to the body. It is therefore essential to cultivate in students a conscious muscle feeling which leads to muscle memory for a perfect arm line in its basic slightly rounded position.

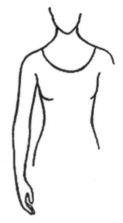

Figure 87: Basic position of the arm. The arm hangs from the shoulder joint in a rounded shape, slightly turned in and bent at the elbow. The elbow points away from the body (sideways-backward) and the palm towards the body. The thumb is directed forward and inward.

Dynamic line of the rounded arm: the dynamic line starts with great activity of the muscles which control the shoulders and the shoulder joint. From here, the muscle tension should decrease until a sensitive, relaxed mobility of the hand and the fingers is achieved. This descending line of muscular tension of the arm is necessary in the basic arm posture and in all movements of the rounded arm. The forearm and the hand have only an accompanying role and should be sensitive and light. It is somewhat different when the arm is stretched and when forearm, hand and fingers actively prolong the movement and direction of the whole arm. In these movements the activity of the shoulders and upper arm is transferred, although on a smaller scale, to the forearm, hand and fingers. *The tension of the forearm, hand and fingers, must never be greater than that of the muscles of the shoulders and upper arm. This is an aesthetic requirement.* Very often quite the reverse can be seen: slackened chest, loose, heavy shoulders, heavy elbow, tense forearm and hard, over-tense hand. This is just as unacceptable for a movement artist as it is for a pianist, violinist or painter; all of them need a sensitive, mobile and light hand, relaxed even in an expression of force and never cramped or tense.

A ROUNDED ARM

Forward raising: starting with a perfect body posture, increase the pressure of the lower abdomen, i.e. the lower segments of the straight abdominal muscle (rectus abdominis) backward and simultaneously lift the arms in their basic rounded position forward until they reach the height of the shoulders. Keep the shoulder width between the upper arms, elbows, wrists and palms. The palms remain facing the body and the elbows turn away from it.

The movement is led by the tip of the fingers, above all by the third finger in the *direction* forward. The directional feeling must be combined with the awareness of the vertical of the body and the horizontal of the shoulders. Feel as if the forearm is being carried up by the upper arm and elbow, which point sideways out. In such a complex feeling lies the visual value of all basic arm movements in the shoulder joint.

Sideways raising of rounded arms: starting with a perfect body posture with an increased pull of the shoulders to the side and down, lift the arms in their basic rounded position to the side up to shoulder height. The rounded elbows are turned backward, the palms forward-downward (in-between direction).

The movement is led by sensitive finger tips, above all by the middle finger, in *the direction* sideways.

Directional feeling: by completing an imaginary curve, slightly bent forward-down and in continuation of the rounded arms.

The upper arms of both arms are in one horizontal line with the shoulders and they must retain this unifying feeling. This must not be disturbed by the slightest deviation of the upper arm in the

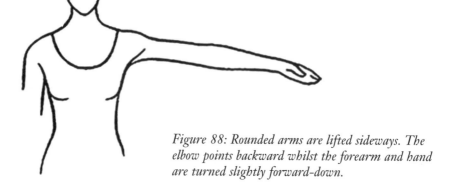

Figure 88: Rounded arms are lifted sideways. The elbow points backward whilst the forearm and hand are turned slightly forward-down.

shoulder joint, whether it be forward, backward, upward or downward. That is the guarantee of the perfect form of the sideways raising of the arms. This requirement is all the more important in connection with the rotation of the chest when the frontal location of the shoulders and the upper arms changes into a diagonal location. Perfect control of the shoulder joint is paramount here to avoid the slightest involuntary deviations, through which the movement loses its visual value and plasticity. Deviations can only be accepted in the movement of a creative dancer when they are intentional and justified.

Backward raising extension: starting with a correct body posture, gradually turn in the shoulders (see COMPOSITE MOVEMENTS OF THE SHOULDERS, p. 156) while lifting the rounded arms in their basic position in the direction backward to the height of approximately one third of the way to the shoulders. The distance between the upper arms corresponds to the shoulder width.

The movement is led by the sensitive tips of the fingers, above all by the third one, in *the direction* backward-downward, contrary to the motion of the sternum which leads forward-upward. The counter direction of the sternum plays an important role in this movement. Keeping the same distance between the arms is also important, even more so because we can only control it through kinaesthetic awareness. Through this action, a directional orientation is also practised. The inward turning of the shoulders must be perfectly controlled, to avoid incorrect execution, resulting in faulty direction of the movement.

Raising upward from a forward raising: from the position of forward-raised arms, continue in an upward direction. The upper arms gradually change their position from slightly turned in to slightly turned out. In contra-motion to the arms, pull the shoulders down with an increased intensity. Keep rounded arms and retain the distance between the upper arms and palms at shoulder width.

The movement is led by the sensitive tips of the fingers, above all by the third one in *the direction* upward. *Directional feeling* culminates in the awareness of the vertical of the body, accentuated by the arms.

Raising upward from the sideways raising: start from the position of sideways-raised arms, where the shoulders and arms are pulled to the sides. While raising the arms, continue gradually turning out the upper arms, forearms and hands until the upward-raising is completed. The arms move closer to each other at the shoulder width, they are rounded in the elbows and the palms almost face each other. In the opposite direction to the arms, pull the shoulders down with an increased intensity. To achieve a beautiful line of the arms in both types of lifting, we must develop sufficient activity in the muscles of the back part of the upper arm. These muscles must be elongated in order to avoid a clumsy and insensitive slackening of the elbows which disturbs the rounded line of the arms.

Recovery to the basic position: lower the arms from any preceding arm movement in the shoulder joint. This is a simple recovery from a basic or a composite movement of the arms in the shoulder joint. The arms, in their relaxed manner, return through the same path to the basic position. The dynamics of such a movement decrease until the final relaxation in the basic position. In the opposite movement to the arms, lift the sternum. This ensures that the movement is carried out with lightness and relaxation.

The movement is led by the sensitive fingertips, above all by the third one, in *the direction* downward.

A modification of the lowering of the arms is an active lowering of the arms with an emphasis on directional orientation. In contrast to the first type, its dynamics are ascending. The arms pass from a roundedness to prolongation, while the upper arm, forearm, wrist and the hand merge together with the accentuated vertical of the body. In the contra-motion to the arms, emphasise the elevation of the sternum and the upward arching of the upper ribs. This will further intensify the end of the ascending dynamics of the active lowering of the arms. This movement has a different expression.

The movement is led by the extended fingers in *the direction* downward.

TURNING THE ARM

Partial turning out: starting with a correct body posture with established shoulders, turn out the upper arms in the shoulder joint slightly without relaxing the elbow. At the same time, maintain a turned-in forearm and hand, with the palm still facing the body. This partial turning out of the upper arm is also a part of an arm movement above the shoulder level, occurring when simultaneously turning in the forearm and the hand. This opposite movement heightens the plasticity of the arms.

The movement is led by the elbow.

Maximal turning out is often complemented by a maximal turning out of the forearm and hand (see BASIC MOVEMENT OF THE FOREARM, p. 170). During maximal turning out of the entire arm in its basic position, the palm turns forward, the elbow remains slightly bent and points backward.

The movement of the upper arm is led by the elbow in *the direction* sideways-inward, *the movement of the forearm is led* by the thumb side of the palm in *the direction* sideways-outward.

Partial turning in of the upper arm in the shoulder joint belongs to the basic position of the rounded arm. It is therefore a part of all its movements as long as they occur at the level, or below the level, of the shoulders.

Maximal turning in of the upper arm: during a sideways-raising of the arms this movement is complemented by either a medium or a maximal turning in of the forearm and hand (for more details see BASIC MOVEMENT OF THE FOREARM, p. 170). In the case of the medium turning in of the forearm (medium pronation), which is most often used, the palm turns backward. However, when the arm is in the basic position, i.e. held along the body in a relaxed manner, the elbow remains slightly bent and points sideways-out. In this basic position, with the maximal turning in of the forearms (maximal pronation), the palm turns sideways-out. The elbow points also sideways-out and remains slightly bent.

The movement is led by the elbow and the thumb side of the hand, the elbow in *the direction* sideways-out, the hand in *the direction* sideways-in. During the turning in of the upper arm in the shoulder joint, keep the shoulder normally turned out, as is required by the established position of the shoulders. The turned out shoulder and the turned in arm are opposing movements which favourably affect plasticity of the upper part of the chest and arm.

Recovery of the basic movements in the shoulder joint is always a return to the initial position, i.e. the basic position with arms hanging in a relaxed manner from established shoulders on the sides of the chest.

All the basic movements of the arm in the shoulder joint can also be executed with a stretched arm.

A STRETCHED ARM

The difference between the basic movements executed by the rounded arm and the same movements executed by a stretched arm is, (1) in shape, (2) in dynamics and (3) in some directional movements.

The difference in shape: all parts of the extended arm are in a straight line because the elbow is stretched, not slightly bent as it is with the rounded arm.

The difference in dynamics: the extended arm does not hang along the body with a sensitively relaxed forearm and hand; the extension of the elbow transfers itself to the forearm and the hand, causing a certain muscular tension in the actively elongated muscles. Even in this case, however, the forearm and hand are not rigidly taut, but sensitively elongated so that the descending tension from the shoulders to the fingertips is preserved.

Directional difference: in the forward, backward, upward stretch and with the arms lowered along the body, the extended arm maintains precisely the directions of the rounded arm, with the exception of the sideways stretch of the arms. When the arm is held naturally in a slightly rounded line, the upper arm, together with the elbow, is a part of the elongated horizontal of the shoulders. The forearm, together with the hand, however, deviates from this direction to sideways-forward-downward while the entire length of the stretched arm (including forearm and hand) points directly to the sides and thus extends, together with the upper arm and elbow, the horizontal of the shoulders. The sideways stretch of the extended arms is intentionally used where the movement of the

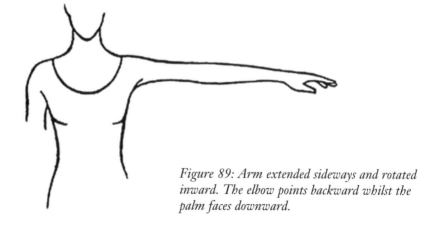

Figure 89: Arm extended sideways and rotated inward. The elbow points backward whilst the palm faces downward.

whole body requires a precise and clear directional leading, as in straight sideways shift of the trunk, a lay-out side etc.

COMPOSITE MOVEMENTS IN THE SHOULDER JOINT

The basic movements of the arm are led by basic, straight directions: forward, sideways, backward, upward, downward. Composite movements are led into between-directions. For example, when one combines a forward-raising with a sideways-raising, a between-direction sideways-forward results, i.e. an oblique (diagonal) direction.

Combination of two basic movements:
   – forward raising of the arms + turning out or in
   – sideways raising of the arms + turning out or in
   – upward raising of the arms + turning out or in
   – backward raising of the arms + turning out or in
The following movements are always in a between-direction or diagonal. Only the movements of the right arm are described:
   – a forward-sideways raising   = a diagonal right-forward.
   – a forward-crosswise raising   = a diagonal crosswise-left-
                                                           forward.
   – a forward-upward raising   = a diagonal, forward-upward.
   – a sideways-upward raising   = a diagonal, sideways-upward.
   – a backward-sideways raising = a diagonal, right-backward.
   – a backward-crosswise raising = a diagonal, left-backward-
                                                           downward
When we add an inward or outward maximal rotation to the basic movements, we obtain a combination of three basic movements.

Combination of three basic movements without rotation:
   – a forward-sideways-upward raising   = diagonally right-
                                                               forward upward
   – a forward-crosswise-upward raising   = diagonally left-
                                                               forward-upward
   – a backward-sideways-upward raising = diagonally right-back-
                                                               upward
When we add an inward or outward maximal rotation to the above three basic movements we obtain a combination of four basic movements.

Combination of four basic movements:
The technical aspect: retain all main characteristics of the basic movements from which they are composed. With all basic and composite movements of the arm it is important to press the shoulder into a correct position so that it does not rise, rotate inward or shift forward. forward.*The movement is led* by sensitive fingertips as it is in basic movements, namely in *between directions*, resulting from the union of two or three basic directions.

CIRCULAR MOVEMENTS IN THE SHOULDER JOINT

We know from the anatomical analysis that the shoulder joint, like the hip joint, has an approximate shape of a hemisphere. The socket of the shoulder joint, however, is smaller and flatter than the socket of the hip joint. The shoulder joint is therefore more mobile and allows the arm a bigger range of movement. The arm can move in all directions and between directions and execute circular movements more consistently than the leg. Its movement is only limited in the direction backward.

Circular movements of the arm are:
– large circles
– small circles
– vertical figures eight
– horizontal figures eight

We execute them with a stretched arm, with extended fingers that draw circular lines in space.

Large circle of the arm facing forward: in a perfect body posture with established shoulders, lead a slightly turned-in, extended arm crosswise forward to the shoulder height. From here (adduction), circumscribe the upper arc through an upward-arms stretch to the sideways stretch (abduction) while the upper arm turns out slightly. From the sideways stretch, circumscribe the lower arc while the upper arm turns slightly in again, finishing in the initial position (adduction) where the circle is completed or a new one begins. The forearm together with the hand, however, keeps its original slight inward turn.

The movement is led by sensitive fingertips, especially by the middle finger. One passes through all *directions* and *counter directions* along the perimeter of the circle.

Large circle of the arm facing the side: in a perfect body posture with established shoulders, lead a slightly turned in, extended arm through a *between-direction* sideways-forward to the shoulder height. From here, circumscribe the upper arc through an upward-sideways arm stretch to a backward-sideways arm stretch while the upper arm turns out slightly. Circumscribe the lower arc while the upper arm turns slightly in again. By reaching the initial position (adduction) the circle is either completed or a new one begins.

The movement is led by sensitive fingertips, especially by the middle fingertip. One passes through all the relevant *directions* and *between-directions* along the perimeter of the circle. Both circles can also be executed with a changed movement of the forearm and the hand, i.e. during the upper arc, the forearm and the hand pass into a medium and maximal pronation (turning in) and during the lower arc they return again into their initial slight pronation (see further text on the movements of the forearms).

CIRCLES ENLARGED BY A MOVEMENT OF THE SPINE AND THE TRUNK

The circle facing forward is enlarged by the rotation of the chest in the direction of the arm movement, as the arm stretches forward-crosswise. We enlarge the upper arc by gradually moving the trunk into a small rounded backward bend, from which we continue into a straight sideways shift of the trunk in the direction of the arm movement. The lower arc is enlarged by a deep, rounded forward bend. While raising the body, we rotate the chest in the direction of the arm movement and return to the initial position.

The circle to the side is enlarged at the beginning by a straight forward-sideways shift of the trunk in the direction of the arm movement. During the upper arc we pass into a small rounded backward bend with torsion of the trunk and when the arm and the trunk, being still in torsion, pass into a straight sideways-backward shift, the upper arc is completed. We proceed into a lower arc which is enlarged by a deep rounded forward bend still in torsion and finish by cancelling torsion, raising and moving into a straight sideways-forward shift in the direction of the arm movement, as we did at the beginning.

The movement is led by the sensitive fingertips, especially the middle one, and passes through all appropriate *directions* and *between-directions* along the perimeter of the enlarged circles. During the practice of the enlarged circles of the arm, the other arm usually counter-balances the movement by elevating to a sideways lift. The participation of the movements of the trunk or the spine is not only a matter of technique, but also a matter of expression. The whole body experiences the path of the circles, drawn by the fingertip into space and yields to the leading of the arm and fingers.

This sensitive participation of the body in movement results from a cultivated movement logic, rather than from rational thought.

Small circles of a stretched arm these can be done both with the arm alongside the body or in connection with directional movements of the arm. When the arm is held alongside the body, the small circles are located low and close to the body. The small circles connected with directional movements begin at a low level, but advance higher and higher along the path of the directional movement or vice-versa. The small circles can differ in size but always with an exact relation to the centre of the circle.

The movement is led by sensitive fingertips, especially by the middle one. It is necessary to be conscious of the centre of the circle and of the path of the circling movement around the centre. Apart from circles, we can draw in space *wavy lines, spirals, sharp lines* with sharp transitions from one direction to the other etc. and connect them with movements of the entire body.

Vertical figure eight*: imagine you are drawing the number eight with your arm in front of your body. In both loops of the figures eight all parts of the arm gradually turn in and out. The vertical figure eight has an upper and a lower loop. Its movement is ascending and descending, following the line of some of the directional movements of the arm, with the point of intersection between the upper and the lower loop in front of the body.

The upper loop: start moving the arm sideways-in (adduction) while ascending. Continue to 'draw' the curve of the upper loop, moving the arm sideways-out while gradually descending until reaching the point of intersection. The upper loop is then completed and the arm is fully turned out.

The lower loop: continue moving the arm sideways-in, simultaneously descending in order to draw the lower loop. At the same time

---

*Translator's note: Movements in the shape of the figure eight are used in swing exercises described in the Appendix.

start turning the arm in while moving it sideways-out. To complete the lower loop, raise the arm to the point of intersection in front of the body.

The movement is led throughout by the outer edge of the hand (the side of the little finger) so that the whole arm and hand is turned in during the diagonal ascent and turned out during the diagonal descent.

Variation: the movement is led throughout by the inner edge of the hand (i.e. the index finger); then we start sideways-out by turning out the whole arm together with the hand and on top it gradually turns in, finishingthe curve, descending diagonally. These figures eight are used in swing movements.

Horizontal figure eight: this has an inner and an outer loop and we lead it from one direction (or between-direction) to the other, in a horizontal line. It can be executed at different heights, below the shoulders, at the shoulder level or above the shoulders. Start to lead with the elongated arm from the forward stretch to the sideways stretch, i.e. 'draw' the lower half of the outer loop, continue to execute the upper half and pass through the point of intersection in front of the body. Execute the lower half of the inner loop and pass to the upper half of this loop and return to the intersection point. The arm remains all the time slightly turned in. It can be combined with a gradual turning out and turning in of the arm starting from the upper arm, as well as with supination and pronation of the arm. There is a possibility of other variations.

The movement is led by the inner edge of the hand (the index finger) starting with the lower curve of the outer loop (supination of the arm). If we *lead* by the outer edge of the hand, we start at the upper curve of the outer loop with a turning in of the arm (pronation). At the point where the loop curves we change from turning in to turning out or vice-versa. With the horizontal figure eight above the shoulder level we retain a slightly turned out upper arm even when, in the course of the movement, we turn in the forearm and hand,

As we complement the large circles of the extended arm by movements of the spine and trunk, so can we enlarge the range of the figure eight with corresponding or contra-directional movements of the spine, trunk or just the head.

All circular movements of the extended arm must be experienced spatially.

BASIC MOVEMENT OF THE FOREARM IN THE ELBOW JOINT AND BOTH RADIO-ULNAR JOINTS

To understand fully the complex mechanism of the movements of the forearm, we must study thoroughly the anatomical analysis of the bone structure of the forearm and its connections. The movements of the forearm are complex because it is not only a matter of bending and straightening, it is above all one of involving two movements, pronation and supination. These distinctly influence the form and direction of the movements of the forearm and hand.(See Figures 74 and 75, p. 142, 143).

Anatomical terminology:
– flexion   = bending
– extension = stretching
– pronation = turning in
– supination = turning out
In movement practice we use the following terms:
– bending of the forearm in the elbow
– straightening of the forearm
– turning in of the forearm and the hand = pronation
– turning out of the forearm and the hand = supination

The basic position from which the movements derive and to which they return is a part of the basic position of the whole arm, which hangs from the established shoulders in a relaxed way, along the body. The elbow is slightly bent (partial flexion) and the arm is consequently rounded. The forearm is slightly turned in (partial pronation) so that the hand turns towards the body. The wrist is extended so that the metacarpal bones, with the forearm, form an almost straight line.

Bending of forearm in the elbow joint is carried out in three degrees as in bending of the lower leg at the knee joint. We distinguish:
(1)   bending to a right angle
(2)   bending to an obtuse angle
(3)   bending to a sharp angle
These three degrees of bending represent three different forms of the arm and have, in complex movements, their specific plastic value.

Bending to right angle: start from the basic position with the arm hanging along the body. [This applies to all the following basic movements of the forearm.] This is to gain an understanding that bending the forearm is a pure, basic movement: i.e. without the participation of the upper arm in the shoulder joint and with immobilised wrist. When bending the forearm, we feel distinctly the muscle work by the front part of the upper arm and at the same time the elongation of the antagonists, which are the muscles of the back part of the upper arm. During bending to different angles, the tension and the elongation changes. When bending to the right angle we feel a medium tension in the muscles of the front part of the upper arm and a medium elongation in the muscles of the back part of the upper arm.

The movement is led by sensitive fingertips, especially by the middle one.

The direction of the bending into a right angle from the basic position of the arm is directly forward.

Bending into an obtuse angle: feel a slight tension of the muscles of the front part of the upper arm and a more pronounced elongation of the muscles of the back part of the upper arm.

The movement is led by the elongated palm of the hand and fingertips.

Direction: forward-down into an obtruse angle.

Bending into a sharp angle: feel a maximal tension of the muscles of the front part of the upper arm and a maximal elongation of the back part of the upper arm.

The movement is led by the sensitive fingertips.

Direction: Forward-upward into a sharp angle.

The recovery movement of the forearm from all three angles is a return to the basic position of the arm alongside the body by a slow relaxation of all participating muscles in the upper arm.

Extension of the elbow joint: holding the arm in the basic position start extending the elbow without any other changes to the basic position of the arm. This extension must not cause the elbow to turn towards the body, but should keep it away, maintaining the arm slightly turned inward in the shoulder joint. We should feel a strong tension in the muscles of the back part of the upper arm, but it is of utmost importance to maintain established shoulders.

The movement is led by sensitive fingertips, especially by the middle fingertip, in the *direction* down, very slightly away from the body.

The movement is part of extension of the arm in its basic position, i.e. arms held along the body. It is also a part of all movements of the arm in the shoulder joint, both basic and composite, as long as they are executed with an extended arm. With arm movements above shoulder level when the upper arm must be slightly turned out (e.g. in an upward-raising), the work of the extensors is even more demanding if we want to avoid the elbow and the whole arm 'growing heavy'. *Only activity of the muscles* of the back part of the upper arm lighten the elbow and keep it in direct connection with the whole arm.

Pronation or turning in of the forearm: in pronation, the radius revolves round the ulna so that it crosses it. Turning in has three degrees: slight, medium and maximal. The hand turns in together with the forearm, the wrist remains extended and immobilised. The degree of pronation can best be identified by the direction of the palm of the hand.

Slight pronation is a part of the basic position of both rounded and extended arms, in which the palm faces the body, i.e. sideways-in. In all basic movements of the arm in the shoulder joint, the palm retains this spatial orientation, except for the sideways-raising of the arm where the palm of both rounded and extended arm points forward-down.

Medium pronation: in the basic position of both rounded and extended arms change the slight pronation into a medium one and turn the palm backward. In the forward and sideways raising of the rounded or extended arm, however, the palm in medium pronation turns downward; in the backward raising it turns back-upward and in the upward-raising it turns forward.

Maximal pronation: in the basic position of both rounded and extended arms we change the slight pronation into a maximal one and the palm turns sideways-out. It is the same when the arms are in a forward, upward or a backward raising. In the sideways-raising the palm turns backward.

The movement is led in the pronation of all degrees by the thumb side of the hand.

The recovery from the pronation involves returning to the initial position through a slow relaxation of the participating muscles.

Supination or turning out of the forearm: in supination both bones of the forearm are in a parallel position, making the maximal the only degree of supination. In the basic position of the arm, i.e. with a slightly turned-in upper arm, the simultaneous supination of the forearm, although a maximal one, has a small range, indicated by the direction of the palm.

The palm of the hand turns only forward-sideways-inward. It is the same in the backward arm-raising. In the forward arm-raising the palm turns sideways-inward-upward, in the sideways-raising it turns forward-upward. In the upward lift, however, in which we also turn out the upper arm slightly, the palm turns sideways-inward-backward. When we add a turned-out upper arm to the supination in all directional movements, we increase the range of the movement. As a consequence, the palm turns fully forward in the basic position; in the forward and sideways-raising it turns fully upward, in the upward-raising fully backward and in the backward-raising it turns fully sideways-out.

The movement is led in the supination of the forearm by the outer edge of the hand.

The recovery from the supination of the forearm is a return to the initial position through a slow relaxation of the participating muscles.

COMPOSITE MOVEMENTS OF THE FOREARM IN THE ELBOW JOINT

We combine two basic movements:

bending + pronation   bending + supination
straightening+ pronation   straightening + supination

Due to the fact that we are able to bend the forearm in the elbow into three distinct angles and also graduate pronation into three degrees, the visual possibilities of the movement of the forearm multiply considerably. When the whole arm is in maximal prona-tion, we are only able to bend the forearm in the direction which corresponds to the mechanism of the elbow joint. For example, when the arm is in a forward raised position and maximally turned in, the forearm bends sideways-inward in the elbow joint. To bend it in an upward direction we would have to turn the upper arm out and reduce the turning in of the forearm from maximal to medium pronation. The teacher and choreographer must distinguish for themselves these possibilities. The direction of the movement is, in this case, an important lead: its technical perfection depends on a correct analysis of the function of each participating joint, to achieve the required direction.

Leading: when the arm is stretched, the movement *is led* by sensitive fingertips. The movement of the arm in pronation *is led* by the thumb side of the hand, during supination by the small-finger side. When the arm is bent, we must be aware of three directions: of the upper arm, of the forearm and also of the palm in pronation or supination.

We must be aware that by adding to the movement of the forearm an arm movement in the shoulder joint, it is not only the direction of the upper arm that changes, but also that of the forearm and the palm. It is an important point for the analysis of complex movements of the arm. For example, the bending of the forearm to the right angle in a maximal pronation executed in a forward raising will have a different direction when executed in a sideways raising.

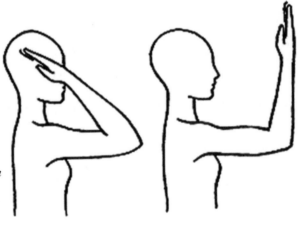

Figure 90: The upper arm and forearm form an acute or right angle. The upper limb is rotated outward.

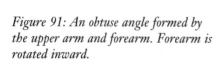

Figure 91: An obtuse angle formed by the upper arm and forearm. Forearm is rotated inward.

6. The Radio-carpal and Metacarpal Joints

BASIC MOVEMENTS OF THE HAND

Anatomical terminology:
- palmar flexion = bending downward
- dorsiflexion = bending upward
- radial deviation = bending towards the thumb side
- ulnar deviation = bending towards the little-finger side

In movement practice we use the following terms:
- tilting of the hand
- raising of the hand
- bending sideways-in
- bending sideways-out

The hand movements occur in both joints simultaneously.

Basic position of the hand: the position from which we start and to which we return when executing a hand movement is as follows. The hand and the forearm are in a straight horizontal line with the upper arm along the body so that their joints are stretched with the relaxed thumb under the index finger, the mid-line of the palm and the middle finger slightly accentuated, i.e. elongated. The hand is sensitive, relaxed but not limp. While holding the forearm horizontally in medium pronation, face the palm downward. The description of the directions of the hand movements is determined in relation to this arm position. In another position, the directions would be different.

Tilting the hand: the hand, in its basic position, bends downward on the palm side of the wrist. The degree of tilting is individual, it should reach the right angle between the hand and the forearm. There are two types of tilting, (i) passive dropping of the hand, (ii) active tilting.

Correct passive dropping of the hand: relax all joints of the hand and fingers completely. The hand hangs passively down from the wrist. The back of the hand is rounded and the fingers are slightly bent.

Active tilting of the hand (palmar flexion): contract maximally the muscles on the palmar side of the wrist and feel distinctly the extension of antagonistic muscles on the back of the hand. Stretch maximally the metacarpo-phalangeal joints to such an extent that hyperextension may occur. Accentuate the mid-line of the palm and the middle finger. The hand is actively extended, even hyperextended, but as a whole it points straight downward.

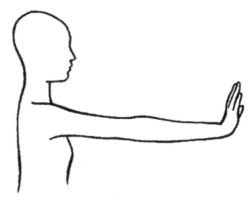

Figure 92: Variation: upper limb lifted forward with hand raised upward. Dorsiflexion of the wrist with extended elbow.

Leading: in the case of passive dropping of the hand, the movement has no lead. In the case of active tilting, the movement *is led* by the middle finger.

Directions: the passively dropped hand points forward-down, the actively tilted hand points directly downward.

Raising the hand (dorsiflexion): in its basic position, the hand bends on the back of the wrist in an upward direction. The degree of the bend is also individual, one can develop it to reach the right angle with the forearm. Raising the hand can only be done actively. Contract maximally the muscles of the back of the wrist and perceive the elongation of the muscles of the palmar side of the wrist. The thumb stays in its basic position under the index finger and together with the hand points upward. Extend the metacarpals and phalanges to hyperextension, especially the middle finger. Feel strongly the mid-line of the palm, together with the middle finger.

The movement is led by sensitively extended fingers, above all the middle one, in the *direction* straight upward.

Bending the hand sideways-out (ulnar deviation): contract the muscles of the little-finger side of the wrist and elongate the antagonist muscles on the thumb side of the wrist. The hand is in basic position with an accentuated mid-line of the palm and the middle finger, with a thumb held under the index finger in a relaxed manner. The bent hand forms an obtuse angle with the forearm and points sideways-out.

The movement is led by the little-finger side of the hand in the *direction* sideways-out.

Bending the hand sideways-in (radial deviation), See Figure 76, p. 143: contract the muscles of the thumb side of the wrist and elongate the antagonists on the little-finger side of the wrist. The bending has a smaller range, the obtuse angle is more open than in the previous movement. The hand is retained in its basic position with an accentuated mid-line of the palm and the middle finger, with the thumb held under the index finger in a relaxed manner.

The movement is led by the thumb side of the hand in *the direction* sideways-in.

The recovery of all basic movements of the hand is a return to the basic position and results from the relaxation of all participating muscles.

Basic movements of the hand change the hand's direction in relation to the forearm; and with a bent arm they also change its direction in relation to the upper arm. To this we must add the direction of the palm, which changes if the movement is combined with pronation or supination. In the case of the hand movement with a stretched arm in pronation, we must perceive the individual directions of the arm, the hand and the palm. In the case of the hand movement with a bent arm, we must be aware of four directions: of the upper arm, forearm, hand and palm. In the hand movements with a stretched arm, the movement of the arm *is led* by the wrist, the movement of the hand *is led* by the fingertips, the pronation of the forearm *is led* by the thumb side of the hand, the supination by the little finger side. So originates a movement in which each part of the arm has its own direction, which we must perceive in complex movements and feel together with the leading. There are *four independently led directions* in the complex movement of the arm. Perception of all four leadings and directions is a pre requisite for the visual value of a complex arm movement, otherwise the movement remains vague and expressionless.

COMPOSITE MOVEMENTS OF THE HAND

We combine two basic movements:
- downward tilt of the hand + bending sideways-out = a *between-direction* downward-sideways-out
- downward tilting of the hand + bending sideways-in = a *between-direction* downward-sideways-in

| – raising of the hand + bending sideways-out | = | a *between-direction* upward-sideways-out |
| – raising of the hand + bending sideways-in | = | a *between-direction* upward-sideways-in |

These composite movements of the hand, which we perceive principally in terms of direction, are used in circular movements of the hand.

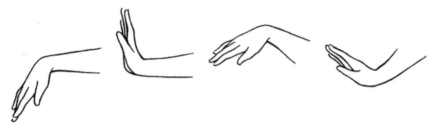

Figure 93
Hand flected down – palmar flexion of the wrist
Hand flected upward – dorsiflexion of the wrist
Lifting of the wrist
Lowering of the wrist

CIRCULAR MOVEMENTS OF THE HAND

– Circling
– The vertical figure eight
– The horizontal figure eight

They arise from basic and composite hand movements, executed gradually in a certain succession.

Circling the hand consists of a downward tilting, bending sideways-out, raising, bending sideways-in or vice-versa. During transition from one movement to another the hand passes through relevant composite movements. At the same time we preserve all specific characteristics of the execution of both basic and composite movements of the hand.

The movement is led by the sensitive fingertips, especially the middle one.

Direction: during the circling we pass through all *directions* and *between-directions* along the perimeter of the circling.

Figures eight of the hand are executed
(I) without pronation or supination of the forearm;
(II) with pronation or supination.

Vertical figure eight of the hand consists of bending sideways-out, raising, bending sideways-in (upper loop), bending sideways-out, tilting downward, bending sideways-in (lower loop).

Horizontal figure eight consists of tilting down, bending sideways-out, raising (outer loop), tilting down, bending sideways-in, raising (inner loop).

The movements are led in both types by sensitive fingertips.

Both circling movements, the vertical and horizontal figures eight, are enlarged and rounded when they are combined with pronation (led by the little finger) and supination (led by the index finger) of the forearm.

The vertical figure eight of the hand with pronation and supination of the forearm differs from the first one by the fact that during ascent we turn out the forearm and the hand (supination) and on the descent we turn them in.

The horizontal figure eight of the hand with pronation and supination of the forearm differs from the first one by the fact that during transition into the outer loop we turn out the forearm and the hand (supination), and during transition into the inner loop we turn them in (pronation). We increase both types of figures eight in size when we combine the pronation and supination of the forearm with bending and stretching of the forearm in the elbow joint. The size will be enlarged even more when we add to it turning-out and turning-in of the shoulder joint.

MOVEMENTS OF THE WRIST

The movements of the wrist are in essence movements of the hand and forearm with the difference that they are led by the wrist. When the wrist moves in space, it happens in the wrist joints and the elbow joint. (Thus, it is a complex movement from the anatomical point of view). During hand movements, the wrist and the elbow stay in the original place; during wrist movements the fingertips and the elbow stay in place but the angle of the forearm towards the upper arm changes.

The anatomists do not classify the movements of the wrist separately. In movement practice we distinguish them from the movements of the hand led by the fingers, because they open to us new possibilities of form.

Basic movements of the wrist are:
- elevation of the wrist
- lowering of the wrist
- shifting sideways-out
- shifting sideways-in

Elevation of the wrist: in the basic position of the hand with the thumb held in a relaxed manner under the index finger and with a fixed position of the fingers, elevate the wrist *above* the fingers. The hand is moderately tilted forward down, and feels the midline of the palm and the middle finger.

The movement is led by the back of the wrist in the *direction* upward.

Lowering the wrist: in the basic position of the hand with the thumb held in a relaxed manner under the index finger and with a fixed position of the fingers, lower the wrist *under* the finger level. Hold the hand actively raised, i.e. hyperextend the metacarpo-pha-langeal joints and stress the midline of the palm and the middle finger.

The movement is led by the palmar side of the wrist in *the direction* downward.

Shifting of the wrist sideways-out (ulnar deviation): in the basic position of the hand with the thumb held in a relaxed man-ner under the index finger and with a fixed position of the fingers, shift the wrist sideways-out at the finger level. The active hand, i.e. extended in the metacarpo-phalangeal joints with a stressed midline of the palm and the middle finger, bends sideways-in.

The movement is led by the little-finger side of the wrist in *the direction* sideways-out.

Shifting of the wrist sideways-in (radial deviation): in the basic position of the hand with the thumb held in a relaxed manner under the index finger and with a fixed position of the fingers, shift the wrist sideways-in at the finger level. The active hand, i.e. extended in the metacarpo-phalangeal joints with a stressed mid-line of the palm and the middle finger, bends sideways-out.

The movement is led by the thumb side of the wrist in *the direction* sideways-in.

COMPOSITE MOVEMENTS OF THE WRIST

We combine two movements:
- – raising + shifting sideways-out
- – raising + shifting sideways-in
- – lowering + shifting sideways-out
- – lowering + shifting sideways-in

The gradual execution of basic and composite movements of the wrist in a definite succession results in circular movements *of the wrist.*
- – Circling
- – The vertical figure eight
- – The horizontal figure eight of the wrist

Circling consists of shifting sideways-in or sideways-out, raising, shifting sideways-out or sideways-in, lowering etc. During transition from one movement to another, the wrist passes through composite movements.

The movement is led always by the relevant side and 'between-side' along the perimeter of the wrist and passes through all *directions* and *between-directions* along the circumference of circling.

Vertical figure eight consists of: shifting sideways-in, raising, shifting sideways-out (upper loop), shifting sideways-in, lowering, shifting sideways-out (lower loop).

The movement is led always by the relevant side and 'between-side' of the back of the wrist, then by the palm side of the wrist and passes through all *directions* and *between directions* along the perimeter of the loops of the figure eight.

Horizontal figure eight consists of raising, shifting sideways-in, lowering (inner loop), raising, shifting sideways-out, lowering (outer loop).

The movement is led always by the relevant side and 'between-side' of the inner half of the wrist, then the relevant side and 'between-side' of the outer half of the wrist and passes thus through all *directions* and *between-directions* along the perimeter of the loops of the figure eight.

In the vertical figures eight, emphasise the back and the palmar side of the wrist. In the horizontal figures eight, the inner and outer parts of the wrist are emphasised in the fluent rounding of the loops.

The recovery movement of all basic and composite movements of the wrist is a return to the basic position of the hand. This happens by relaxing all participating muscles.

BASIC MOVEMENTS OF THE THUMB IN THE CARPO-METACARPAL JOINT

Anatomical terminology:
– abduction = pulling away of the thumb
– adduction = drawing the thumb towards the index finger
– opposition = drawing the thumb towards the middle finger and towards the last two fingers
– reposition = return to the initial position.

In movement practice:
– pulling the thumb away sideways-out or pulling away downward
– drawing of the thumb towards the index finger
– drawing the thumb under the middle finger and towards the last two fingers.
– return to the initial position (under the index finger).

Abduction of the thumb sideways-out and down: from the basic position of the hand with the thumb held in a relaxed manner under the index finger, pull the thumb sideways-out or downward, until all the muscles between the metacarpal of the index finger and the metacarpal of the thumb are tightly elongated.

The movement is led by an extended thumb in the *direction* sideways-out or downward.

Adduction of the thumb towards the index finger: from the basic position of the hand, with the thumb held in a relaxed manner under the index finger, draw the thumb towards the index finger by a maximal contraction of the muscles between the metacarpal of the index finger and the metacarpal of the thumb. The thumb is parallel with the index finger.

The movement is led by an extended thumb in the *direction* upward.

Drawing the thumb under the middle finger: from the basic position of the hand with the thumb held in a relaxed manner under the index finger, draw the thumb under the middle finger by a maximal contraction of the muscles of the thumb mound (*thenar eminence*).

The movement is led by the metacarpal of the thumb in *the direction* sideways-inward.

The recovery of the thumb: relax all muscles participating in this movement and return the thumb to the basic position.

It is also possible to draw the thumb under the fourth or fifth finger.

COMPOSITE MOVEMENTS OF THE THUMB IN THE CARPO-METACARPAL JOINT

We combine two movements:
- pulling away sideways-out + pulling away downward = *between-direction* sideways-out-down
- drawing under + pulling away downward = *between-direction* sideways-in-downward

Circular Movements *result from a gradual execution of basic and composite movements in a definite succession. These are:*
- Circling
- The vertical figure eight
- The horizontal figure eight

Circling of the thumb: from the basic position of the relaxed thumb under the index finger, pull away the thumb sideways-out, then down, draw the thumb under the middle finger and pull up alongside the index finger.

The movement is led by an extended thumb and passes through all *directions* and *between-directions* along the circumference of the circling.

Vertical figure eight: from the basic position of the relaxed thumb under the index finger pull away the thumb sideways-out, then down, then draw it under the middle finger (lower loop) Again, pull away the thumb sideways-out, pull alongside the index finger and again draw under the middle finger (upper loop).

The movement is led by an extended thumb and passes through all *directions* and *between-directions* along the perimeter of the loops.

Horizontal figure eight: from the basic position of the relaxed thumb under the index finger, pull away the thumb downward, draw under the middle finger and pull alongside the index finger (inner loop), again pull away the thumb downward, then sideways-out and pull alongside the index finger (outer loop).

The movement is led by an extended thumb and passes through all *directions* and *between-directions* along the perimeter of the loops.

The described basic and composite movements of the thumb are used above all as exercises to develop the sensitivity of the hand muscles. After each active movement of the thumb, return to the basic relaxed position of the thumb. It is necessary because the thumb is often involuntarily stretched, sticking out undesirably into space and damaging the harmonious line of the movements of the hand.

Thumb movements are distinct and can be utilised in both mime and expressive dance.

BASIC MOVEMENTS OF THE FINGERS IN THE METACARPO-PHALANGEAL JOINTS

Anatomical terminology:

| flexion | = bending | abduction | = pulling away |
| extension | = stretching | adduction | = pulling towards |

In movement practice we use these terms:
– bending of the whole finger   = tilting down
– stretching of the whole finger = raising
– pulling of the whole finger sideways-out
– pulling of the whole finger sideways-inward.

Bending and stretching the thumb: from the basic position of the relaxed thumb under the index finger, contract the thenar muscles of the thumb and bend both phalanges of the thumb, so that the thumb crosses the palm under the index finger. Return the thumb under the index finger, not in a relaxed manner, however, but actively elongated. Only when the movement is completed, it returns into the initial relaxed position.

Bending and stretching the fingers: from the basic position of the hand, bend elongated fingers in their metacarpo-phalangeal joints by a maximal contraction of the muscles of the palm and by elongating the muscles of the back of the hand which are their antagonists. The bending forms a right angle with the back of the hand. Return the fingers to a maximal stretch (not the basic relaxed position), so that the hand becomes overextended, the fingers point diagonally upward and form small grooves on the backs of the metacarpo-phalangeal joints. In this movement, we contract the muscles of the back of the hand and elongate the muscles of the palm. Then we ease the tension of the muscles and return the hand into its basic position.

The movements are led by the elongated fingers in the *direction* downward and then diagonally upward. The movements are executed by all fingers together or separately.

Abduction and adduction of the fingers and thumb: from the basic position of the hand, at first pull away (abduct) the little finger from the rest of the fingers which are held together and return it to the initial position. Then pull the little finger together with the ring finger away from the middle finger and return, then the little finger, ring finger and middle finger are pulled away from the index finger and return again and finally execute abduction by all four fingers together, i.e. tilting sideways-out, then adduction, i.e. tilting sideways-in. Then pull away the thumb (while the metacarpal of the thumb remains under the index finger) and with two phalanges of the extended thumb pull away from the rest of the fingers. Then spread all the fingers apart with the middle finger staying in the centre. There are two ways of actively pulling the fingers back together. *Firstly*, the middle finger stays raised and the other fingers draw together into a position under the elevated middle finger. *Secondly*, slightly depress the middle finger and the rest of the fingers join above it. Make sure the fingers are always actively extended throughout this exercise. *Thirdly*, relax the fingers.

The movement is led by extended fingers in the *direction* sideways-out and sideways-in.

COMPOSITE MOVEMENTS OF THE FINGERS IN METACARPO-PHALANGEAL JOINTS

We combine two basic movements:
- extension to hyperextension + abduction
- partial tilting down + abduction (a complete downward tilting in these joints with spreading of the fingers is not feasible)
- extension to hyperextension + adduction
- partial tilting + adduction

The movements are led by the extended fingers in the *between-directions* sideways-out-upward, sideways-out-downward, sideways-in-upward and sideways-in-downward.

CIRCULAR MOVEMENTS

The gradual execution of basic and composite movements in a definite sequence results in circling movements of the fingers:
  – Circling
  – The vertical figure eight
  – The horizontal figure eight

Circling: from the basic position of the hand, the thumb and the rest of the fingers elongate the joined fingers and tilt them down together, i.e. bend, then abduct in the direction sideways-out, raise, i.e. hyperextend and adduct sideways-inward. A circle, or rather an ellipse, results. Circling of the thumb is executed separately.

The movement is led by extended fingers and they pass through all *directions* and *between-directions* along the perimeter of the ellipse. The circling is done either by all fingers joined together except for the thumb, or separately by each finger.

Vertical figure eight: this consists of abduction sideways-out, raising and adduction sideways-in (upper loop). The lower loop consists of abduction sideways-out, downward tilt and adduction sideways-in.

Horizontal figure eight: this consists of raising, abduction sideways-out and downward tilt (outer loop). The inner loop consists of raising, adduction sideways-in and downward tilt.

The movements are led by elongated fingers, which pass through all *directions* and *between-directions* along the path of the figures eight.

BASIC MOVEMENTS OF THE FINGERS IN THE INTER-PHALANGEAL JOINTS

Anatomical terminology: flexion and extension.

In movement practice we use the terms bending and stretching of the fingers.

Bending and stretching the thumb: from the basic position of the hand with the thumb held in a relaxed manner under the index finger, bend the second phalanx of the thumb in its only inter-phalangeal joint so that the first and the second phalanges form a right angle and at the same time the metacarpo-phalangeal joint remains stretched. Return the second phalanx of the thumb into its basic position so that the inter-phalangeal joint stretches again.

The movements are led by the second phalanx of the thumb in the *direction* sideways-in and back.

Bending and stretching the fingers: from the basic position of the hand and fingers, separately bend the fingers both in the first and second inter-phalangeal joints. Bend the second phalanx in the first inter-phalangeal joint and keep both the metacarpo-phalangeal joints and the second inter-phalangeal joint stretched. The fingers bend either in a right, obtuse or sharp angle. When bending the last, i.e. third, phalanx of the fingers one can bend it in the second inter-phalangeal joint only to an obtuse angle, at the most to a right angle. Bend each finger separately as well as all fingers together. After each bending, there follows a maximal stretch, to hyperextension. After that, relax the fingers.

The movement is led by the second and third phalanx in the *direction* downward and upward.

It is difficult to control the fingers in this way and it requires patience while practising. For eloquence of the dancing hands, however, this ability is desirable particularly in mime. In any case, exercising of the introduced movements contributes to suppleness of the hand and relieves it of unacceptable cramped tension.

CLENCHING AND EXTENDING THE HAND

From a horizontal, supinated position of the forearm with the palm facing upward, bend the third, second and first phalanx of all fingers (one by one) until the tips come close to the palm. Bury them into the palm where the metacarpo-phalangeal joints are located and bend the thumb across the fingers, forming a clenched fist.

Recovery I: gradually stretch the hand, finger by finger, into a maximal extension to hyperextension.

The movements are led gradually by all phalanges into a maximal bending in the direction upward and then downward-in. When unrolling, gradually stretch all joints starting with the thumb from the metacarpo-phalangeal joint and finishing with the last inter-phalangeal joint until reaching maximal extension or even hyperextension of the fingers in the *direction* forward.

Recovery II: from the fist to the basic relaxed position of the hand

and fingers: after forming the fist with maximal contraction of all muscles of the hand and fingers, relax these muscles without trying to stretch them. Due to relaxation, the hand slowly opens by itself and ends in a relaxed and slightly bent position of all joints of the hand and fingers. The hand is in a supine position together with the forearm.

THE SIGNIFICANCE OF THE ANALYSIS FOR SPATIAL FEELING

The purity of execution of all described movements depends on one's ability to articulate, through kinaesthetic awareness, the hand and fingers and to feel intensively through both the leading and direction of the movements of the entire finger and each of its parts, separately. The movements can only be eloquent if they are directionally distinguished and felt through, otherwise definition becomes lost. In circling movements, the awareness of the spatial path of the movements, no matter how short, needs to be experienced as well.

In complex movements of the arm which need multi-directional orientation, such an articulated feeling is very demanding for both dance and mime artists, and for choreographers and educators. However, we need to realise that the visual sense of all these creators is always deeply linked with their relationship to space.

Spatial feeling is one of the leading components of movement and dance aesthetics.

I

ANATOMY: SUMMARY OF MUSCLE ACTIONS

The names of the various muscles which cooperate with one another to produce movement at certain joints are named below; the muscles are mentioned in the order of their importance in the particular movement described.

MOVEMENTS OF THE CERVICAL PART OF THE VERTEBRAL COLUMN

(i)   Flexion: the sternomastoids, longi colli and scaleni.
(ii) Extension: the splenii capitis, splenii cervicis, trapezii and upper part of the long muscles of the spine.
(iii) Lateral flexion: the sternomastoid, scaleni, levator scapulae, trapezius and upper part of long spinal muscles all of one side.

(iv) Rotation: the sternomastoid of the opposite side, the small rotators of the cervical part of the vertebral column and the upper part of the long spinal muscles.

Respiration
(i)   Quiet respiration: the diaphragm, recti abdominis, oblique and transverse muscles and the intercostals.
(ii) Deep respiration: all the muscles under (i), assisted by the sternomastoid, scaleni, pectorals, latissimus dorsi and quadratus lumborum of both sides.

Movements of the thoracic and lumbar parts of vertebral column
(i)   Flexion: the recti abdominis, oblique muscles of the abdomen and psoas and iliacus of both sides. Gravity performs most of this action in the erect position.
(ii) Extension: the long spinal muscles. The latissimus dorsi and trapezius of both sides can assist this movement when the shoulder girdle is fixed.
(iii) Lateral flexion: the oblique muscles, rectus abdominis, spinal muscles, latissimus dorsi, quadratus lumborum and psoas, all of one side.
(iv) Rotation: the external oblique of one side with the internal oblique of the opposite side assisted by the long and short spinal muscles.

Movements of the shoulder girdle*
(i)   Backward rotation or bracing the shoulders back: the trapezius, rhomboideus major and rhomboideus minor.
(ii) Forward rotation: the serratus anterior, pectoralis major and pectoralis minor.
(iii) Elevation or shrugging the shoulders: the trapezius and levator scapulae.
(iv) Depression: latissimus dorsi and lower fibres of the trapezius.

Movements of the shoulder joint
(i)   Flexion or forward elevation of the upper arm: the pectoralis major (clavicular portion), the anterior fibres of the deltoid, the biceps and the coracobrachialis.
(ii) Extension: the posterior fibres of the deltoid, the latissimus dorsi, the long head of triceps and the teres major.

---

*The movements described refer to one half of the shoulder girdle.

(iii) Abduction: through the first 10 or 15 degrees, the deltoid assisted by the supraspinatus; from 15 to approximately 90 degrees, the deltoid alone; from 90 to 145 degrees, the serratus anterior with the trapezius assisting and controlling rotation of the scapula while the deltoid, supraspinatus and small muscles of the shoulder keep the shoulder joint fixed. At this point the humerus must be externally rotated, if that has not already been done, in order to raise the arm vertically above the head. This final movement is completed by the deltoid, mainly by its anterior fibres.

(iv) Adduction: the pectoralis major, latissimus dorsi, infraspinatus, teres major and minor, subscapularis and long head of triceps.

(v) External rotation: the infraspinatus and teres minor.

(vi) Internal rotation: the pectoralis major (sternal portion), subscapularis, latissimus dorsi and teres major.

Movements at the elbow joint

(i) Flexion: the brachialis, biceps brachialis, brachioradialis, and the flexor group of the forearm muscles.

(ii) Extension: the triceps.

Movements of the forearm

(i) Pronation: the pronator teres and pronator quadratus.

(ii) Supination: the biceps and short supinator muscle.

Movements at the wrist

(i) Palmar flexion: the flexors of the wrist and the long flexors of the fingers and thumb.

(ii) Dorsiflexion: the extensors of the wrist and the long extensors of the fingers and thumb.

(iii) Radial deviation: the flexor and extensor of the wrist, which are inserted on the radial side of the carpus, and the long abductor and extensors of the thumb.

(iv) Ulnar deviation: the flexor and extensor of the wrist which are inserted into the ulnar side of the carpus.

Movements at the hip joint

(i) Flexion: the rectus femoris (of the quadriceps), psoas, iliacus, sartorius, and adductores.

(ii) Extension: the gluteus maximus, biceps femoris, semimembranosus, semitendinosus and the fibres of the adductor magnus which arise from the ischium.

(iii) Abduction: the gluteus medius, gluteus minimus, sartorius and tensor fasciae latae.

(iv) External rotation: the small muscles arising from the hip bone and inserted into the back of the upper end of the femur; also the sartorius.

(v) Internal rotation: the gluteus medius, gluteus minimus, tensor fasciae latae and psoas.

Movements at the knee joint

(i) Flexion: the biceps femoris, semimembranosus, semitend nosus, sartorius and gastrocnemius.

(ii) Extension: the quadriceps.

Movements at the ankle joint

(i) Dorsiflexion: the anterior tibial muscle and long extensors of the toes.

(ii) Plantar flexion: the gastocnemius, soleus, posterior tibial muscle and long flexors of the toes.

Movements at the joints between the talus and calcaneus and the talus and the navicular bone

(i) Inversion: the posterior tibial and anterior tibial muscles.

(ii) Eversion: the peroneus longus and peroneus brevis.

(See Figures 94, p. 205; 95 and 96, p. 206; 97 and 98, p. 207; 99 and 100, p. 208.)

3

ANATOMICAL FIGURES

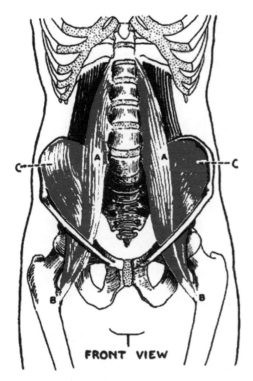

Figure 11: The psoas and iliacus
muscles
A – Psoas major
B – Insertion of Psoas and iliacus
into lesser trochanter
C – Iliacus

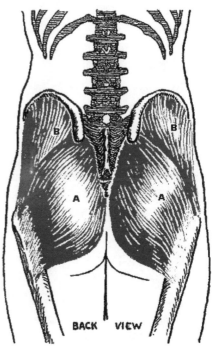

Figure 12: The gluteus maximus
and medius muscles
A – Gluteus maximus
B – Gluteus medius

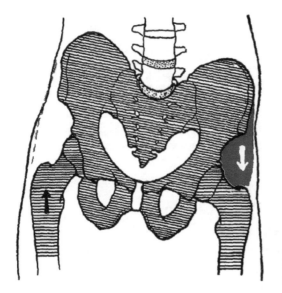

Figure 13: The left gluteus medius and minimus tilting the pelvis

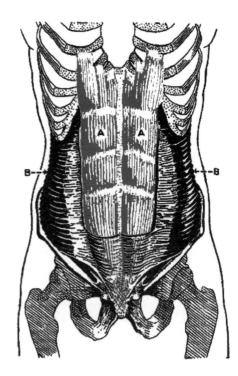

Figure 14
A – The rectus abdominis muscle
B – The transverse muscle

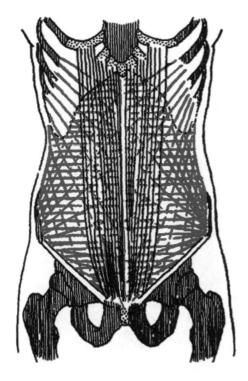

Figure 15: Direction of fibres of the oblique, transverse and recti abdominis muscles

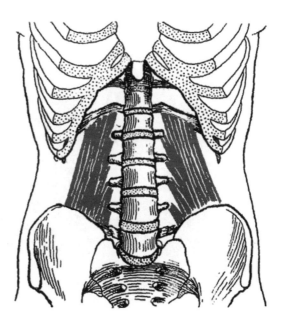

Figure 16: The quadrati lumborum

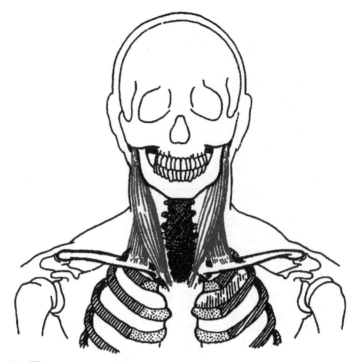

Figure 31: The sternomastoids

FRONT   VIEW

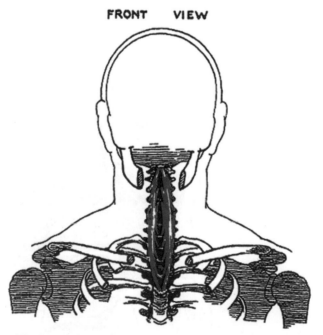

Figure 32: The longi colli (part of the ribs, sternum, clavicles and jawbone have been cut out)

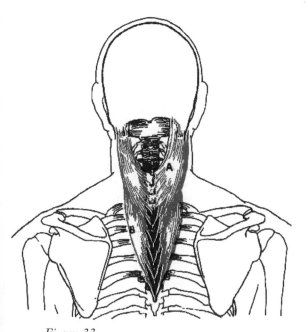

Figure 33:
A – Splenius capitis
B – Splenius cervicis

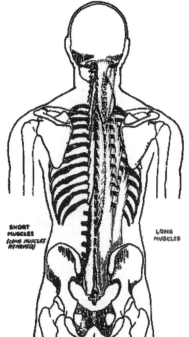

Figure 34: Attachment of
long and short spinal muscles

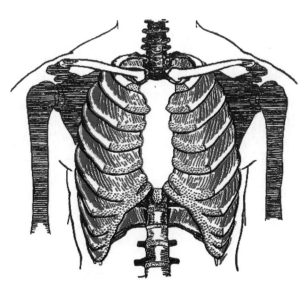

Figure 35: The intercostal muscles from the front

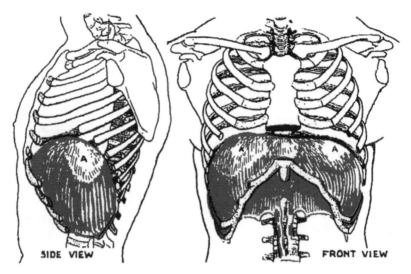

Figure 36: The diaphragm
A – Tendon
(The ribs and sternum have been partly removed)

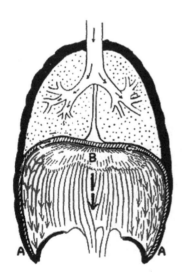

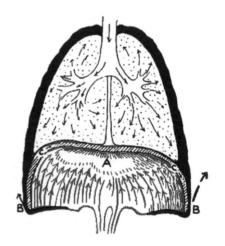

Figure 50: Early inspiration. The
diaphragm contracting from the
ribs as fixed point.
A – Lower ribs
B – Diaphragm moving down
C – Cut edge of diaphragm

Figure 51: Late inspiration. The
diaphragm contracting from its central
tendon as fixed point.
A – Diaphragm
B – Lower ribs moving upward and
outward

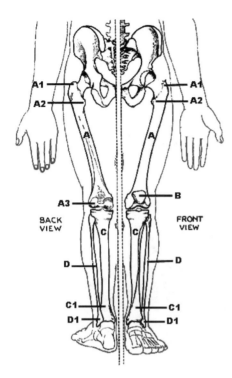

Figure 52: The bones of the leg
A – Femur
A1 – Greater trochanter
A2 – Lesser trochanter
A3 – Condyles
B – Patella
C – Tibia
C1 – Internal malleolus
D – Fibula
D1 – External malleolus

Figure 53: The bones of the foot
The skeleton of the foot is made up of: the seven bones
of the main part of the foot which together make up
the
tarsus; the five bones of the fore-foot called the
metatarsals; the bones of the toes or phalanges
A – Tarsus
B – Metatarsals
C – Phalanges
D – Talus
E – Calcaneus
F – Navicular (which means boot shaped)
G – Cuneiform
H – Cuboid

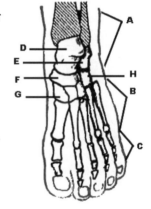

Figure 54: The longitudinal and
transverse arches of the foot
A – Calcaneus
B – Talus
C – Navicular
D – Cuneiform
E – Inner three metatarsals
F – Phalanges of inner three toes
G – Cuboid
H – Outer two metatarsals
J – Phalanges of outer two toes

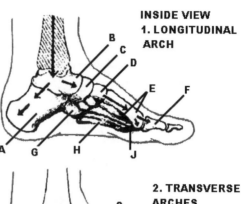

INSIDE VIEW
1. LONGITUDINAL
   ARCH

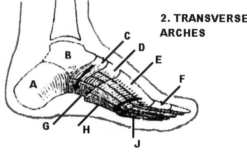

2. TRANSVERSE
   ARCHES

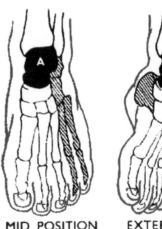

Figure 57: Inversion of
the left foot
A – Talus

MID POSITION
B

EXTERNAL ROTATION
C

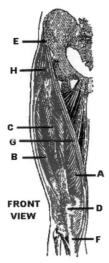

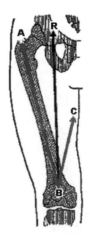

Figure 58: Anterior muscles of the thigh
A – Inner head of quadriceps
B – Outer head of quadriceps
C – Rectus femoris
D – Patella (enclosed in tendon)
E – Anterior portion of the ilium
F – Upper end of the tibia
G – Sartorius
H – Tensor of the broad fascia

Figure 59: Resultant direction of pull
on the patella
BA – The direction of pull of rectus
femoris and the outer and intermediate heads of quadriceps
BC – Direction of pull of the inner
head of quadriceps
BR – Direction of the resultant pull
B – Patella

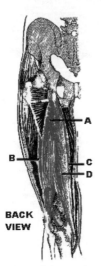

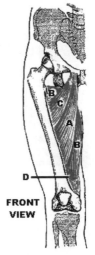

Figure 60: The left biceps femoris, semi-
membranosus and semitendinosus
A – Long head of biceps femoris
B – Short head of the biceps femoris
C – Semimembranosus
D – Semitendinosus

Figure 61: The right adductor
longus, magnus and brevis
A – Adductor longus
B – Adductor magnus
C – Adductor brevis – opening for
main blood vessels

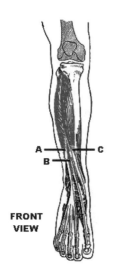

FRONT
VIEW

Figure 62: The long extensors
of the toes and the anterior
tibial muscle (right leg)
A – Long extensor of lesser toes
B – Long extensor of big toes
C – Anterior tibial muscles

Figure 63: The calf muscles of
the left leg
A – Gastrocnemius
B – Soleus (Outer and inner
edges only are visible)
C – Achilles tendon

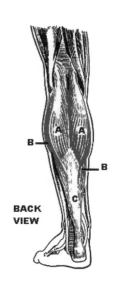

BACK
VIEW

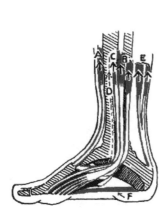

Figure 64: Muscles supporting
the arch of the foot
A – Anterior tibial muscles
B – Long flexors of the toes
C – Posterior tibial muscles
D – Peroneus longus (obscured
by the bones)
E – Calf muscles
F – Small muscles of the foot

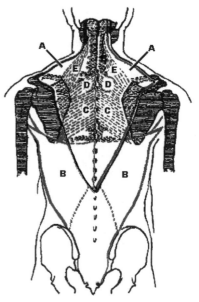

Figure 77: Muscles connecting the
upper limbs to the vertebral column;
viewed from behind
A – Trapezius
B – Latissimus dorsi
C – Rhomboideus major
D – Rhomboideus minor
E – Levator scapulae

Figure 78: Section through the upper part of the thorax, viewed from above showing muscles connecting the thorax to the upper limbs
A – Pectoralis major
B – Pectoralis minor
C – Serratus anterior

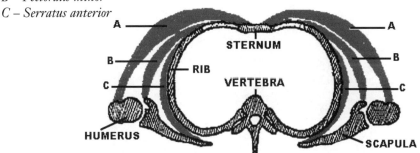

Figure 79: Muscles of the left shoulder girdle viewed from behind
A – Deltoid
B – Supraspinatus
C – Infraspinatus
D – Teres minor
E – Teres major

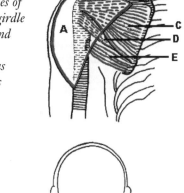

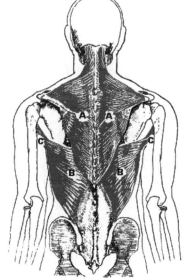

Figure 80
A – Trapezius
B – Latissimus dorsi
C – Twisting of the muscle fibres near insertion

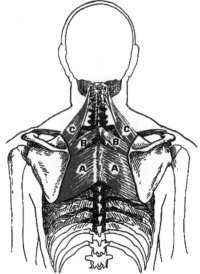

Figure 81
A – Rhomboideus major
B – Rhomboideus minor
C – Levator scapulae

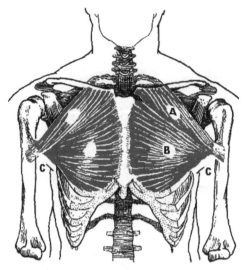

Figure 82
A – Clavicular part of pectoralis major
B – Sternal part of pectoralis major
C – Twisting of muscle fibres near the insertion
of sternal part

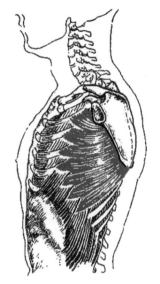

Figure 83: The left serratus
anterior

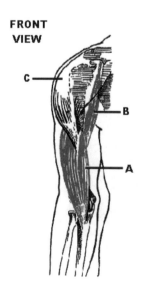

Figure 84
A – Brachialis
B – Coracobrachialis
C – Deltoid

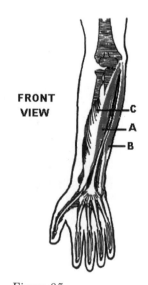

Figure 85
A –
B – } Flexors of the wrist
C – Part of superficial
flexor of the fingers

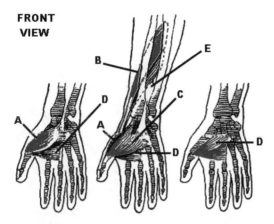

Figure 86: The superficial muscles of the thumb (the long abductor and short extensor of the thumb are shown in the middle of the group because they belong to it functionally)
A – Muscle of opposition
B – Long abductor (short abductor not shown)
C – Short flexor
D – Adductor
E – Short extensor

ILLUSTRATIONS OF THE SUPERFICIAL MUSCLES

Figure 94: The muscles of the trunk and shoulder girdle viewed from the front
A – Sternomastoid
B – Trapezius
C – Clavicle
D – Deltoid
E – Pectoralis major
F – Serratus anterior
G – External oblique
H – Sternum
J – Latissimus dorsi
K – Brachialis
L – Biceps brachialis
M – Triceps (long head)
N – Coracobrachialis
O – Rectus abdominis covered by aponeurosis
P – Inguinal ligament

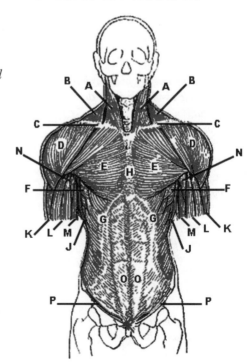

Figure 95: The muscles of the
trunk and shoulder girdle viewed
from behind
A – Trapezius
B – Latissimus dorsi
C – Prominence due to underlying
sacrospinalis
D – External oblique
E – Infrasinatus
F – Teres major
G – Rhomboideus major
H – Teres minor
J – Deltoid
K – Triceps
L – Brachialis
M – Biceps brachialis
N – Sternomastoid
(In the living body with the left
arm raised, the left scapula will be
approximately 25mm higher than
shown in the diagram)

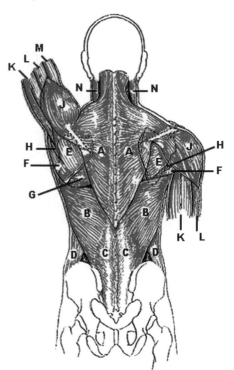

Figure 96: The muscles of the trunk and
shoulder girdle as viewed from the side
A – Deltoid
B – Trapezius
C – Infraspinatus
D – Teres major
E – Teres minor
F – Rhomboideus major
G – Latissimus dorsi
H – Pectoralis major
J – Serratus anterior
K – Triceps (long head)
L – Brachialis
M – Biceps brachialis
N – Coracobrachialis
O – Latissimus dorsi
P – Rectus abdominis
Q – External oblique

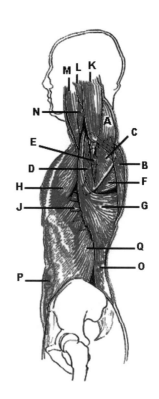

*Figure 97: The muscles of the arm and
forearm viewed from the side*
A – Deltoid
B – Biceps brachialis
C – Brachialis
D – Triceps
E – Brachioradialis
F and G – Extensors of the wrist
H – Long extensor of the fingers
J – Extensor of the wrist
K – Long abductor of the thumb
L – Short extensor of the thumb
M – Long extensor of the thumb
N – Anconaeus

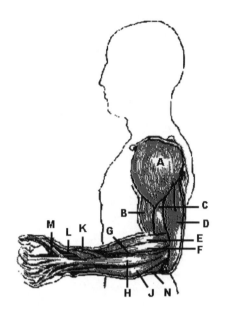

*Figure 98: The muscles of the thigh and leg viewed from
the front*
A – Tensor fasciae latae
B – Sartorius
C – Rectus femoris of quadriceps
D – Outer head of quadriceps
E – Inner head of quadriceps
F – Patella
G – Anterior tibial muscle
H – Long extensor of the toes
J – Peroneus longus
K – Long extensor of the big toe
L – Inner edge of gastrocnemius
M – Inner edge of soleus
N – Ligament maintaining extensor tendons in position
O – Psoas
P – Iliacus
Q – Pectineus
R – Adductor longus
S – Adductor magnus

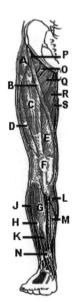

Figure 99: The muscles of the thigh and leg viewed from behind
A – *Gluteus medius*
B – *Gluteus maximus*
C – *Broad fascia of the thigh*
D – *short head of biceps femoris*
E – *long head of biceps femoris*
F – *Semitendinosus*
G – *Semimembranosus*
H – *Adductor magnus*
J – *Gracilis*
K – *Sartorius*
L – *Gastrocnemius*
M – *Soleus*
N – *Peroneus longus*
O – *Peroneus brevis*
P – *Long flexor of the toes*
Q – *Posterior tibial muscle*
R – *Long flexor of the big toe*

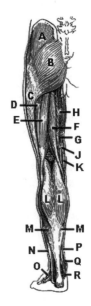

Figure 100: The muscles of the thigh and leg viewed from the side
A – *Tensor fasciae latae*
B – *Gluteus medius*
C – *Gluteus maximus*
D – *Sartorius*
E – *Rectus femoris of quadriceps*
F – *Outer head of quadriceps*
G – *Broad fascia of the thigh*
H – *Long head of biceps*
J – *Semitendinosus*
K – *Patella*
L – *Anterior tibial muscle*
M – *Long extensor of the toes*
N – *Peroneus longus*
O – *Peroneus brevis*
P – *Gastrocnemius*
Q – *Soleus*
R – *Peroneus tertius*

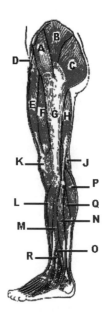

4
SYNTHESIS OF MOVEMENT

Synthesis is the opposite of analysis. Through analysis we articulated the human body into individual parts and ascertained their movement possibilities. Thus we obtained an outline of the basic and composite movements of all parts of the body executed in a particular joint or joint unit. We removed irrelevant and incidental movements and were left with certain raw material of single movements from which we can create entire or complex movements. We arrived at a solid movement line felt deeply as an indivisible whole, in which the body parts (each in its own way) participated and merged into unity.

By combining single movements into one unit, we fulfilled only one requirement of the synthesis of the movement, i.e. synthesis of form. Movement synthesis is, however, complicated and multiform, and must embrace other components if it is to become a means of artistic expression. Besides the synthesis of form, it also requires a spatial, rhythmical and dynamic synthesis. This places considerable demands on the future dancer. To fulfil these demands the dancer must develop mental ability and movement skills, which are summarised as 'higher movement technique'. This technique not only requires bodily discipline but assumes, in the first place, a mental discipline. Without it the artist would not gain the ability to concentrate deeply, a skill which is so important for the dancer.

Concentration is a complicated process through which the artist takes possession of him/herself. Above all he or she must be in a state of perfect body balance which enables them to perceive the bodily architecture and experience it as a structure in space. In this way the dancer gains a permanent relationship with both the inner and outer space in which he/she lives. The persuasiveness of the movement depends on this perception.

The structure of the human body is based on a vertical line, a horizontal line and an arch. The body is symmetrical about each side of the spine which forms its vertical axis ('the vertical'). The shoulders and the hips intersect this axis and point to the sides ('the horizontal'). The ribs curve along both sides of the spine sideways-forward and form with the sternum the vault of the chest ('the arch'). The pelvis arches along the sides of the sacrum and the vault of the skull ends the spinal axis.

I

COORDINATION OF MOVEMENTS

To coordinate movements means to bring them into a logical and organic relation. We can also call it an *interplay of movements*.

From the chapter, ANALYSIS OF MOVEMENT, we know that every part of the body has its own movement possibilities, its own basic and composite movements. To coordinate movements of all these parts may seem logical and easy, but it is not so. From birth children learn to achieve either good or less than good coordination according to their intelligence and physical abilities. When the movements serve a particular purpose (for example a game in which the child is interested, or later, a favourite task) the purpose coordinates the movements more and more perfectly until we reach control of all the movements necessary to that purpose. Any specialised work must coordinate individual tasks in the same way. A perfection in coordination reveals mastery in the field. What technical refinement must a pianist or violinist, for example, have so that their shoulders, arms, wrists, hands and fingers serve their art smoothly and precisely without any visible effort? The technical perfection and polish of their performance is a result of absolute interplay of all movements necessary for the mastery of their instrument. For the movement artist, technical mastery concerns an interplay of the movements of all parts of the body. That is why the movement interplay in its finest detail must, from the beginning of the tuition, be a conscious aim of the teacher.

The beginner acquires a basic awareness of the interplay of the movements while working on the elevated dance posture. All parts of the body, having their own specific task and function, must be involved. The mutual interplay of these functions is the foundation of a sensitive dance posture and the basis of technical perfection. From here, dancers rise toward a perfect form of coordination by learning gradually to balance their bodies correctly, not only in a calm standing position but also while exercising. Thus they slowly adopt the ability to coordinate the movements of both smaller and larger units of complex movements as well as their own improvised movements. At the same time, they discover the independence of all bodily parts and their mutual coherence and interplay.

In each complex movement we have a particular coordination problem. Students solve it only when they acquire the feeling of unity and wholeness on a psycho-physical basis. That means that they do not feel movements only as certain forms but they also perceive the spatial, rhythmical and dynamic component of the movements, i.e. they both perceive and live through their content. Movement form speaks, but only when the dancer is in harmony and unison with its contents. Deep immersion in movement and union between the inner space of the dancer and the surrounding space (summarised in the term '*inner tension*') is a primary factor in the effort of movement coordination which is part of movement synthesis.

The illustration of the Dancing Shiva (Figure 123, p. 270), the Indian sculpture from the fifteenth century, is an example of perfect coordination of single movements within a complex movement. It is in all respects a perfect movement synthesis. The body posture is faultless, all five rules of elevated dance posture are respected, the body is perfectly balanced and it has a spatial span starting from inside and radiating towards the outside. Although there is a broken line in the supporting leg, the body is so perfectly balanced that we see, and recognise through our own body awareness, the span of the vertical line up to the crown of the head and even higher. We can feel the connection with the cosmos both in the head and trunk postures, whose lightness and elevation are exemplary. The spreading of the shoulders balances the vertical line of the body with a calming horizontal line. The arching of the chest is spontaneous and in perfect relation to its loftiness. The free leg and the triple arm balance this already harmonious posture. The arm in front follows and emphasises the span of the arch of the chest, the right upper arm and the left hand prolong the horizontal of the shoulders and both the right and front hand emphasise the vertical of the body. The posture of the Dancing Shiva is enlivened from within in its immobility just the same way as the posture of the deer finding the scent. This posture continues but it seems that at any moment it will unfold itself into another movement, just as perfectly balanced and coordinated.

Despite the rich break-up of this movement we feel its cohesion. It flows out in the first place from a unified emotional content to which all single movements are subordinated. It is unity within plurality for which we strive in dance.

A beginner usually does not coordinate the movements correctly. Movements are linked randomly, i.e. inaccurately and without any inwardly justified guideline. Let us clarify this with a simple example. The starting position is an erect kneeling position. Lower the pelvis into the position of sitting on the heels, while simultaneously lifting the arms sideways, then again raise the body into the initial position while lowering the arms along the body. To be able to coordinate these simple movements perfectly, we must feel that our body is sensitively balanced and perceive it as an entire unit. It is, of course, essential to control the technical basis of all single movements, to know the conditions of the rounding of the lower spine while keeping the upper spine 'immobilised' and to control a faultless shoulder posture during the lifting of the arms sideways.

The same control must be retained on recovery, i.e. while rising from the sitting position on the heels to an erect kneeling position, simultaneously lowering the arms to their initial position. Each of these four movements demands that we maintain certain technical rules and that we know and exactly observe the leading of the movement and fully perceive their spatial orientation.

To coordinate all these single movements so that they give the impression of unity is more difficult than it seems. The accuracy of the starting and ending of both simultaneous movements causes particular problems. It is not a matter of approximate timing, but of timing that is precise to a split second. At the beginning, one movement usually lags behind the other, stops or speeds up and finishes sooner. This inaccuracy of the interplay is caused by an initial inability to perceive both movements as one undivided movement with a common emotional content.

In the last example I used the expression 'immobilised spine', which is explained in the chapter ANALYSIS OF MOVEMENT. This label must not be taken literally. It means that the upper spine does not have any visible changes in movement; it remains in the basic erect posture. It should not be understood that the spine becomes rigid and stiffens in its upright position. A movement expert knows that the upright posture is a live movement, in which the spine is elastically elongated and ready to react to the slightest impulse for movement. It is, therefore, a sensitive part of the whole.

The apparent non-participation of a certain body part which is not directly involved in the movement becomes a real non-participation the moment we lose its sensitive link with the other parts and so exclude it from the entire feeling. Every beginner must have experienced the disagreeable feeling of overstrained hands, heavy shoulders or a flabby abdomen in the moments when attention was focused on the visibly working body part, abandoning the feeling of wholeness. It takes some time for the student to realise that the body as a whole must be constantly enlivened from within, so that all its parts are capable of participation in the slightest single movement of any one part. *The feeling of wholeness of the simultaneously occurring movements and their union in one emotional experience is the coordination and mutual interplay for which we strive.*

II

BINDING OF MOVEMENT UNITS

All the components of expressive movement (form, space, rhythmic and dynamic feeling) are a part of movement synthesis. Each participate in the binding of the integrated unit. Each in its own specific way so that we can distinguish between them. There is a bond of form, spatial, rhythmic and dynamic bonds.

BINDING OF FORM

By the binding of form we mean an effortless linking of one movement to another. Dance composition is a summary of many movements, which are linked like the tones and chords of a musical composition. The movements pass from one to another and flow together in a fluent movement stream. The visual aspect of the movements is, at the same time, an essential condition of success. The dance student must, therefore, gain and increase their experience in a conscious linkage of movements and the teacher must support and guide this endeavour.

Firstly the student must learn about and be conscious of the basic binding of forms without which the other bindings cannot be realised. That means that a transition from one movement to another must not be blurred or inaccurate, but precise and clear.

The students must get used to adhering to a precise beginning and ending of the movement, be familiar with a faultless execution of all single movements and their leading in space, be experienced in controlling the inner tension and be able to coordinate movements in order to feel their cohesion and unity. Only then are they prepared for work on accurate and pure linkage of forms.

The main emphasis during binding of form should be on the leading of the movement. The refined feeling of the body part which leads the movement (e.g. in fingertips during certain arm movements, or delicate feeling of the left or right temple during the rounded sideways bend of the neck and head, or sensitivity in the chest area during the trunk elevation) is the basic condition of the binding of form. The student must practise evoking the refined feeling before starting the movement. A gentle sensitivity must be cultivated to leading with perseverance until the movement reaches its goal in space. When, in execution, the leading passes to another part of the body, the student must immediately evoke a refined feeling of similar quality and intensity in this new part and allow the first awareness to slowly fade away. This evoking of feeling in one small, but leading part of the body, while the feeling in the previous leading part is simultaneously disappearing, is technically demanding and must be cultivated.

The leading of connecting movements can sometimes remain unchanged during two and even more movements, For example, we lead the arm by the fingertips into a crosswise forward position and from here into a sideways stretch with the same leading. The second movement must start exactly from the place where the previous one ended, with changed direction but the same leading. When the leading of the second movement changes, e.g. if we lead with the palm and then with the wrist, the movement would of course start from the place where the first one finished, but this time with a change in direction and leading. The link-up from the precise point where the previous movement ended is one of the primary conditions of the binding of form. If this accuracy is overlooked the transition from one movement to another is blurry. In the same way, a weakened leading and a loss of sensitivity will cause vagueness and lack of clarity in the transition and so erode the entire movement form.

In the leading of a complex movement a number of single movements are simultaneously executed involving several parts of the body. A good example is a *rounded backward bend of the spine* combined with *raising the arms*. The initial position is a straight elevated posture. As we know from the chapter ANALYSIS OF MOVEMENT, the rounded backward bend consists of several single movements, a forward shift of the pelvis (led by the groins), an elongation of the anterior part of the trunk forward-upward (led by the sternum) and an extension of the upper spine (led by the crown of the head). Added to this is the upward movement of the arms (led by the fingertips). All this leading begins and ends simultaneously (see COORDINATION OF MOVEMENTS, p. 210). Delicate sensitivity must, therefore, be evoked in all named parts of the body at the same time. The refinement and intensity must remain until the completion of the complex movement, in our case the rounded backward bend with the upward raising of the arms. If we wanted to link this with another complex movement, e.g. *lay-out-side* to the right involving a sideways raising of the arms and rotation of the neck and head in the direction of the lay-out, we would leave the leading to the fingertips while raising the arms to the side and to the sternum, while maintaining the upward direction.

We would, however, change the leading of the remaining parts of the body as the new movement demands it. We would transfer the leading from the groins to the right half of the abdominal wall in order to lead the trunk into a straight sideways tilt. At the same time, the tip of the left foot would sensitively lead the left leg in the sideways raising and we would transfer the leading from the crown of the head to the right ear so that it can lead during the rotation of the neck and head to the right. One part of the body passes the leading onto another and only then frees itself by a gradual, slight relaxation. Of course, we must not neglect the technical aspect of the single movements, e.g. in the transition of pelvis from the forward shift to a shift to the left we must push in the right hip joint; or during the leg lift to the side we must elongate the inner left thigh etc. This means that we must preserve all the specific features of the basic and composite movements described in the chapter ANALYSIS OF MOVEMENT.

The combined leading of single movements occurs often in complex movements. Without correct coordination and correct interplay in leading, the dancer cannot achieve a perfect binding of form. And without a perfect binding of form, the spatial bond will also suffer.

SPATIAL BOND (BINDING)

Spatial bonding is tightly connected with binding of forms for the very reason that the movements are almost always led by something and somewhere into space or they fade into it. The directional feeling, as we have learned, makes the movement shape more accurate and the spatial bond is, therefore, also a visual element.

Contrary to the binding of form, the spatial bond is a response by the dancer's inner self. Although the dancer perceives space with kinaesthetic awareness, he/she transforms this perception immediately into a strong emotional experience. Only this kind of perception of space is valid in expressive dance. Space, rhythm and dynamics are components of expressive movement, which evoke in the dancer emotions strong enough to transfer to the spectator. When these emotions are truthful and not simulated they connect the dancer with the spectators in a shared experience.

Let us return to the example of the two complex movements scrutinised from the point of view of binding of form. They were a *rounded backward bend* with raised arms, followed by a *lay-out* to the right with arms raised to the side and rotation of the neck and head in the direction of the lay-out. We discovered how the transition from one movement to another can be made pure in form. Now let us discover how to best link the two movements from the point of view of space. The spatial experience of the rounded backward bend is the arching of the spine upward and through high release, backward. The arms form an accordant arch with the body and together they perceive its path, i.e. the arch in space. This feeling of the whole body does not, however, end where the crown of the head and the fingertips have reached but physically exceeds that point in space, uniting the dancer with the surrounding space. It is a powerful experience and differs markedly from a movement with the same form, yet without such a perception of space and without the emotion that flows out of it, and which gives the movement an emotional content. During the transition into a lay-out sideways, the dancers abandon the arch in space, but their connection with the outer space lasts. It outgrows all directional changes and even the changes in the leading; and its permanency links one spatial perception to another. In our example, the dancer's feeling of the curved path transforms into one of a horizontal between two straight directions, right and left. This change in feeling must be immediate and must precede the physical movement. The trunk, the right arm and the head submit to the right direction, and the pelvis, the left arm and the left leg to the left. The whole body has passed from a distinct arc into a horizontal with a strong contra-directional feeling. This feeling of direction does not end at the fingertips of both hands and the toes of the left foot, but again exceeds the physically defined space by perceiving the space beyond.

In another complex movement, the dancer follows a certain goal in space. Reaching the goal does not, however, mean an inter-rupted contact with the space which surrounds the dancer. The goal can be near or far. If it is far, the path to it can be extended by a movement from the spot—e.g. by a step—executed by another part of the body, thus reinforcing the directional feeling, involving this process more than one bodily part.

Example: the fingers lead forward to the goal but are not able to reach that far. That is why the leading of one leg joins in by per-forming a forward lunge and at the same time the sternum joins in by leading the trunk into a straight forward tilt and so brings the fingers closer to the goal. While performing this movement, the dancer must not lose his or her relationship with the surrounding space. Here, one leading follows the other in their common goal forward and the dancer remains in it until the moment all the lead-ings are united by one spatial experience and until there is a change in direction and leading in the next complex movement.

So far we have paid attention to movements which led us from the centre of the body into space. Now let us turn our attention to the spatial bond of a movement which, on the contrary, brings us closer to the centre of the body and joins us with it.

Example: perform a lunge forward on the right leg, combined with an extension of the spine, simultaneously raising the arms for-ward (the first movement). Shift the body weight onto the back leg and bend it while bending and lifting the front, free leg with the knee pointing towards the chest. At the same time, pass from the extension of the spine to the rounded forward bend in axis, the arms turned in and bent both in the elbows and wrists so that the fingers point towards the chest (the second movement). The first move-ment points into the space out of the centre of the body; the other one, on the contraty, points towards the centre of the body. The first movement is 'contra-directory': the right knee, the groins and the fingers of the turned-out arms lead the movement forward, the sternum leads forward-upward and the crown of the head leads the neck with the head backward through a high release. The backward direction is also emphasised by the heel of the leg which is stretched backward. The arc of the body spanning through a high release backward is counter-balanced by the arms, groins and the knee pointing forward (the right knee). The movement goes in both directions from the centre of the body outward and the relevant principles, described earlier, must be applied here. The second movement is another case, its direction is towards the centre of the body. For a dancer this means a transition from a spatial feeling extending beyond space and defined by movement, to a feeling of space which is, on the contrary, drawn towards the centre of the body. This withdrawal from a wide-spread to a narrowed space is a strong experience during which the dancer lives through completely antagonistic emotions. The dancer feels as if the surrounding space is folding in and shutting itself up. The connection of the dancer with the outer space has not been interrupted but changed in character. The dancer feels it as something alive which penetrates his/her dance.

Sculptures scrutinised in terms of body balance and coordination of movements reveal, through the dynamically executed complex and single movements, an unconditional link with space. In this imaginary unfolding of movements, this form of art cannot lose its spatial connection. It lives, not only in its immortalised form, but also in its possible metamorphoses.

RHYTHMIC BOND (BINDING)

Dance composition is a summary of many complex movements linked in sequence like the tones or chords in a musical composition. The components of its movement synthesis are pure form and a strong experience of space with which the movement form is closely linked. Another indispensable component is rhythm, or rather a rhythmic feeling. Whether evoked by the music or the theme, it must evoke in the dancer a vivid rhythmic response. When the rhythmic feeling is too weak, the dance performance lacks one of the important components of the synthesis without which dance is not dance.

Folk and society dances of all nations are built on rhythm. National temperament as well as manners and customs of the period in which the dances originated manifest themselves through rhythm. In the first place, however, they reveal zest for life, joy from rhythmic movement and the need to share it with others. Expressive dance, on the other hand, communicates the emotional content of the music or story and is designed for the spectator.

The role of rhythm in stage dance is multi-faceted. A stage dancer must know individual components of rhythm, distinguish them and work with them. These components are: tempo, metre, rhythmic values and dynamic shading. The dancer's rhythmic feeling must in its totality combine all the components into one unit. The stage dance makes heavy demands on the dancer who must be capable of living through the rhythm of different characters and of feeling the stormy excitement as well as the majestic calm of movements. The dancer who plays Romeo lives with quite a different rhythm from that of Tybalt; the composer Prokofiev expressed the two characters in two distinct ways. But it would not suffice if the dancer were governed solely by the music; the dancer must also know and respect the content. Not only music, but also the theme, defines the rhythm of dance.

The task of the teacher at the outset must be to consider all the demands put on the dance artist, including that of rhythm, which must be pursued uncompromisingly.

In movement practice we often meet with an understanding of rhythm which does not correspond to its role in stage dance. Emphasis is put on maintaining the time values (which are of course very important); but the emotional experience of rhythm is not sufficiently taken into account. This is not a full-blooded rhythm, but rather a kind of rhythmic plan. We know, however, that the very emotional relationship to rhythm is lifeblood to a dancer. The effort of the educator, therefore, must be directed towards awakening and developing not just rhythmic accuracy but the superior, all-embracing rhythmic feeling.

This can be done in a number of ways. Firstly, the teacher must ensure that the rhythm with which he/she chooses to enrich the excercises musically (even if they are exclusively technical) adheres precisely to the movement. It must also have its full expressive value, i.e. that it is dynamically shaded. Dynamic shading is not just an addition, on the contrary, it is an important part of rhythm which conveys its emotional content. It is above all the dynamic shading which transforms a rhythmic plan into full-blooded rhythm.

To cultivate the rhythmic feeling during exercises a sung rhythm, or a rhythm played on an instrument which is capable of singing out a pure melody—e.g. a flute—is the most useful. To use just a small drum is not appropriate because it cannot express the duration of movement. Also, the usual piano accompaniment often used in a mechanical and spiritless way, is not, from my experience, a suitable musical supplement. Melody, rhythm and dynamics do not sound, through this kind of accompaniment, as purely and clearly as in singing. Especially in the beginning of teaching, when the students are supposed to develop an accurate movement form, it is necessary for the musical counterpart to be unambiguously truthful. A melody sung by the teacher has been proven the best. The quality of the voice does not matter as much as the accuracy of rhythm and the expression of rhythmic and dynamic shades, with which the practised movement deals. The teacher can best of all achieve this because he/she leads the exercise and knows what the movement requires.

Metre is a certain frame into which we write the rhythm. Expression of the movement rhythm can be accurate only when the rhythmic values are supported by another component of rhythmic feeling, i.e. a metric feeling. That is why the teacher, together with the sung rhythm, indicates on her drum the metre of the bar in which the melody is sung. The students perceive both metre and rhythm and they gradually learn to join in one rhythmic experience and thus gain rhythmic accuracy. This manifests itself in accurate starting and ending of movements in given time, as consistently required of them by the teacher.

Feeling of tempo: this is another important component of rhythmic feeling. The teacher cultivates it by practising the same movements, the same exercises at different speeds. A tempo is chosen according to the kinds of movements, as well as according to their rhythmic character. At first, the teacher practises differences in tempo with students by setting and accompanying it. Later the teacher sets the tempo but does not accompany the exercise either by singing or by drum. The teacher creates different variations of such exercises and it is not easy to grasp the tempo, to adjust the given movement to it and then maintain the tempo to the end, according to the need. The students must learn not only to distinguish between metre, tempo and rhythm, but also to be able to join all of them into an entire rhythmic feeling.

Rhythmic bond of movements requires that one continuously lives through the rhythm in all its breadth and significance, so that the individual parts are not detached from one another, but are linked together. It is exactly this undying rhythmic feeling which bonds the movements most efficiently, even when there is a short stop or a pause in the rhythm. We grasp it when we experience for the first time that the pause is not a breather, relaxation or a removal from the rhythmic stream, but that it can be, on the contrary, its climax. In the pause, the dancer maintains the muscle tension of the preceding movement and expresses the pause by holding the movement and the breath, keeping the intensity of the inner tension unchanged. Inner tension is the pillar of rhythmic bonding without which the rhythmic feeling would be unstable, as can be observed in students who are not yet capable of a deep concentration.

Movement rhythm is created by movements of uneven range and uneven duration. They form different rhythmic relationships and together they create a smaller or a bigger unit. Rhythmic bonding into such a unit presumes a perception of the unit and its structure, which makes it important to develop in students a feeling for a form. The teacher must, from the very beginning, head towards this goal by presenting students with increasingly complicated exercises (even purely technical ones) in an accurate form, well balanced in terms of movement and rhythm. The pedagogue must be aware that the perfect composition of exercises is, for students, an example that influences the development of their feeling for form, although they themselves may not realise it. An exercise enhanced by perfect form has its educational role: it must be entire, rhythmically accurate, dynamically shaded and, when it is a larger unit, it must have its dynamic climax and should reach a logical conclusion. This way the students experience directly the movement unit and gradually learn that a sequence of movements not chosen incidentally, but has an order which binds them into an entire, self-contained form. They experience, and later understand, the basic structure of a simple form of even the smallest unit, i.e. exposition, development and recapitulation. One movement, with its rhythmic element passes into another, develops, culminates on the first beat of a second bar and heads towards the conclusion. Without a feeling for form and for unity, the dance cannot bind the movements together. When the students have understood this not only through intellect but through their full emotional response to a small rhythmic form, they have also grasped the principle of the rhythmic bond of a large movement unit. They have understood that the rhythmic bond, or the link-up of rhythms, is the same in a small or a large unit and that the feeling for form helps them strengthen their rhythmic cohesion. If they work on rhythm in a state of keen perception, it will be clear to them that rhythm is not a matter of abstraction but of feeling and a life-like nature; and that it unconditionally belongs to a synthesis of the movement unit.

DYNAMIC BOND

In discussing dynamic bonding, we need to distinguish dynamic shading of a single rhythm from the dynamic line of a dance unit, even the smallest one. The dynamic line passes through the smallest movement unit as well as the larger dance composition, and creates the dynamic form of the whole. At the same time, it is a dynamic bond, i.e. a part of movement synthesis of the entire dance performance.

Dynamic form is a very expressive component of dance composition. It has two dynamic peaks, the upper and lower, i.e. the dynamically strongest and dynamically weakest point. It has its dynamic curves, the ascents and descents, and its accents, i.e. accentuated moments which stand out conspicuously from the total dynamic line.

In the dancer, the dynamic form of the composition, whether it be connected with music or not, is a reflection and a portrait of his or her inner experience. When the dance has a pure musical base the dancer follows the dynamic form of the score. When, however, the dancer wants to express both the music and an idea connected with it, then he/she independently intervenes: the dynamic form of the music is slightly changed according to his/her own conception of the theme without disturbing its basic contents. For example, the dynamic climax is strengthened by syncopation or becomes immobilised in places where it responds to the theme while the music flows on. Alternatively one movement can embrace one whole melodic phrase. The dynamic form of the dance will then be the dancer's independent creation, all the more if the dance is created without the music.

The dynamic line links the movements into one whole and binds them with its emotional content. Out of all the components of the movement synthesis which take part in the total composition, the dynamic component is the most expressive and effective one.

Just like the rhythmic and spatial bonds, the dynamic bond is, above all, a matter of the dancer's inner self, it is most closely connected with the emotional content of the dance. The bond is brought to life by the fact that the dancer maintains the intensity of the inner tension, does not disturb and/or break the dynamic flow, but devotes him/herself to it as he/she does to the rhythmic stream. This commitment must be felt even more deeply because the dynamics directly touch the soul.

Movement synthesis is a culmination of movement; it is superior to movement analysis from which it draws. Without movement analysis, there would be no movement synthesis because purity and conclusive evidence of synthesis depend on purity and conclusive evidence of analysis. For dance art, movement analysis is indispensable. A detailed analysis of the movements of the human body reveals to the choreographer the possibilities of conveying shades of expression through movement details which, without a close analysis, would remain obscure. The synthesis, however, is a creative process and the freedom of choice of expressive means, of which the possibilities are inexhaustible, must be left to the creator. The movement possibilities discovered through analysis bound by firm rules, but in synthesis we have the freedom to explore our own combinations, variations and flight.

Higher movement technique culminates in movement synthesis. Having mastered it, the dance student is prepared for creative movement work, i.e. dance composition*

III

SOME METHODICAL ADVICE

Exercises for developing awareness
Material obtained by movement analysis, i.e. analysis of correct body posture, of basic and composite movements of all body parts, is processed into exercises which vary from each other in terms of both purpose and form. Exercises for developing awareness have

*Jarmila Kröschlová *Výrazový Tanec*, (Expressive Dance). Praha: Orbis 1964.

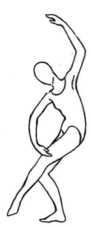

Figure 101

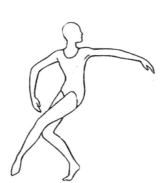

Figure 102

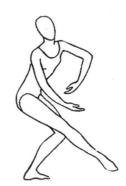

Figure 103

Figure 101: The complex movement does not unfold in space, but rather closes in towards the centre of the body. The pelvis creates the centre where all the single movements converge. This includes the left arm because it is bent in the elbow and the wrist, and so is directed towards the body.

Figure 102: The body has a similar shape but has an opposite effect. Here the body weight is shifted onto the toes thus the body movement is carried expressively forward into space. The feeling forwards dominates, although this is tempered by the rotation of the head and upper trunk into space, backwards. The rounded left arm moderates the backward direction.

Figure 103: In this movement the directional feeling forwards-down is unusually strong and clear. The whole body is flowing into forward space, although the pelvis is drawn backwards while the trunk is held in a straight forward tilt. The right arm emphasizes the drawing forwards of the body, conforming with the feeling created by the movement of the left forearm and hand.

Figure 104: The whole body is involved in a wavelike shape. The arms complete the movement without emphasizing a conflict of directions.

Figure 105: The position on high demi-pointe with maximal elongation upwards of the whole body and right arm together with the elongated left upper arm, all contribute to the feeling of tension. Although the head deviates sharply in a tilt and rotation to the right, it does not detract from the upward directional experience.

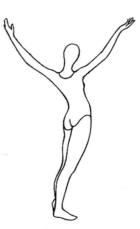

Figure 104

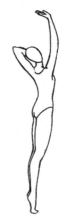

Figure 105

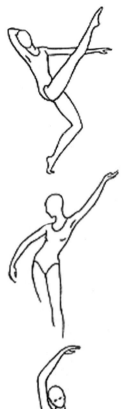

Figure 106: The dynamic tension of the movement is in the crossing of directions. The position on high demi-point of the left foot represents the centre of the movement. The trunk, in a straight backward tilt together with the thigh of the left leg, is in a contra-direction to the maximally extended right leg which is aimed upward. Both directions form an acute angle with each other. The arms balance this movement by an unaccented action.

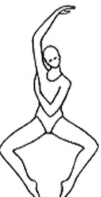

Figure 107: Straight lateral shift-tilt of the lower trunk to the left is moderated by a small rounded bend of the upper trunk to the right. Thus, the spatial experience of the straight lateral shift-tilt is weakened. The head with its rotation to the right emphasizes the predominance of the right side of the body over the left. The arms maintain the spatial bilateral balance.

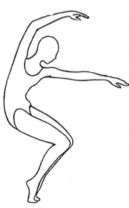

Figure 108: The horizontal of both legs turned out in a partial squat of high demi-point is balanced by the vertical of the body and arms, although the right arm is rounded and not extended upward. This results in an expressive movement, which is not directed upward, but toward the body. This feeling is further strengthened by the movement of the head and leading elbow of the left arm. Both emphasize the contra-direction downward.

Figure 109: Standing on high demi-pointe with knees bent forward, with a rounded trunk (pelvis tucked under). The line of the movement is formed by the clear spatial relationship of the whole body from feet to head. The right arm completes the curve with the help of thoracic rotation to the right. The head merges with the expressive curve of the movement whose direction incorporates the left arm. The left arm balances the position.

the simplest form: their main purpose is expressed in their name. By means of these exercises, the students become aware of:

(1) the muscle work and single movements of the elevated body posture;

(2) the muscle work during basic and composite movements of all parts of the body, their specific characteristics, leading and direction.

The categories of muscle work (contraction, extension and relaxation), are discovered by the students during a detailed acquisition of all components of a correct body posture. This demands a clear differentiation of muscle activity.

Exercises for developing awareness have the simplest form containing these parts:

– Initial position or posture
– Main movement
– Recovery movement.

Besides these, I also indicate in the descriptions the direction, tempo, rhythm, dynamics and purpose of the exercises as well as mistakes in or difficulties faced by the exercise. All these are issues of which the student must be aware.

In all these exercises we become aware through our body sensations of a muscular contraction, extension and relaxation (kinesthetic awareness), as a perfect execution demands it. The exercises may be best conducted through singing or words, not just by the use of a drum or piano, as was mentioned earlier. The voice, using words like: 'con-trac-tion, re-lax-a-tion', indicates the fluency and length of the movement, as well as its dynamic shading; and a gentle strike on the drum gives time, its metre and tempo. The striking must be quiet and unobtrusive. In these exercises for developing awareness, it is best to choose the measures: 4/4, 3/4 or 5/4 in a slow tempo.

IV

AWARENESS EXERCISES FOR CORRECT BODY POSTURE

The main pillar of technical teaching is the sequence of exercises for developing awareness of correct body posture. Adherence to its five principles consists of many components of many single movements. At first we work through all the components separately, each one of them individually so that they sink deep into the students' movement memory and only then do we unite them gradually into a perfect posture. The most suitable position for this purpose is lying on the back.

Lying on the back: the whole area of the back, the posterior part of the acromions and the pelvis, and the legs touch the floor. The legs, slightly turned out and closed together, lie in the same plane as the trunk, and the turned-in arms rest in a relaxed manner along the body, supported by the outer sides of the hands with the palms facing the body and the elbows slightly turned away from the body and directed to the sides. The arms are slightly rounded, not stiffly stretched or excessively bent. The head rests on the back of the skull and the chin forms an approximate right angle with the front of the neck. (Move the sacrum closer to the floor.)

The teacher should make sure that the students learn to control this position. It will help them become aware of the mid-line which divides the body into two symmetrical halves. The mid-line runs through the crown of the head, the spine, sacrum and between the legs. When in a standing position on both feet, the mid-line also becomes the axis of the body. Before starting to practise with the students, the teacher must make sure that the body is symmetrically positioned around this mid-line: for example, that the head does not incline sideways, that one shoulder is not lower or higher, that one side of the ribs is not more arched than the other, that both hips lie on the floor in the horizontal line so that both legs are alongside each other and the arms are in the described position exactly along the body.

The initial position, lying on the back, should not be a rest but a position which is concentrated and felt through, in which each part of the body is in a correct relationship to the other. The hip joints are above the centre of the insteps, shoulder joints above the hip joints and the outer openings of the ears above the shoulders. The students should remain freshly aware of how one part of the body is connected to another and how they inter-relate. They need to cultivate this sensation so they can recognise a deviation and correct it. This basic sensation of the body balance should be cultivated and consolidated. That is why we incorporate the following preparation time and time again in the awareness exercises of correct body posture.

Relaxation and sensitisation of the muscles and joints of the whole body

Initial position: lying on the back.

Main movement: gradually relax all bodily units and their parts as named by the teacher. Relax until completely loose.

Recovery: inapplicable, because we remain in complete relaxation.

Direction: downward towards the floor to which the whole body clings.

Tempo, rhythm, dynamics are indicated by the teacher in a soft, guiding voice in order not to disturb the students' concentration. Calmly and gradually the teacher names all the bodily parts of which students should be kinaesthetically aware; and softly indicates on the drum a slow tempo.

The purpose of the exercise is to achieve the ability to concentrate and awaken the bodily sensation (kinaesthetic awareness) of all named units and their parts.

The teacher must try to detect faults firstly by observing an uncontrolled initial position and occasionally in the restlessness of the student, revealed in involuntary movements. The body should be absolutely calm and almost motionless during this exercise.

The teacher repeats this exercise from time to time during the course of learning. Later on he/she will require the process of relaxation to stop at a certain level, allowing a sensitive readiness for movement with a minimal muscle effort.

Establishment of the pelvis—abdominal muscles

Initial position: lying on the back.

Main movement: develop pressure from the front in the direction backward onto the pelvis by contracting the lower segments of the straight abdominal muscles - *rectus abdomini* (under belly), and firmly press the sacrum to the floor. At the same time, keep the whole body relaxed.

Recovery: relax the tension of the abdominal muscles so that the sacrum moves slightly away from the floor.

Direction: backward-downward, led by both hips and sacrum.

Tempo, rhythm, dynamics: four slow beats for contraction of the muscles (crescendo), four for relaxation (decrescendo).

The purpose of the exercise is to be aware of the participation of the abdominal muscles in the establishment of the pelvis and to awaken in them kinaesthetic awareness.

Mistakes:
- lying on the back without being conscious of the mid-line of the body, i.e. without being aware of the axis.
- holding the breath.

Establishment of the pelvis—buttock muscles

Initial position: lying on the back.

Main movement: contract the buttock (gluteal) muscles over the hip joints and hips toward the sacrum. Thus we exert pressure on the pelvis from the back while keeping the body relaxed.

Recovery: relax the tension of the buttock muscles and the pelvis returns to the initial position.

Direction: forward-upward, led by the groins.

Tempo, rhythm, dynamics: four slow beats for contraction (crescendo), four for relaxation of muscles (decrescendo).

The purpose of the exercise is to be aware of the participation of the buttock muscles in the establishment of the pelvis and to awaken in them kinaesthetic awareness.

Mistakes:
- as in the previous exercise.

The teacher should point out to the students how the pelvis lightens through the activity of the gluteal muscles and the thighs turn out moderately in the hip joints.

The establishment of the pelvis by both abdominal and gluteal muscles

Initial position: lying on the back.

Main movement: combine the pressure of the abdominal muscles with the contraction of the gluteal muscles, i.e. the pressure on the pelvis from the front together with the pressure on the pelvis from the back by which the pelvis becomes established. The pressures counter-balance each other.

Recovery: gradually relax the muscle tension and the pelvis will return into the initial position.

Direction: the forward-upward direction *is led* by the groins, the backward one *is led* by the hips and the sacrum.

Tempo, rhythm, dynamics: 4/4 signature; four slow beats for establishing, four for relaxation, two beats for establishing, three for relaxation, one beat for establishing, three beats to hold, four beats for relaxation. The teacher must insist on maintaining the value of the beat.

The purpose of the exercise is to be aware of the counter-balancing pressure on the pelvis from the front and back, by which the pelvis becomes established in its basic position.

Mistakes:

- as in the previous exercises.

The instruction to 'establish the pelvis' should always prompt a common counter-balancing activity of the abdominal and gluteal muscles described in the previous exercises.

Levelling excessive lumbar lordosis

First exercise

Initial position: lying on the back.

Main movement: establish the pelvis while relaxing the intercostal muscles so that the lower ribs do not protrude excessively.

Recovery: relax the tension of the abdominal and gluteal muscles and contract them again. Make sure that during the exercise, the intercostal muscles remain relaxed.

Direction of the movement of the rib arches is a sinking and a levelling with the mid-line of the body.

Tempo, rhythm, dynamics: 4/4 time signature, two slow beats for establishing the pelvis, two beats for relaxing without letting the intercostal muscles tense up, then one beat for establishing and one for relaxation.

The purpose of the exercise is to undo any habitual tension in the intercostal muscles and to achieve their sensitivity.

Mistakes:

- inability to relax the tension in the area of the rib arches.
- imperfect coordination of the pelvic and intercostal muscles which should always be flexible, yet relaxed and not rigid.
- holding the breath.

Both the teacher and the students must realise that there is a connection between a protruding rib cage and excessive lumbar lordosis.

Second exercise

Initial position: lying on the back.

Main movement: by contracting the straight abdominal muscles (*rectus abdomini*) pull the relaxed rib arches downward, closer to the pubic bone, without lowering the sternum. On the contrary, exert a 'contra-pull' of the sternum upward. The pull and the 'contra-pull' must not be forcible but delicately felt.

Recovery: relax the pull of the rectus abdomini without letting go the established pelvis. Both the sacrum and the hips stay pressed to the floor.

Direction of the rib arches is downward and the contra-direction of the sternum upward.

Tempo, rhythm, dynamics: the teacher indicates 4/4 measure in slow tempo for the movement of the ribs.

The purpose of the exercise is to become aware that by a downward pulling of the rib arches, excessive lordosis of the lumbar spine flattens out. The students learn at the same time the coordination of the muscular activity, i.e. a simultaneous tensing of the rectus abdomini and a relaxing of the intercostal muscles of the relevant rib arches. It is an important skill for further technical training.

Mistakes:
- insufficient relaxation of the muscles of the rib arches which consequently resist the contraction of the rectus abdomini.
- holding the breath.

Levelling excessive chest kyphosis
Initial position: lying on the back or sitting down.

Main movement: concentrate your attention on the part of the thoracic spine between the shoulder blades. Through kinaesthetic awareness, perceive the spinal processes of the vertebrae and pull them together. Thus the support point of the neck and head is established. The sternum and the neck and head become elevated as a consequence of this muscle activity.

Recovery: sensitively relax the tension of the muscles of the thoracic spine. The relaxation of the muscles exists only to an extent where the muscle is still ready for movement.

Direction is upward and *is led* by the sternum.

Tempo, rhythm, dynamics: time signature 4/4, four beats of medium speed for establishing of support point, four beats for relaxation, gradually changing the intervals in between.

Purpose of the exercise: to flatten out the excessive kyphosis of the thoracic spine and to realise the connection between the support point of neck, head and sternum.

The establishment of the support point also helps to level the excessive neck (cervical) lordosis.

Mistakes:
- Pulling together the shoulder blades instead of pulling

together the spinous processes, revealing insufficient sensitivity of thoracic spine.
- tension of inappropriate muscles, preventing a spatial sensation of upward direction of the sternum.
- Excessive relaxation during recovery. Students sometimes slacken instead of just reaching the initial balanced body tension.

A complete levelling of lordosis of the neck

First exercise
Initial position: lying on the back.

Main movement: elongate the neck and concentrate attention on the seventh neck (cervical) vertebra. Using the elongated neck muscles as much as possible push it back into line with the other neck vertebrae, so that the cervical spine is almost flattened out.

Recovery: relax the tension of the muscles around the seventh cervical vertebra without slackening them, still maintaining a balanced body tone.

Direction: the upward direction of the neck *is led* by the crown of the head.

Tempo, rhythm, dynamics: time signature 4/4 in a slow tempo, one beat for pushing the seventh cervical vertebra inward, one beat to hold, two beats to relax. When repeating this exercise, gradually lengthen the time for each movement until the relaxation takes four beats.

Purpose of the exercise is to become aware that a perfect elongation of the neck cannot be achieved without consciously pushing the seventh cervical vertebra almost into line with the others. This is important also during a backward bend of the neck and head (hyperextension), because it prevents an uncontrolled dropping of the head.

Mistakes:
- lack of refined sensitivity.
- exaggerated muscular tension which destroys the interplay with other parts of the body. If the seventh cervical vertebra protrudes exceedingly, there appears an indentation in place of the sixth cervical vertebra which will disappear with correct work. This mistake is usually connected with swollen upper parts of the trapezius muscle.

Second exercise

Initial position: lying on the back.

Main movement: connect all movements which counterbalance the excessive lordosis and kyphosis of the spine. At the same time, pull the relaxed lower rib arches down, establish the support point of the neck and head resulting in a contra-directional elevation of the sternum upward and pull in the seventh cervical vertebra by elongated neck muscles. Thus the excessive S-shaped curvature of the spine has been flattened.

Recovery: relax the tension of all participating muscles only to the point where the muscle is still ready for movement.

Elongation of the spine

First exercise

Initial position: lying on the back, later also in the sitting position.

Main movement: maximally elongate the spine by a gradual contraction of the muscles along the spine and the back from the coccyx to the support point of the neck and head and from this point, extend the neck as far as the skull. Simultaneously, counterbalance the excessive curvature of the spine.

Recovery: relax the maximal elongation of the spine as well as the increased activity of the other participating muscles. However, do not exceed the limit where the relaxed muscles still remain sensitive and ready for movement.

Direction is upward along the whole spine as far as the skull and *is led* by the sternum and the crown of the head.

Tempo, rhythm, dynamics: time signature 4/4, four slow beats for increased activity - hold, four for release - hold.

The purpose of the exercise is to become aware of the difference between the increased activity of the muscles and their relaxed, sensitive activity coordinated within the framework of an elevated carriage of the spine.

Mistakes:
 • an imperfectly coordinated muscle activity.

Second exercise

Initial position: lying on the back.

Main movement: with a minimal muscular effort but with a refined bodily sense, separate the vertebrae from each other in the direction from the sacrum towards the skull. The difference between the elongation of the spine in the previous exercise and this refined feeling lies in a lightness, a lightened spine. In both cases it is a matter of straightening the spine, but with a difference in expression.

Recovery: through a slight relaxation, the spine, in a way, slides down without changing its basic correct posture.

Direction: upward, and *is led* by the crown of the head.

Tempo, rhythm, dynamics: the time signature is 4/4 in pianissimo.

The purpose of the exercise is to cultivate the feeling of lightness and elevation with the least muscular effort, which has to be replaced by inner tension, accompanying the experience of space and lightness.

Mistakes:

• an incorrect relation between the inner and muscular tension.

This kind of a lightened, erect spine is suitable for an elevated dance movement.

Establishing widely spread shoulders

First exercise

Initial position: lying on the back, later in a sitting position with the back to the teacher.

Main movement: relax the upper part of the trapezius and around the acromioclavicular joints. By contracting the sub-clavicular muscles, press the clavicles towards the upper ribs and by contracting the lower part of the trapezius pull the shoulder blades down. Elevate the sternum in a 'contra-pull'. The back muscles work to a maximum. Thus the downward pull of the shoulders is executed.

Recovery: relax the maximal tension of the muscles into a normal one, i.e. a sensitively relaxed posture.

A pull of the shoulders downward and of the sternum upward is one of the three functions of which the establishment of the shoulders consists.

Direction: the shoulders downward and the sternum upward.

Tempo, rhythm, dynamics: time signature is 4/4 in a slow tempo. two beats to pull the shoulders downward, two beats to hold and four beats to relax.

The purpose of the exercise is to realise the difference between a maximal downward pull of the shoulders, necessary for example in the rounded backward bend of the spine and between the normal pull which occurs when we relax the maximal tension. As we know,

this is a part of the normal relaxed elevated body posture.
Mistakes:
- incorrect tension of the upper trapezius and around the acromioclavicular joints.
- shoulder blades pulled together instead of being pulled downward. The teacher's supervision and correction here are especially necessary.

Second exercise

Initial position: lying on the back; later in a sitting position with back to the teacher.

Main movement: simultaneously with a maximal pull of the shoulders downward, stretch the pectorals maximally to the sides by involving the rhomboids. The shoulders broaden through this active extension.

Recovery: relax the maximal tension of the muscles into a normal one so that the muscles remain sensitive and ready for movement.

Direction of the shoulders sideways and downward *is led* by the acromions and the lower angles of the shoulder blades.

Tempo, rhythm, dynamics: the time signature 4/4, three beats to pull, one beat to hold, four beats to relax; then one beat to pull, three beats to hold and four beats to relax. Slowly at first, then faster, with crescendo.

The purpose of the exercise is to realise the interplay of the muscles during the simultaneous pull downward and sideways; to achieve the activity and sensitivity of the pectorals.

Mistakes:
- incorrect muscular function during which the shoulder blades draw together instead of downward
- allowing the acromions to deviate from the side of the chest instead of remaining above the hip joints, so that the trunk is not perfectly balanced. This results in an incorrect coordination of the movement.

The pull of the shoulders to the sides is another one of the three functions for establishment of the shoulders.

Third exercise

Initial position: lie on the back; later in a sitting or standing position with the back to the teacher.

Main movement: while pulling the shoulders downward and sideways, press the shoulder blades towards the ribs by contracting serratus anterior muscles. The lower angles of the shoulders move slightly sideways away from the spine and the acromions shift slightly backward. Thus we turn out the shoulders and therefore we complete their establishment.

Recovery: relax the maximal tension of the muscles into a normal one when the muscles remain fully sensitive and ready for movement.

The turning out of the shoulders, i.e. pressing the shoulder blades towards the ribs, is the last one of the three functions of which the establishment of shoulders consists.

Direction: in the general establishment of the shoulders, the shoulders pull downward, the pectorals to the sides, the lower angles of the shoulder blades forward towards the ribs and the acromions backward. This combined feeling is possible only during a perfect coordination of single movements.

Tempo, rhythm, dynamics: the time signature is 4/4 of a medium tempo, one bar for the main movement, second bar to hold, third bar recovery, fourth for hold, avoiding a slackening of the body posture.

The purpose of the exercise is to cultivate the habit of the established shoulders during both maximal and normal muscular tension while the arms remain relaxed. With minimal muscular effort, but with a refined kinaesthetic awareness and with the presence of inner tension, this aim is achieved.

Mistakes:
- insufficient coordination and over-straining of muscles.
- losing kinaesthetic awareness.
- transferring muscular tension to inappropriate places such as the arms.
- holding the breath.

Elongation of straight legs to the toes and heels in a parallel position

Initial position: lying on the back.

Main movement: with the legs in a parallel position, elongate one leg as if you wanted to separate the thigh in the hip joint from the pelvis, the lower leg in the knee joint from the thigh, and the foot in the ankle joint from the lower leg. The muscles of the whole leg elongate elastically to the tip of the toe. The movement is then repeated by the other leg and by both legs together. The movement of the legs in a parallel position runs from the hip joint to the tip of the toe. The same is practised later with a moderate turning out.

Recovery: relax the joints either simultaneously or in sequence.

Direction: into space in a straight line along the axis of the body, and *led* by the tip of the toe.

Tempo, rhythm, dynamics: time signature is 4/4 in a slow tempo, indicated by a dynamically ascendant voice during the extension, and by a dynamically descendant voice during recovery. Use one bar for each movement, without interruptions. Link the movements of one leg to the movements of the other, and to the movements of both legs simultaneously. Practise them as one rhythmical unit.

The purpose of the exercise is a preparation for directional movements of the non-weight-bearing leg directed into distance; and to become aware of a stretching of all three joints during directional movements of the legs.

Mistakes:
- incorrect leg position.
- deviations from the parallel line and insufficient refinement of feeling of supple, elongated joints.
- unconvincing distance perception which fails to extend beyond the point reached by the tip of the toe.

Later, perform this exercise with an elongation of the heel (resulting in dorsiflexion) to experience the feeling of lightened elongation of the leg into the heel; and to increase the mobility and sensitivity of the heel as well as the ability of heel elongation. If the ankle joint is not relaxed enough, the elongation of the heel is insufficient. This is a common fault which curbs the elasticity of walking, running, skipping and jumping*

Extension of maximally turned out legs to the toes and heels

Initial position: lying on the back, legs parallel.

Main movement: turn out the legs in the hip joints by a strong contraction of the buttock (gluteal) muscles and by the outer rotators of the thighs; and elongate into distance in the same manner as in previous exercises. The extended tips of the toes, however, move closer to the floor on their little-toe side.

Recovery : by easing the gluteal muscles and the outer rotators,

---

*Translator's note: In the standing position a lack of relaxation in the ankle joints prevents correct location of the body weight and therefore the body axis.

return the legs into their initial position. At the same time, relax their three main joints.

Direction: is into the distance and *is led* by the tip of the toe.

Tempo, rhythm, dynamics: as in previous exercise.

The purpose of the exercise is to prepare students for directional movements of parallel or maximally turned out legs, led into distance.

Mistakes:

- incorrect initial position, e.g. hyperlordosis.
- transferring tension on inappropriate muscles.
- insufficient sensitivity of the work of the joints and an insufficient spatial awareness beyond the limit of the physically reached movement.

Perform this exercise later with an elongation of the heels. This is to prepare students for extending legs to heels, in a maximal turning out, which they will apply later in a standing position but in a reverse order: i.e. detaching the shins in the ankle joints from the feet; the thighs in the knee joint from the shins; and the pelvis in the hip joints from the thighs.

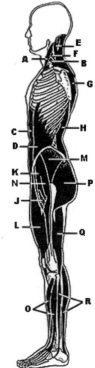

Figure 110: The muscles (of one side only) which maintain the upright position
Muscles of the trunk—Anterior:
(A) sternomastoid
(B) longus colli
(C) rectus abdominis
(D) oblique muscles of the abdomen
Posterior:
(E) splenius capitis
(F) splenius cervicis
(G) trapezius
(H) lower part of long spinal muscles
Muscles of the lower limb
Anterior:
(J) psoas
(K) iliacus
(L) quadriceps
(M) gluteus medius and minimus
(N) tensor fasciae latae
(O) long extensors of toes and the anterior tibial muscle
(ii) Posterior:
(P) gluteus maximus
(Q) hamstring muscles
(R) Long flexors of toes, the calf and posterior tibial muscle

Turning out the shins at the ankles

Initial position: lying on the back with one leg bent in a right angle and supported with a firm sole on the wall ahead. The thigh is positioned directly forward, not turned out. Another option is in a sitting position on a chair with the legs bent to a right angle, parallel feet resting on the floor at the width of the hip joints.

Main movement: press the sole of the foot of the bent leg firmly to the wall (or the floor). Turn out the shin and establish the ankle so that it does not deviate sideways. As a result, the instep rises and arches. It is also possible to perform this exercise with both feet at once. (see ANALYSIS OF MOVEMENT, p. 15).

Recovery: relax the muscular tension until slack; the feeling of firm ankles disappears and the instep lowers.

Direction: turning out of the foreleg is sideways-out-backward, led by the outer ankle.

Tempo, rhythm, dynamics: time signature is 4/4 of a medium tempo, two beats for turning out, two beats to hold, four beats to relax.

The purpose of the exercise is to become aware of the bodily sensation of the reinforced ankles as a result of the turned-out shins. Also, to perceive elevation of the instep arc and the sole of the foot clinging to the wall or floor. It is an essential part of a firm elevated posture and an essential part of leg movements which require the immediate establishment of stability and balance.

Mistakes:
- not adhering to all the described details of the working leg. Very consistent supervision and correction is necessary.

Turning out of the leg in the joints is one of the most important single movements of the elevated posture as well as of all movements of the weight-bearing leg.

V

ANATOMY: THE MUSCLES OF POSTURE

The muscles of posture are situated mainly on the anterior and posterior aspects of the body. It is necessary to realise that all the muscles involved in maintaining the erect posture take their fixed points from below and endeavour to balance one bone upon another. The muscles of the foot steady the arch to form a firm basis; the muscles in front of and behind the tibia, steady the tibia on the foot; the femur is balanced on the tibia by the quadriceps in front and the

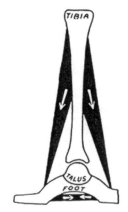

Figure 111: Muscles of posture acting from fixed point below

gastrocnemius behind; the position of the pelvis is fixed by the abdominal muscles, the rectus femoris (part of the quadriceps), the psoas, iliacus and by the sartorius, all of which act on the front of the pelvis, and by the gluteus maximus and hamstring muscles, which exert their pull on the back of the pelvis; the gluteus medius, gluteus minimus and tensor fasciae latae prevent the pelvis from tilting sideways; the vertebral column is balanced upon the steady pelvic base by the extensor muscles of the spine, the muscles of the abdominal wall and the muscles of the neck.

VI

SYNTHESIS OF ALL COMPONENTS OF CORRECT BODY POSTURE

An elevated dance posture can be expressed by pulling and contra-pulling and by pressures and contra-pressures perceived by the dancer while feeling the entirety of the body and the posture.

From the soles of the feet planted firmly on the floor, with the body weight located correctly, pull upward over the ankle, knee and hip joints and continue pulling along the spine to the crown of the head and across the abdominal wall as far as the sternum. The contra-pulling of the lower rib arches and the shoulders occurs downward while the shoulders are simultaneously being pulled to the sides. Apply pressure on the abdominal muscles from the front and contra-pressure of the buttock muscles on the pelvis from the back. Then apply pressure on the seventh cervical vertebra and pressure of the shoulder blades on the back of the ribs. Moderately turned-in arms hang with their own weight from the shoulder joints along the sides of the chest. The axis of the centre of gravity runs through the crown of the head, the sacrum and the centre of the closed-up feet. The same applies to standing on one leg with the difference that the axis runs through the crown of the head, the hip joint and the middle of the supporting leg.

A perfect coordination of all components of a correct body posture, prac-
tised separately in awareness exercises, is a synthesis of an elevated dance
posture. The dancer perceives the structural synthesis (architecture) of
his/her body and a mutual balance of all its parts. The hip joints are in a
vertical plane above the middle of the forefeet, the shoulder joints above
the hip joints and outer openings of the ears above the shoulders.

SOME INITIAL POSITIONS USED TO PRACTISE THE SYNTHESIS OF CORRECT BEARING

Lying on the back: the whole surface of the back and the posterior part of the acromions and pelvis touch the floor. The
closed-up feet lie in the same plane as the trunk and the turned-in
arms rest loosely along the body, supported by the little-finger
edge of the hands and with palms facing the body. The elbows are
away from the body, pointing to the sides. The arms are slightly
rounded, not stiffly stretched or bent. The base of the skull rests on
the floor and the chin forms a right angle with the front of the
neck. Pull the sacrum as close to the floor as possible.

We use lying on the back as the first initial position when
practising the awareness exercises of correct body posture
because it creates the conditions for feeling and awareness of the
body axis, also needed later in raising the arms and legs forward,
upward etc.

Lying on the right side: the right leg, including the side and the
hip, the right side of the trunk and the raised right arm with its
palm rest on the floor. The right ear rests on the arm. The left leg
is placed alongside the right and the bent left arm is supported on
the palm on the floor in front of the chest.

In this position the activity of the abdominal and buttock muscles is particularly important and difficult because of their pressure
on the pelvis from the front and back. Establishing the pelvis, the
support point of the neck and head and of the shoulders demands
in this position an increased muscular activity.

Lying on the abdomen: the front of the extended legs, abdomen and
the forearms and palms of the bent arms rest on the floor and the forehead supports itself on the back of the fingers (the heels are together).

Levelling the excessive curvature of the spine is especially difficult in this position. To reduce lumbar lordosis it is necessary to

increase the activity of abdominal muscles. The chest kyphosis is usually enlarged in this position and we must therefore concentrate on the work of the muscles which establish the support point of the head; and the relaxation of the intercostal muscles under the increased pressure of the shoulder blades on the ribs. It is also essential to establish the shoulders.

Sitting on the heels: in sitting, with feet tilted down and extended to the tips of the toes (plantar flexion) the shins support themselves along their whole length on the floor. The legs are maximally bent in both knee and hip joints so that the pelvis in its maximally tucked-under position sits on the heels. The lower spine is rounded, the upper spine is, on the contrary, upright from the support point of the neck and head. The relaxed and slightly turned-in arms hang from perfectly established shoulders exactly along the sides of the chest. In this initial position, the teacher must examine whether the body is perfectly balanced, with shoulder joints in a vertical plane above the hip joints and with the ear openings above the

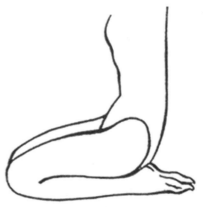

Figure 112: Sitting on the heels with pelvis tucked under

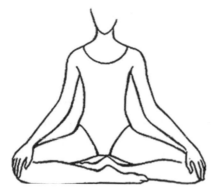

Figure 113: Sitting cross-legged. The thighs are widely spread apart and turned out. The knees are bent at an acute angle. The knees point sideways-forward, the heels are in one line and close to the crotch.

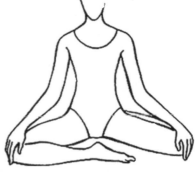

Figure 114: A variation on Figure 113. Both lower limbs are spread widely apart, bent in a sharp angle at the knees and supported by the floor. The bent limb in front of the body is turned out. The bent limb behind the body is turned in.

shoulders while the pelvis is maximally tucked under. (see POSITIONS OF THE PELVIS, p. 30).

Sitting upright on the floor: the trunk forms a right angle with fully extended legs while sitting with both feet together or apart. The pelvis has an almost vertical (levelled) position, the spine is erected from the coccyx upward. In a contra-motion to the elevated sternum, the shoulders and rib arches are pulled downward. The chest is extended to the sides. Slightly turned-in arms hang from established shoulders, exactly on the side of the thorax. In order to achieve the right angle between the trunk and the legs in this position, it is particularly important to increase pressure by the buttock muscles from the back and abdominal muscles from the front onto the pelvis. The shoulders should be above the hip joints.

Sitting with legs crossed: the legs, maximally turned out in the hip joints, are bent in both the hip and knee joints; the thighs are maximally open sideways and the legs are turned out in the knee joints, so that knees rest on the floor and the lower legs lie on the floor along their whole length. The feet have plantar flexion, the instep is elongated. They are crossed in such a manner that the heel of one foot rests on the floor in front of the instep of the other foot, both as close as possible to the body. The pelvis is either in a levelled (almost vertical) or a tucked-under position, as the following exercise demands. The upper spine and sternum are erected in a contra-movement to the established shoulders and to the rib arches which are pulled downward. The palms of the relaxed arms rest on the knees and the elbows are suspended. The shoulder joints are in a vertical plane above the hip joints; the outer ear openings are above the shoulders with the chin approximately at a right angle to the front of the neck.

Balance of this initial body position depends mainly on the ability to turn out the thighs maximally in the hip joints, the lower legs in the knee joints, and to maximally relax both joints in the direction of the turning out. It is important to achieve a maximal opening of the thighs sideways, so that the lower legs lie along their whole length on the floor. At the same time, the longitudinal axis of the feet must not deviate from the longitudinal axis of the lower legs. This fault occurs very often due to an insufficient turning out and opening of the thighs.

Upright kneeling: synthesis of all components of the elevated posture must be applied also in upright kneeling. A particular emphasis must be placed on establishing and lightening the pelvis by elongation of the hip joints upward, followed by an elongation up the spine as far as the skull (head) and across the abdominal wall to the sternum. The arms hang in a relaxed manner along the sides of the chest in their basic, slightly turned-in position. The balance of the body in the upright kneeling position is an important element in this initial position. This is achieved when the shoulder joints are above the hip joints and outer ear openings above the shoulders.

Kneeling 'on all fours' (supported by the hands on the floor): the body weight rests on the knees, upper legs and arms, which are turned in the shoulder joints so that the fingers on the floor turn towards each other and the palms are on the floor. The distance between the hands and knees is consistent with the width of the shoulders and hips and the forearms are maximally turned in. The trunk is in a straight forward tilt, with an elongated and levelled spine; the chest kyphosis decreases by moving closer the spinous processes in the support point from which the neck and head are elongated or slightly elevated.

A necessary condition of correct execution is a levelling of the lumbar lordosis by establishing the pelvis and pulling the lower rib arches towards the pubic bone. It is essential to maintain the right angle between the thighs and trunk, between the arms and trunk, and between the chin and front of the neck (except in the elevation of the head). The spine must not sink between the shoulders; the shoulders must be drawn towards the sides and the thoracic muscles should 'thrust out' the chest and lighten it.

Variation: kneeling 'on all fours' with a curved back. In this position the trunk is in a forward bend, with the pelvis tucked under, so that the spine arches upward.

Figure 115: Kneeling on 'all fours'. Body weight rests on the knees and hands, which are in dorsiflexion with the fingertips facing each other. Whole arms are turned in and stretched at the elbow.

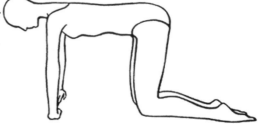

Kneeling 'on all fours' in a deeper forward tilt: stretched arms support themselves with the palms of the hands on the floor so far in front that the sternum moves quite close to the floor (the hip joints are above the knees and the head is in rotation to the right or left). The trunk is elongated in a relaxed manner while striving to push down towards the floor in the support point and the widely-established shoulders should not rise towards the ears.

In this initial position, it is difficult but important to turn out and pull the shoulders sideways in order to establish them. They easily lift and become narrowed, causing the neck to sink between them and to interfere with the free mobility of the neck and head. Even in this low position, the chest should be held higher than the arms and must not unnecessarily burden them with its own weight.

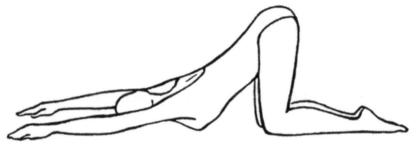

Figure 116: Kneeling on both knees. A deeper straight-forward tilt of the trunk. Elongated arms together with the palms resting on the floor in front of the body. The hyperextension of the trunk is emphasized in the 'support point' section of the thoracic spine. The sternum moves close to the floor and the hip joints are above the knees.

Standing with a straight forward tilt while supporting the body with hands on the barre: the weight rests on the extended legs, which are at a right angle to the straight forward-tilted trunk and on the extended arms with the fingers lightly supporting themselves on the barre. The pelvis tilts forward at a right angle to the legs, the trunk is lightened by an elongation as far as the sternum so that the abdominal and buttock muscles do not slacken, the neck and head are elongated from the support point. The perfectly established shoulders maintain their width and the chest is held slightly above the shoulders so that the arms are not unnecessarily burdened by the weight of the trunk.

The forward pull of the trunk and the simultaneous contra-pull of the pelvis backward are essential components of this initial position because they are the source of its activity and lightness. The technical prerequisites of this activity and lightness are the establishment of the pelvis and shoulders, together with the chest, held in an elevated manner. That is the difficulty of this initial position.

Standing with one side to the barre: the prerequisite is an elevated dance posture. The inner arm is lightly raised forward-sideways, with the fingers lightly resting on the barre so that it can glide along the barre as required. The other arm is raised sideways in its basic position (i.e. rounded).

The teacher must examine whether the body is perfectly balanced, with the hip joints in a vertical plane above the middle of the forefeet, the shoulder joints above the hip joints, the outer ear openings above the shoulders and the axis of the centre of gravity running through the crown of the head, sacrum and the middle of the closed-up feet. In this position, we execute the basic and composite movements of the legs before advancing to practising them without support.

Standing on one leg facing the barre, the other leg raised forward onto the barre: stand in an elevated dance posture on one leg slightly turned out, the other leg, turned out, elongated and raised forward with the tip of the toe lightly on the barre. In raising the leg, the contra-pull of the hip is in the direction backward, and a conscious elongation of the muscles on the back of the same leg, especially of the thigh, are equally important. The foot of the raised leg is in plantar flexion, with an extended instep. The position of the arms is selected by the teacher according to the need of the exercise.

The teacher needs to check the balance of this posture as in the previous initial position, firstly to ascertain if the axis of the centre of gravity runs correctly through the hip joint and the knee of the stationary leg, ensuring that the hip and the ankle of this leg do not deviate from the axis. Make sure the instep arch is elevated.

Standing on one leg facing the barre, the other leg raised sideways onto the barre: stand in an elevated dance posture on one leg slightly turned out, the other leg turned out more and elongated, resting the tip of the toe lightly on the barre in a sideways-raised position. The position of the arms is selected by the teacher according to the need of the following exercise.

Firstly, the teacher must check the balance of the posture, as in the previous position. The difficulty of this initial position lies in the fact that the hip joint of the sideways-raised leg must be maximally turned out and relaxed in the direction of turning out. The hip does not lift; on the contrary, it is kept in a horizontal line with the hip of the weight-bearing leg so that it does not deviate from the axis of the centre of gravity. The muscles on the inside of the raised leg must be actively and maximally extended, the foot tilted down (plantar flexion), with an arched and extended instep. A frequent fault is having a slack ankle joint causing the heel to drop.

ARM POSITIONS IN THE INITIAL POSITIONS OF THE BODY

The position of freely hanging arms alongside the chest: this arm position has already been described in the chapter ANALYSIS OF MOVEMENT as a basic position of the arms. It is also a position of the arms while standing and lying on the back. Difficulty arises with the inability to relax the appropriate ligaments of the shoulder joints, and to relax the arms themselves. This prevents the arms from hanging freely and causes the elbows to bend moderately backward. It is also difficult to maintain the contra-direction of the palms facing the body and of the elbows away from the body sideways-out, which should result in slightly rounded arms.

The position of the arms with the hands clasped at the back of the head: the first condition of this arm position is to establish the shoulders, giving emphasis to the turning out and downward pull of the shoulders against the contra-pull of the sternum upward. Next,

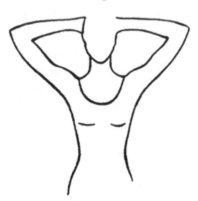

turn out the upper arms, while turning in the forearms with palms supporting the back of the head. This arm position demands a link between an elongated trunk and upper arms, from the hips over the muscles marking the armpits and over the posterior muscles of the upper arms to the elbows. The elbows point sideways-up and slightly forward (not directly to the sides).

Figure 117: Clasped hands support the back of the head. The upper arm is rotated out, the forearm rotated in and the elbow points to the sides.

This position of the arms, if executed correctly, helps to erect the upper part of the chest. When it is incorrectly executed, i.e. if the shoulders and upper arms are not turned out but turned in, then the neck and the head are pushed forward and squeezed as in a vice between the turned-in shoulders. According to the level of correct execution, the teacher can estimate the degree of control the student has over the upper part of the chest. An insufficiently developed kinaesthetic awareness of the upper chest makes this control difficult to grasp and the teacher will achieve success only through patient and repeated correction.

The position of raised arms, linked above the head, with palms turned upward: pull the lifted arms, fingers clenched together and, with the palms turned upward in a contra-pull to the established shoulders, pull downward. The pull of the arms originates from the upward pull of the trunk from the hips with an erected sternum. The contra-pull of the shoulders is reinforced by the pull of the rib arches downward.

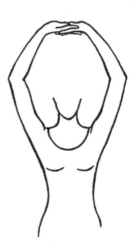

The difficulty of this position of the arms lies in a correct balance of pulls and very strong contra-pulls. This is at the same time its main purpose.

Figure 118: The upper limbs create an arch above the head. The palms of clasped hands are facing upwards. Upper arms rotated out, forearms and hands in.

The position of the arms with hands on the hips: the turned-out shoulders are in a contra-movement to the turned-in upper arms and forearms. The elbows are bent at a sharp angle pointing precisely sideways. The hands, in dorsiflexion at a right angle at the wrist, lean firmly with their palms on the hips. The sternum is erected in a contra-movement to the shoulders drawn downward.

The main difficulty of this arm position lies in the fact that it is absolutely necessary to maintain accurately all the pulls and contra-pulls, movements and contra-movements. Otherwise, the line of the movement is unsatisfactory. Common faults are elbows pointing sideways-back instead of exactly sideways, which is a sign of established shoulders pointing sideways-forward instead of exactly sideways. The line of the neck, from the support point, is then distorted so that this position loses its form and purpose.

The position of stretched arms, raised sideways (see Figure 89, p. 164): in a contra-movement to the turned-out (established) shoulders, the upper arms are turned in. The elbows are stretched and the moderately turned-in forearms, with palms turned downward, point with stretched fingers exactly sideways. The horizontal of the shoulders, prolonged by the arms, is emphasised against the vertical of the body through spatial awareness. For this position, it is important to have awareness of continuity from the shoulders, over the shoulder joints and over the elbows to the middle fingers. This is unfortunately not always observed.

Arm position similar to that for carrying loads on the crown of the head: perfectly established shoulders and turned-out upper arms with elbows pointing sideways-upward create a consistent and firm lines. The forearms, turned out and bent in the elbows to a sharp angle, are extended in the wrists to the fingers which rest lightly on the crown of the head. The upper part of the chest, including the sternum, neck and head, is erect and emphasises the vertical of the body. The connection of the trunk and arms must be unconditionally maintained and is achieved by an upward pull from the hips, across the abdominal wall, over muscles defining the back of the armpits and the muscles of the posterior part of the upper arms, as far as the elbows. This is an arm position used by girls or women carrying a load on their heads, e.g. a basketful of grapes at vintage. Grace, elevation and firmness of this position depend on the continuity and coordination of muscle work between the trunk and arms. The extension of the line from the hips up to the elbows must not be affected by anything.

The position of arms forming an arch above the head: the arms are lifted, the upper arms are moderately turned out in the shoulder joints, the forearms and hands are maximally turned out with palms turned downward. The fingers of the bent hands are extended and almost touch each other with their fingertips. The arms are slightly bent at the elbows so that together they form a rounded oval above the head. The pull of the whole trunk from the hips

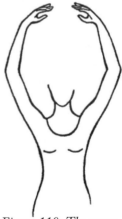

Figure 119: The arms form an arch above the head.

upward across the arms, as far as the wrists, is in contrast to the contra-pull of the shoulders and rib arches downward.

Variation: the palms and forearms may also be turned upwards.
The main difficulty of this position is the necessity of maintaining established shoulders and not losing the connection between the trunk and arms, above all the upper arms. This is achieved by continuity of muscle work, i.e. an upward pull and a contra-pull of the shoulders and rib arches downward.

PROBLEMS WHEN NEGLECTING BODY BALANCE DURING WORK ON COMPLEX MOVEMENTS

Awareness exercises for correct body posture are an indispensable part of movement and dance tuition. We cannot neglect them without consequences, if we want to make systematic progress in acquiring technical skills. Through these exercises we acquire and heighten the sensitivity of the body. The teacher must always return to them in order to achieve a student's body balance. This is one of the main conditions of movement synthesis. Only through repeating, and feeling through, again and again, all the details of the elevated body posture through kinaesthetic awareness can one achieve those essential body sensations. Body sensations, awakened by practice, become embedded in one's memory and stay there permanently. That is also why the teacher carefully observes the students, no matter how advanced, to ensure that their movement does not in some way deviate from the five rules of the elevated body posture. As soon as a fault is discovered, the teacher should return instantly to the appropriate awareness exercise, knowing that this will improve the technical performance of the whole unit.

For example, during the complex movement of swinging the legs crosswise in front with half turn, finishing with a lay-out side, the teacher may find unsteady balance in students because they have not kept the axis of the centre of gravity in the position on one leg. Awareness exercises are reintroduced for reinforcing the pelvis and for elongation of all joints and muscles of the legs, at first while lying on the back. These are then repeated in different positions, i.e. standing on both legs with the students focussing their attention on the awareness of the axis of the centre of gravity; and finally standing on one leg, while making sure that the students are aware of, and cope with, the changed centre of gravity. To consolidate this, the teacher must practise the swing of the free leg crosswise in front and to the side a few times with the students and only then return to the initial complex movement. Such a consolidation of correct 'muscle-memory' gradually increases technical perfection.

If we want to achieve a correct body posture in all movements, we cannot limit ourselves during practice to the simplest initial position (e.g. lying on the back), but must again practise these exercises in various positions. It is a preparation for acquiring all five rules of correct body posture in every position and in every movement. Take the example of establishing the pelvis. It is a movement divided into two separate exercises which finally unite into one coordinated movement. i.e. establishment of the pelvis. The concept must become a certain reality to dance students, a certain experience, always distinguishable from other bodily sensations. This occurs only by practising in different positions of the body.

Each of the initial positions has its own level of workload. When we work on establishment of the pelvis we select, for example, an erect sitting position with legs together as an initial position. The difficulty of this position is in the requirement that the trunk be at a right angle to the legs; the difficulty varies according to the individual. The position demands an increased pressure of the buttock muscles on the pelvis from the back, so that the pelvis maintains the required vertical position in the right angle with the trunk and becomes established in this position. In the effort to achieve this, the muscles on the back of the legs must extend maximally, which can cause considerable pain. It is, however, a position which flattens out excessive lumbar lordosis and also prevents the established pelvis from 'falling back'. We need to combine our effort for establishing the pelvis with an erect hold of the chest, neck and head. In this way we relieve the pelvis and so achieve more easily the required right-angled position of the trunk towards the legs. In the recovery movement (relaxation of the buttock and abdominal muscles), we must not reduce the elongation of the trunk and the spine. It has to be maintained even during multiple repetitions of both the main and the recovery movements.

Awareness exercises for the correct body posture can also be made more difficult by selecting different arm positions. *For example*, first work on establishment of the pelvis in the position of lying on the abdomen with the forehead resting on the fingers of the bent arm, as described in SOME INITIAL POSITIONS OF CORRECT BEARING. *Exercise:* lying on the abdomen, p. 241. This is much easier for establishing the pelvis than with the hands on the back of the head. The increased difficulty lies, above all, in the fact that the upper chest, from the support point up, must be maximally active. This cannot be achieved without a simultaneous extension of the trunk from the hips upward, across the muscles defining the posterior part of the armpits and across the muscles of the back of the upper arms as far as the elbows. The pull of the muscles of the outer contour of the trunk and arms must be realised, felt through and maintained, together with the contra-pull of the shoulders and rib arches downward. The established pelvis exerts a contra-pull in relation to the chest, whose upper part lightens and lifts slightly from the floor. Co-ordination and synthesis of all components of the correct body posture is rather difficult in this position and makes the main task, i.e. the establishment of the pelvis and the involvement of the abdominal muscles in particular, more difficult. Co-ordination and synthesis of the single movements are, however, inevitable; without that the following movement would have unstable foundations.

When we connect a certain single movement of the correct body posture with some basic or composite movement, the awareness exercise becomes more difficult: for example, establishment of the pelvis in an erect kneeling position with the torsion of the trunk. To establish the pelvis in an erect kneeling position, it is necessary to increase the activity of the abdominal and buttock muscles so that the pelvis is kept in a vertical line with the thighs and thorax and does not 'fall backward'. However, to combine the erect kneeling position with the rotation of the thorax, e.g. to the right, we must increase even more the activity of the left side of the abdominal wall (the opposite side to rotation): the pelvis does not turn with the thorax but puts up resistance to it. By an increased pressure from the front on the left hip, we maintain the horizontal of the hips and so achieve active elongation of the oblique abdominal muscles. This firms up the abdominal wall during normal work of the buttock muscles. The pelvis is established in its basic position. It is, of course, a more difficult movement than when establishing the pelvis without the thorax rotation, but the body sensation which accompanies it is all the more pronounced.

VII
AWARENESS OF DETAILS

Awareness exercises originating in the combination of an initial position with a basic or a composite movement are more demanding. They represent a higher level of tuition. They have the same structure as the first grouping of the awareness exercises: that is, the initial position, the main movement and the recovery movement. The main purpose of both kinds of grouping is to develop our awareness and give all our attention to it. The main demand is to master the initial position as perfectly as possible. In the awareness exercises of the basic and composite movements, the teacher must constantly monitor the synthesis of all components of correct body posture and their balance. This applies to unusual positions which the teacher creates as a necessary part of increasing the difficulty of execution. It is always necessary to master technically the initial position first and only then to add the practised movement. All resulting movements must be precisely executed, as we have learned in the chapter ANALYSIS OF MOVEMENT. A logical conclusion is that the second grouping of the awareness exercises must be introduced at a later stage of tuition. Exceptionally, we can make the awareness exercises of a single movement of correct body posture more difficult by adding a certain basic movement. Basic and composite movements, described in ANALYSIS OF MOVEMENT, originated from elevated dance posture. In practice, however, we cannot be satisfied with only this initial position if the training is to be versatile. Every new position brings a new problem in carrying out a basic or composite movement, a change in execution or just a change in bodily sensation, evoked by a change in position. *For example*, a straight forward tilt of the trunk while standing with legs together and a straight forward tilt with legs astride: the legs in the first case are extended and turned out and in the second case they are extended, turned out and astride. Here we must emphasise turning out in the 'astride' position, as the establishing of the pelvis during the forward tilt with legs 'astride' demands more muscular effort.

Another example: the initial position is standing on the left leg, the right leg is elongated, raised sideways and rests with the tip of the toe on the barre. There is a problem when rotating the chest to the left because the right leg must turn very intensively out to the right, while the chest rotates to the left in order to keep the hips in a frontal-horizontal position and to prevent the right hip from lifting. To do this, we must relax the hip joint of the right leg maximally in the direction of turning out. When we do not succeed, the balance of this position will be impaired and cause an imperfect rotation of the chest. This is because the oblique abdominal muscles will not extend and their activity will not be sufficient during the establishment of the pelvis.

Another example: exercising directional movements of the leg while lying on the side—the most difficult position for establishing the pelvis. We must execute basic directional movements, i.e. a forward, sideways and a backward raising of the leg with a controlled, established pelvis, with hips in a vertical line, one above the other. The problem set by this exercise is in the fact that even the slightest slackening of abdominal and buttock muscles causes a deviation from the vertical line of the hips and so also a deviation in the direction of the practised directional movements. When the legs work correctly (i.e. when the posterior parts of the thighs are actively elongated during the forward-raising of the leg, the inner thighs during the sideways-raising of the leg, and the front parts of the thighs during the backward-raising of the leg), the control of the pelvis becomes easier. The correctly led activity lightens the leg. An interplay of abdominal, buttock and thigh muscles is absolutely essential here.

The teacher must control simultaneously both the technique of the initial position and the execution of basic movements. The teacher checks if the initial position is really balanced and if the basic movements are executed exactly, particularly in this demanding position. *Each fault in the initial position causes a number of imperfections affecting negatively the movement itself and each imperfect execution of basic or composite movements threatens the balance of the initial position.*

Not all students have the same talent and diligence and a teacher is sometimes forced to return to the exercises in which the initial positions have not been mastered perfectly. However, this effort will not be in vain: the renewed attempt at execution will bring the student a small step closer to achievement. The process of overcoming the difficulties helps the students become more aware of the important role the single movements of the correct body posture play in the technical perfection of the position, as well as of the movement itself. When the teacher is well-disciplined and does not rush, but corrects patiently and repetitively, the student will gradually conquer all technical hurdles.

The teacher must then create more initial positions, it is a methodical necessity. Possibilities of creating new positions are numerous, when we realise that *each body movement which we can stop at a certain phase, i.e. 'freeze' in it without losing balance, can become an initial position for awareness and other exercises.*

For example: one of the basic movements of the pelvis is a maximal forward tilt with a passive trunk (see ANALYSIS OF MOVEMENT of which the final section can become a useful initial position of the body for various exercises). We can connect this well-balanced position, for example, with basic movements of the neck and head, i.e. with a rounded forward bend, a lateral shift, backward lean and rotation. The correct posture of the shoulders must be maintained, (they must not drop towards the ears) while maximally relaxing the whole spine and particularly the neck and head. Just as in the erect standing position, the shoulders must not slacken. The problem, and at the same time the benefit, of this position is in the fact that the neck and head are not in the usual erect posture but hang down. This places higher demands on the sense of orientation in students. Through this unusual position, they are forced to follow more carefully the work of the neck muscles in order to maintain the direction of the movement. They must perceive the muscular activity and direction and constantly be aware of them.

The initial position is often a 'frozen' complex movement, i.e. it consists of basic and composite movements in various body parts, in various joints or systems of joints. As an example, let us clarify a forward lunge with a bent and maximally turned-out leg, while the back leg, held straight, remains extended. When we remain in this position, the forward lunge can become an initial position of the body when practising various basic or composite movements, for example straight movements of the trunk. The exception is a straight backward lean which in this initial position of the body, is unworkable.

The initial position in a sideways-forward lunge: in its basic position, the pelvis is in a vertical plane with the erect trunk. The hips and shoulders are horizontal. The right hip joint is bent to a right or sharp angle, the thigh is maximally turned out and points forward-sideways out. The knee and the ankle joints are bent to a sharp angle, the shin is turned out at both joints. The foot forms a sharp angle with the shin and the ankle joint is in a dorsiflexion with abduction. The thigh, the lower leg and the foot have the same direction forward-right. The left leg is extended left-backward, turned out in the hip joint and resting on the whole sole of the foot. Its lower leg forms a direct line with the thigh, the foot is turned out and bent in maximal dorsiflexion. The weight of the body rests in the middle of both forefeet (the left instep must not lower itself). Both legs are equally weighted by the erect trunk. The forward lunge differs from the described lunge by the fact that the heel of the front foot is in a straight line with the heel of he back foot. Both knee caps (patellas) point in the same direction as the lengthwise axes of the feet, the front thigh deviates slightly from the direction forward, the back one points directly backward. Again, both legs are equally weighted by the trunk.

Instructions about a perfect execution of basic and composite movements can be found in ANALYSIS OF MOVEMENT. This also informs us about their characteristic features, as well as about bodily sensations, which accompany correct muscle work. The bodily sensations (kinaesthetic awareness) are also a reliable self-control when striving for technical perfection of the movements.

ANALYSIS OF MOVEMENT advises us also the direction of each movement and what leads it, which also belongs to technical perfection. While creating the awareness exercises, we can draw from the chapter both basic and composite movements which we want to practise, and the information about technical perfection of the initial positions. Each single movement of any initial position is introduced and described in this chapter together with its correct execution. The teacher must, therefore, learn to analyse complex movements and become aware from which single movements they are composed. An initial position, as we already know, is often a complex movement.

The choice of initial positions during exercises should be deliberate. It is necessary to work out why the new initial position makes the movement more difficult, whether the degree of difficulty is proportional and whether it meets the immediate needs of the students and tuition. The more advanced the students are, the more the teacher can take advantage of various positions and intensify their difficulty.

A REQUIREMENT DURING THE CREATION OF MOVEMENT UNITS

While practising complex movements we create small movement units in which, for the first time, there is a requirement for coordination and binding in connection with a feeling for form. Begin by repeating with students three times the practised basic or composite movement and recovery to the initial position; and require them to feel these three repeated movements as a unit. It is important that they feel the first couple of movements as an introductory part (exposition), the second couple as a middle part (development), the third couple as the conclusion. At the same time, the singing accompaniment provokes feeling by binding together all three parts rhythmically and melodically, dynamically ascending into the second part and descending in the final part.

Altogether there are six movements which the dance student links into one by means of coordination, bond and feeling for form. Movements are linked to the others through form, space, rhythm and dynamics. During these six movements none of the bonds must weaken, even for a moment, and they must reach the conclusion together. In this way we cultivate the main condition for formal feeling (i.e. graded inner tension) and for the first time the teacher requires its longer duration. Inner tension must embrace all three parts of the small, simple movement forms.

The following, more demanding, movement unit includes various basic or composite movements.

Initial position: stand upright with hands at the back of the head.

1. *Main movement*: a small, rounded backward bend (extension).
   Recovery: return to initial position.
2. *Main movement*: a straight sideways shift to the right.
   Recovery: return to initial position.
3. *Main movement*: a straight sideways shift to the left.
   Recovery: return to initial position.
4. *Main movement*: rotation of the chest, neck and head to the right.
   Recovery: return to initial position.
5. *Main movement*: rotation of the chest, neck and head to the left.
   Recovery: return to initial position.
6. *Main movement*: open the arms to the sides *leading* with the little finger edge. Lower them to the normal position along the body, *leading* with the inner part of the wrist.

The movements pass in slow, 3/4 time signature. The teacher creates, through accompaniment by singing or playing, a dynamic form of the whole: expressing on the one hand, the dynamic ascent of the main movements and the descent of the recovery movements; and on the other hand, when the transition from the first part to the middle part occurs and from here to the last part by a gradual heightening and then lowering of the volume of the voice towards the conclusion. Because of constant returns to the initial position, it is not quite possible to create satisfactorily a total, undivided form, in terms of shape or space. That is why it is the dynamic form that creates the whole. The purpose of this exercise is, above all, to increase the ability to maintain an uninterrupted inner tension through coordination and movement bonds. The arms and legs remain still.

In a more complicated unit, composed of various basic or composite movements, the recovery movements are substituted by a direct transition from one movement to another. Each movement has a 3/4 time signature in a slow tempo.

Initial position: standing upright with arms raised sideways.

1. *Main movement*: a backward bend of the spine (hyperextension) combined with a rotation of the chest, neck and head to the left.
2. *Main movement*: a straight sideways shift of the trunk to the right.
3. *Main movement*: a rounded sideways bend (i.e. lateral flexion) of the spine to the left.
4. *Main movement*: a rounded backward bend of the spine combined with rotation of the chest, neck and head to the right.
5. *Closing movement*: elevation and recovery to the initial position.

It is demanding and difficult to find correct binding of form in an exercise composed in this way. Transitions from one movement to another require a very sensitive leading of both the pelvis and the chest in each basic and composite movement and with a full spatial experience. The students train themselves in the binding of form and space at first without any arm movements. This composition of movements without constant recovery to the initial position also enables them to feel the form of a certain ascent of movement succeeding each other into a movement climax. This would be in the fourth main movement in the extension of the spine with rotation. Spatial bond together with the binding of form, supported by rhythmic and, above all, dynamic bond arrives at the same culmination. The movement and the dynamic peaks merge together. From the point of view of composition, one can regard the first main movement as an introduction which develops into a climax in the fourth main movement and passes into the conclusion. As the students progress in these exercises, the teacher can also heighten their feeling for form by rhythmic and melodic development. The first main movement with the introductory melody would last two bars; the second and the third, with a melodic and rhythmic graduation until the fourth movement, would each last for three bars; and the recovery to the initial position, with a descending tune and decreased dynamics, would last four bars. In the process the students would also acquire the feeling for changes in the duration of the movement.

VIII
CREATING COMPLEX MOVEMENTS

This is a demanding stage of tuition, a refined formation of complex movements, because it concerns a versatile movement synthesis. Demands are increased on coordination and on a heightened and prolonged inner tension of students, as well as a more developed feeling for form.

All experiences and knowledge gained from the awareness exercises are fully applied in this further stage of tuition. The teacher's attention must continue to focus consistently on both the perfect balance of the body in movement and the perfect execution of single movements from which the complex movements are composed. The teacher must ensure their coordination in complex movements as well as to the formal, spatial, rhythmic and dynamic bonds. Without these there is no movement synthesis. Thus we create units from complex movements in which the formal aspect is increasingly important.

The structure of these exercises is more complicated than the awareness exercises because we add to the main and recovery movements one or more secondary movements, i.e. to the movements of the trunk and spine we add movements of the legs and arms.

A simple complex movement lay-out forward

Initial position: stand in the first position, the arms along the body in a relaxed manner

Main movement: a straight forward tilt of the trunk.
1. Secondary movement: (simultaneously with the main one) a high backward lift of the stretched leg.
2. Secondary movement: (simultaneously with the main one) raise the arms sideways.

Recovery: return to the initial position of the main and secondary movements.

The forward *direction* of the trunk *is led* by the sternum, the backward lifting leg *is led* by the tip of the toe, the contra-direction forward, backward is intensively felt.

Tempo, rhythm, dynamics: one bar of 3/4 time signature in a slow tempo for the main movement, accompanied simultaneously by the secondary ones, second bar for recovery. Crescendo - decrescendo.

Purpose of the exercise: a perfect interplay, awareness and practice of all kinds of bonds, increased ability to concentrate.

Mistakes:
• incorrectly balanced body while standing on one leg
• imperfect coordination
• interrupted linkage
• lack of inner tension.

The teacher must develop a critical eye for detail.

Complex movements of a higher degree: a sequence of two main movements and four secondary ones in which the last two secondary movements are part of the recovery.

Initial position: standing on one leg, with the other leg elongated, raised forward, turned out and resting on the barre. The arms hang along the body in a relaxed manner.
1. *Main movement*: a deep rounded forward bend above the raised, elongated leg on the barre.

Secondary movement: raise your arms through the sideways lift.
2. *Main movement*: a deep rounded backward bend with the arms held upward.

Secondary movement: the leg on the barre bends to a sharp angle in the hip, knee and ankle joints and turns out.

Recovery: rise from the backward bend, followed by returning the arms from their raised position through the sideways lift to the initial position, simultaneously stretching the leg into its initial elongation.

Directions in the rounded forward bend: the lower spine *is led* by the sacrum backward, the upper spine *is led* by the forehead forward-down. Directions in the extension: the lower spine forward-upward *is led* by the hips and the groins, the upper spine upward-backward *is led* by the sternum and the crown of the head. *Rising*: the lower spine in the direction backward-upward *is led* by the sacrum and hips, the upper spine forward-upward *is led* by the sternum and the crown of the head. The directional feeling of the arms merges with the directions of the upper spine. The knee points right-forward.

Tempo, rhythm, dynamics: three bars of 3/4 time signature. The first two bars have an emphasis on the first beat for those complex movements that are executed in a swing character, the third bar accommodates the evenly flowing, legato character of the movement in decrescendo. This closes the whole composition.

Purpose of the exercise: work on perfect coordination and bonding of the movement unit.

Mistakes: the teacher must check and correct inefficiencies of the initial position, the execution of the single movements and their interplay with both the main movements as well as with their recovery. Attention must be paid to the bonds of the complex movements as well as of the whole, requiring from the students a feeling for the form of the composition: introduction, development and conclusion.

COORDINATION

Again we become aware of the coordination principle. It is, on the whole, unchangeable, being always a matter of an exact beginningand an exact ending of simultaneously flowing movements. In the more complicated forms of exercise, the secondary movement can be added, with delay to the whole, ending together or with a delay. The delayed beginning, however, must always be exactly defined, rhythmically, and accurately kept. The leading of the movements plays the main role here. The binding of movements is, in principle, more complicated because it changes. This applies particularly to the binding of form. The deep rounded forward bend into the rounded backward bend is different from the link of the rounded sideways bend with the rounded backward bend or when we make a transition from the straight sideways shift into a rounded sideways bend. In the introduction to SYNTHESIS OF MOVEMENT we discussed the movement bond and its components, the binding of form, space, rhythm and dynamics; but it would still be beneficial to clarify this last exercise from this point of view.

Binding of form: the exercise consists of two complex movements:
  (a) a deep rounded forward bend,
  (b) a deep rounded backward bend while standing on one leg with the other leg raised forward and resting on the barre.

Both main movements follow each other directly. The sacrum leads the movement backward into the deep rounded forward bend of the lower spine. Simultaneously increased pressure of abdominal muscles on the pelvis from the front, and the movement of the upper spine forward-downward, *is led* by the forehead. During the deep backward bend, the leading of the lower spine is taken over by the hips and the groins in the forward-upward direction. The leading of the upper spine is transferred to the sternum and the crown of the head in an upward-backward direction, with a simultaneously increased pressure of the buttock muscles on the pelvis, from the back. The arms, led by the fingers, complement the movement of the spine in accordance with its movements and directions, even though the movement of the arms starts in another direction, i.e. sideways-upward. If the movement of the arms were a main movement, it would be decisive, but when it is a secondary movement, their directional orientation recedes into the background and asserts itself only in the conclusion. This is when the arms, together with the upper spine, point forward-downward. In the hyperextension the fingers of the upward lifted arms have the same upward-backward direction as the main movement. During recovery to the vertical of the body, the arms are lowering through the sideways lift down to the initial position. The direction of the whole body dominates again, the direction of the arms recedes and slowly becomes identical with the vertical as the movement approaches the end. The secondary movements of the leg raised forward and supported on the barre by the tip of the foot, are a reaction to the pressure of the buttock muscles on the pelvis from the back (this results in all three joints of the leg bending to a maximum). During recovery, the joints of the leg react to the pressure of the abdominal muscles on the pelvis from the front by a regressive maximum extension of the leg joints.

Binding of form requires that the change of leading as well as the change of muscle activity, follow each other smoothly. They do not become disturbed, e.g. by a weakened leading in the moment of transition or by a sudden interruption of the muscle work during any change of the activity (abdominal or buttock muscles). Any change in leading and new muscle activity must link up immediately after the ending of the first movement so that the next movement can begin purely and accurately. Similarly, during the transition from the backward bend to the recovery, the leading of the lower spine is taken over by the hips and the sacrum in the direction backward-upward, and the leading of the upper spine during recovery is transferred to the sternum and crown of the head in the direction forward-upward. During all three phases of the movement unit, we must retain the continuity of the leading as well as of the muscle activity.

Spatial bond: this requires that the directions of the movement from the centre of the body into the space are drawn to the end, especially by those parts of the body which lead the movement. The spatial sensation continues 'to radiate' in the given direction, although the movement has already reached its destination in space. In this way, the dancer connects with the surrounding space. The spatial bond of the secondary movements, in this case arm movements, is realised by the fact that the secondary movements above all take over the directions and aims of the main and recovery movements, also supporting and intensifying them.

Rhythmic bond: links secondary and main movements so that they flow simultaneously and undivided. The same rhythm bonds them together in such a way that different forms (of arms and trunk) merge into unity. Together they form three 3/4 bars. The first two bars start with an accent and are used by both complex movements executed in a swing character with an impulse and fading into space. The third complex movement, which is the recovery to the initial position, has a legato character without any accent, and it slows down and weakens in the final phase of this movement unit.

Dynamic bond: is simple. It binds the two first parts, i.e. both complex movements, by ascending dynamics and the third part by descending dynamics until a complete calm.

The binding of form, space, rhythm and dynamics follow a common aim. They do not contradict but complement each other, and help each other to accomplish the main pre requisite of the dance creation, a movement synthesis. The formal feeling of the whole and its structure (introduction, development and conclusion) supports this process.

In these exercises the dance students deepen their ability to maintain their inner tension alive and gain experiences of a higher movement technique. Creation of complex movements in these exercises, presented and worked out in this manner, is a teacher's concern and is a preparation for future independent creation by the student.*

In the last exercises, the movements of the arms and legs were secondary movements. This is not always the case. Movements of the trunk, spine, neck and head can become secondary movements and the movements of the arms and legs become main movements. One such example is the enlarged circles of the arms, described in ANALYSIS OF MOVEMENT, in the section about circling movements of the arms in the shoulder joint. These movements, in which the circle of the arm is a main movement, and the secondary movements are those of the trunk, spine, neck and head which complement the circle and enlarge its range.

They are entirely subordinate to the leading of the extended fingers of the circling arm. Leg movements also can be main movements.

Example:

Initial position: kneeling on one leg which is turned out in the hip joint to a maximum with the bent knee pointing to the side. The kneeling leg is bent in the knee joint to a sharp angle, turned out and placed with the foreleg on the floor. The foot is extended (plantar flexion) so that it lies on the floor in the same line as the lower leg and its heel pointing upward is exactly under the centre of the vertically positioned pelvis. The other leg is stretched in the knee and extended to the side, it is maximally turned out in the hip joint where it is bent at an obtuse angle to the body. The foot is also plantar flexed (tilted down) and forms a straight line with the leg. The body weight rests on the knee of the kneeling leg and on the heel of the extended leg. The trunk has an elevated posture, the elongated arms are raised sideways.

---

*J. K. Výrazový Tanec, *Expressive Dance* Orbis, Prague, 1964.

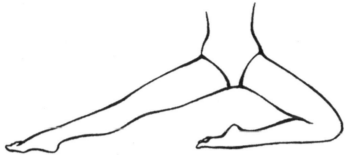

Figure 120: Kneeling on one leg with extension of the other leg sideways. Both legs are maximally turned out at the hip joints.

Main movement: the elongated leg slides along the floor with an extended instep. The weight of the body must not shift towards the big-toe side of the foot. During the movement the hip joints bend more and more. The vertically positioned pelvis with the raised trunk sinks gradually to the heel of the kneeling leg.

Secondary movement: the hands are led by the extended fingers, and the arm movement is completed by forming an arch above the head with palms facing the ceiling (the hands are in dorsiflexion).

Recovery: by contracting the inner thigh muscles, the thighs move closer together again and the trunk, led by the hips and sternum, lifts into the initial position. The arms led by the inner side of the wrists lower themselves and the hands, led by the elongated fingers, complete the return to the initial position.

Directions: the near horizontal of the legs against the vertical of the body and the arc of the arms with forearms in pronation.

Tempo, rhythm, dynamics of the whole: this is a slow legato rhythm with a 4/4 time signature, where the main and secondary movements have a crescendo and the recovery of both main and secondary movements have a decrescendo.

The purpose of the exercise is a summary of all movements and exact feeling for the binding of form, space, rhythm and dynamics, which must merge into one total experience.

Mistakes of a technical kind are caused mainly by an insufficient turning out of both thighs in the hip joints and by an insufficient relaxation during the movement, so that both the initial position and the movement cannot be properly balanced. The horizontal of the hips and the shoulders is important so that the axis of the trunk is not disturbed and the vertical of the body can be perceived. The teacher must check for faulty binding of form, space, rhythm and dynamics.

The described exercise can be varied, e.g. the initial position of the arms can be a natural hold along the body. From there the arms will move into a sideways lift at the same time as the main movement. Both the arms and the legs will, at the peak of the main movement, reach the horizontal. As a result, the main directional experience will have changed.

Another *variation* can be achieved by adding to the main movement of the leg another main movement, e.g. a straight sideways shift. Both main movements flow together, i.e. they merge into one whole but neither is subordinate to the other. Each movement retains its independence, its leading and its direction. They are independent in all aspects, except for the rhythm, which they share. The teacher can join the main movement of the legs with other main and composite movements of the trunk or spine, e.g. with a backward rounded bend + rotation etc. Complexity can also be graduated by increasing the number of secondary movements. For example, if we add to the two main movements (that of the legs and a straight sideways shift of the trunk), another secondary movement (rotation of the neck and head), the rotation of the neck and head intensifies one of the main movements, whose direction it takes over. That means that if the neck and head turn to the right in the straight shift to the right, the secondary movement will emphasise the sideways shift of the trunk. When the neck and head rotate, however, in a contra-direction to the sideways shift, that is in the direction of the stretched leg, the rotation will emphasise the movement and direction of the leg. In form and expression they are two different movements. We can also achieve an expression change through a rhythmic and dynamic change of this unit.

For example, if we execute rotation of the neck and head only on the fourth beat of the first bar, the secondary movement (rotation) will be accentuated and we shall achieve a rhythmic, dynamic and finally an expressive change to the whole unit. In the second bar, all the movements return simultaneously to the initial position, while the dynamic feeling subsides. Each such change carries with it a technical problem, as well as coordination and bond difficulties, which must be checked and corrected by the teacher. The feeling for form of a small unit must not be neglected, either. Movement fantasy of both teacher and choreographer can grow in these exercises into ever richer forms and can guide the students to more complicated forms and larger units.

IX
COMPLEX MOVEMENTS FROM THE SPOT

These are movements by which one advances in a certain direction through space, direct or indirect: a step, walk, run etc. A step is part of the normal walk and as such is simple. Complicated dance steps build on the basis of simple dance steps, with an addition of various secondary movements. Complicated dance steps can also be created from a combination of various types of movements from the spot, resulting in a step which is richer from the point of view of form and rhythm.

Simple dance step (walk)
A normal step becomes a simple dance step under these conditions:
1) if the executed dance posture is a perfectly balanced state of body in movement
2) if the student masters a perfect execution of single movements
3) if the step is coordinated, i.e. if the single movements of the legs, pelvis, spine and arms are in perfect harmony
4) if the steps in walking and running are linked uninterruptedly from every aspect, including rhythm, dynamics and space
5) if by means of these components movement synthesis of the dance step, walk or run is achieved.

As we see, the dance quality is not a question of complexity of form, but a question of execution. We can create a dance movement out of every natural one. The most important points for the technical mastery of a dance step are an established pelvis, an established support point of the neck and head, established shoulders and a horizontal level of the hips and shoulders. As for the legs, the important points are an elastic elongation and adequate turning out, a correct placement of the body weight without losing balance, prompt turning out of the shins at the ankle joints and a resulting firming of the ankles. The foot of the weight-bearing leg must be planted on the floor so that the body obtains a firm support in the standing position on one leg, with the axis passing through the crown of the head, the hip joint and the centre of the weight-bearing leg. This is a very important condition because a dance walk and run always has weight on only one foot at a time. In simple dance walk, one never stands on both feet at the same time.

CONCLUSION

Each of the complex movements, including movements on the spot, has its own definite form, its single movements and their spcial leading, and its own technical features. Technical mastery of each complex movement is the primary condition for both coordination and bonding of the movement. Here, the students' artistic instinct and sensitive body is needed. Their inner activity, i.e. a capacity for deep concentration based on inner tension, comes to the fore. Without it we can reach no movement coordination or bonding of any kind and therefore no movement synthesis. Inner tension joins all kinds of bonds and it is only in this final union that we can achieve movement synthesis. The teacher must strive for every complex movement to be experienced as a whole entity.

In my introduction I outlined what I wanted to achieve in modern dance education. It was a fusion of two abilities: to gain knowledge about movement and apply it; and to develop a high sensitivity in the body and each of its parts. I have learnt that application of knowledge must be unobtrusive and must have a natural effect. Sensitivity of the body must interpret the contents of the movement. It is a matter of two equal factors and it depends on their perfect balance. Expressing the contents without a perfect technical execution would lose the artistic value. A perfect form without emotional content cannot awaken the spectator to an artistic experience. We must, therefore, cultivate both and join them in a whole. Only then will the students reach mastery of modern dance technique.

Work by the great masters clearly confirms a synthesis in the way they observe people and movement. An artistic recognition of the laws of movement has developed through the ages and modern perceptions are still governed by them. These laws are unchangeable because they derive from an understanding of our physical and mental substance. They can become refined, cultivated or damaged, but deep down they remain the same. The efforts of educators of artistic movement must, therefore, aim toward a continuous and increasing emotional participation in the laws of movement. That is why we must keep alive our response to works of art; and in our own performance sustain the emotion, allowing it to be reborn afresh each time.

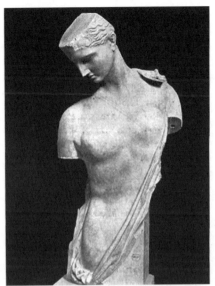

*Figure 121: Psyche of Capua. Museum
in Naples end of fourth century. Elie
Faure,* History of Art: Ancient Art.
*London: John Lane, the Bodley Head,
1921.*

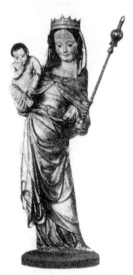

*Figure 122: Madonna of Zahražany:
Most parish church, fourteenth century.
Albert Kutal,* Czech Gothic Art

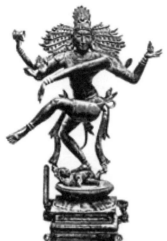

Figure 123: Statue of the Dancing Shiva: Indian sculpture from fifteenth century. The perfect balance of all body parts and the feeling of an axis at the centre of the multiplicity of movement forms is very striking. Each movement is consciously felt in every detail. All directions and contradirections are clearly led thus resulting in unusual lightness and vivacity of movement. Some Indian dancers are also today reaching this highly developed excellence which is testament to an immensely cultured sensitivity of the muscles. The sculptor of this work must have possessed this kind of sensitivity to be able to portray this unusual refinement of movement form.

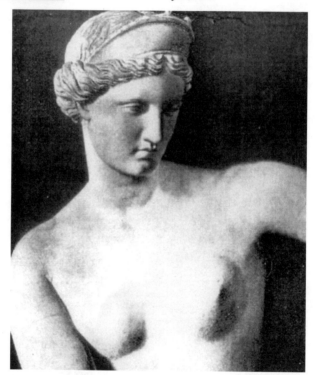

Figure 124: Venus of Capua, Greece from the height of Greek culture. An ideally formed upper chest with widespread shoulders, elevated sternum and perfectly held head. The neck is elongated, the head turns slightly to the left tilting forwards at the same time. The movement is led from the back of the neck, the muscles at the front of the neck are relaxed. The line from the right ear to the right shoulder is elongated, the other shoulder with the arm is moving in the opposite direction. The leading of the movement into space is consciously felt and is therefore very expressive. It can communicate with us more than the expression on the face.

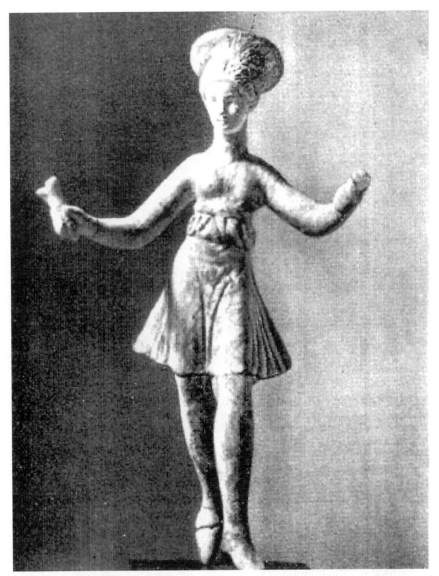

Figure 125: Greek dancer in terracotta Here the artist did not see proportion as a priority. Indeed, the dancer has unsuitably long and solid legs and arms, short body and narrow shoulders. In spite of this, in her carriage there is so much lightness and grace. Although disproportionate, the movement is balanced and consciously felt. The sensation of the axis is very intensive. There is no unnecessary tension. The moderately turned out legs are active and sensitively led from the hips. The pelvis is established. The arms together with the upper trunk and head balance the movement of the legs. One realises how a beautifully formed body alone is unimportant for the dancer. On the other hand a delicately cultured and refined muscular sensation combined with inner tension is the all-important factor through which the dancer communicates feelings with the audience.

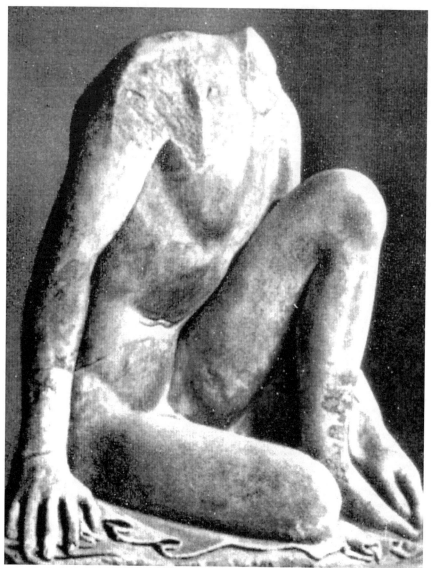

Figure 126: Statue of a Youth. Later ancient period, Greece. The vertical position of the pelvis and the pulling of the abdomen backward in relation to the contra-motion of the chest forwards, is typical of the correct elevated posture of the trunk in a sitting position. The body otherwise is relaxed, resting. Although at rest, the muscles are poised to react immediately on impulse. What a noble example of natural motion of this youth from a folk background.

APPENDIX I

STAGE MOVEMENT

excerpts from *Jevištini Pohyb* by Eva Kröschlová

WALKING

Walking is the most complex movement of the human body, perhaps even the most individual one, but definitely the most difficult to cultivate. When someone wants to refine their walk, to give it variability and to enable it to reflect a character in a variety of situations they must undergo an entire movement training and begin by seeking natural sources of movement.

An untrained person who presumes it is enough to examine a manner of walking to be able to adopt it, is gravely mistaken. Not even a specialist can help by analysing in detail all the faults a person makes during walking. Only the student who acquires a wide range of tempo-rhythmical changes and transformations of the form of walking can do this; but even then it is just a presumption of success. Success depends on the ability to feel deeply the inner and external life of the character which is reflected in the manner of the walk.

Some actors can manage without any extensive movement training; but they will not succeed in portraying the characteristic walk of another if they do not immerse themselves emotionally. The actor who has developed, by special schooling, a sensitivity for refined movement nuances, will probably have in their subconscious a richer resource for the depiction of different characters.

Let us present, as an introduction, what is written about walk in *Anatomy for Visual Artists* by J. Zrzavý (Prague: 1957).

> *Walk is, after breathing, the most coordinated movement in the human body. Everybody has a characteristic walk whether it be the length of stride, tempo or speed in individual phases of the step, or in the bearing of the body. This distinctive walk changes within the same individual, either consciously or subconsciously as the need arises, eg. silent walk and walking on a soft, uneven or smooth base. An expert can draw conclusions from a person's style of walk as to his occupation,*

habits and past illnesses. Some of the deviations in the walk are conditioned by the physical characteristics of the legs (length, weight and shape of individual parts, location of the legs).

There are several phases of a double step which occur in a definite succession:

1) *The phase of 'peeling off'*
2) *The phase of the 'swing'*
3) *The phase of 'double support'*

During 'peeling off' the leg, which is just behind, bends in the ankle joint towards the forefoot and stretches in the knee joint. The heel lifts first and then the whole foot peels gradually off the floor. By pressing the forefoot and the toes on the floor, this leg pushes the body forward and transfers the body weight onto the forward leg. The forward leg continues to place itself into a more vertical position and eventually becomes a weight-bearing leg.

The phase of the 'swing' begins after the complete 'peeling off' of the propelling leg from the floor. At the same time, the propelling leg is partly bent in all joints so that the vertical fluctuations are as small as possible. The leg swings forward, then gradually stretches and touches the floor, first with its heel and then takes over the support of the body from the other leg which starts to peel off the floor. When both feet touch the floor the phase of double support begins. The front leg (the supporting leg) touches at the heel and the back leg (the propelling leg) at the tip of the toe. This phase is the most unstable of all but is luckily very short-lived. The shorter the phase, the quicker the walk. Both lower legs are tilted forward, slightly more in the back leg than in the forward or stepping-out leg. At this moment the lower limbs are most 'shortened' and the centre of gravity is at its lowest.

During walking the centre of gravity alternately rises and lowers in correlation with the extension in the knee joint of the leg, which is at that moment weight-bearing. The centre of gravity is at its highest at this moment when the hanging leg passes the weight-bearing one (in the middle of the step). The deviation of the centre of gravity in the vertical direction can reach as much as 32mm and the larger it is, the longer the step.

As the weight of the trunk is transferred during walking alternately from the right leg to the left leg, the centre of gravity is also being shifted from side to side (on average 120mm). In some people with a wide pelvis this shift is excessive (people with a 'waddling' style of walk) and in others the movement is small (the upright walk), especially during a fast walk.

The length and time of a step is dependant on the length of the lower limbs and is, therefore, guided by the laws of swing. The longer the lower limbs, the longer are the steps. Admittedly, a slow step is shorter and a quick step is longer but at a high speed it shortens again. High heels do not permit a long step, carrying a load also shortens the step and lengthens the phase of the double support. Walk is also influenced by fatigue, during which the vertical shift of the centre of gravity of individual parts of the body, as well as the centre of gravity of the whole body, is small. Bending of the knees increases and the step is shortened - thus the phase of double support is lengthened. Mental fatigue has the same effect on the walk creating a shuffling walk. Walk, however, is also subject to fashion.

The process of walking is not a matter of a free swing, but of the work of the massive pelvic and leg muscles. During walking, these muscles work semi-automatically. The power needed for individual steps distributes itself into several muscles of 'synergic' groups (i.e. groups of muscles working together) so that it is not necessary for individual muscles to give maximum performance during walking. For this reason one does not normally tire excessively even after a long walk. This is also assisted by the circumstance that movements of both legs occur rhythmically, so that groups of muscles during each double-step are once contracted and once relaxed. This fact has a large effect on the shapes of the legs during walking. There is not a single phase during which the same muscles on both legs are contracted at the same time - i.e. symmetrically.

On the weight-bearing leg the buttock muscles (mainly gluteus medius and gluteus minimus) and the thigh adductors contract to ensure support for the pelvis. The large buttock muscle (gluteus maximus) pushes the pelvis with the trunk forward and gradually carries out extension in the hip joint. The extensors on the front part of the thigh stretch the weight-bearing leg. The calf muscles and the fibular muscles are responsible for pushing off the body and lifting the heels, and subsequently the whole body, upward. Flexors on the back of the thigh contract towards the end of the peeling- off phase and tilt the lower leg at the moment the heel leaves the floor.

Extensors on the front of the lower part of the swinging leg bend the foot so that the tip of the toes does not brush the floor. Flexors on the back of the thigh and calf muscles keep the lower legs tilted. Flexors in the hip joint shift the thigh and therefore the whole leg forward. In the second half of the swing the extensors contract vehemently on the front part of the thigh and give it the impulse for a big step forward. Before the stepping-out foot touches the floor, all muscles are already relaxed.

During normal walking, the non-weight-bearing leg rotates in the hip joint slightly outward with its own weight while it stretches. That is why, when finishing the step, the tip of the toe deviates from the middle plane. This way of walking is common during a slow, serious walk. During walking with bent knees and bent trunk (so-called 'stooped walk') the outward rotation in the hip joint does not occur and the sole of the foot, suddenly landing with all its surface on the floor, points with its longitudinal axis straight forward. Admittedly, a walk of this kind is fast but unnatural and unattractive, the same as tip-toeing and walking with extended tips of the toes. During running, the footsteps are even behind each other. During walk, the head performs rocking movements on one hand, a rotation to the side of the weight-bearing leg on the other hand and finally vertical fluctuations in accordance with the vertical oscillations of the centre of gravity of the whole body. While standing on the weight-bearing leg the head is at its highest; in the phase of the double support it is at its lowest.

The trunk, during the swing of the stepping-out leg, is drawn to the weight-bearing leg and together with the pelvis tilts slightly to the side of this leg, so that the centre of gravity moves above the supporting plane of the foot. However, it also tilts slightly forward and backward, in the first half of the step forward, in the second half tilting backward. This tilting is not obvious during a normal walk but is very pronounced with fatigue.

In regards to form, the rotations of the trunk are the most important. The trunk rotates, during the swing of the stepping-out leg in the hip joint of the weight-bearing leg, around its vertical axis forward. These rotations are especially large in women with a wide pelvis and in short, fat people. The shoulder on the side of the swinging leg shifts, however, slightly backward in order to compensate the rotation of the pelvis (i.e. the lower part of the trunk). Together with the shoulders, the upper limbs also move during the walk in a corresponding way, i.e. forward and backward, but in the opposite direction to the legs. As in the legs, it is not a free pendulum-like movement, but an active movement which prevents greater rotation of the trunk during walking. This swinging occurs only with a small amount of force. Short people with wide shoul-

ders usually have their arms drawn slightly away from the body in order to simultaneously balance deviations of the trunk to the side of the weight-bearing leg. During slow walking the arms swing freely along the body. During fast walking the arms bend in the elbows so that the length of the arms is shortened and the bending of the arms can adjust to the fast swinging of the legs.

During walking, being an outer expression of life, all parts of the body are in action. The spine is a sort of distributor and a compensator of the forces transferred from the lower limbs to the trunk and from here to the upper limbs and to the head. Thus, it adds to the walk harmony, fluency and grace.

Age influences walk—at first by developmental elements, in old age by the retrogressive change factors. The development of walk in a child is given by morphological influences (i.e. structure and form of the body without regard to function*). The contact of the foot with the base (floor) develops gradually; rhythm and stability of the leg increase and the balance, dependant on the changing proportions of growth, becomes established. Hormonal crises in puberty can cause an undisciplined (clumsy) walk.

Walking in old age is stiff and less automatic. Even small sideways deviations of the centre of gravity must be meticulously corrected. The aged lose the capacity to correct backward deviations and are prone to falling backward. Their steps are short and quick. Although the foot treads down with its whole sole, the walk is unstable. This why the aged often use a walking stick, especially when they have a considerable stoop. Rotation of the body does not result from a swing but from the fact that the external limb goes around the internal limb.

Sexual differences in walk are considerable and are closely connected with differences in proportions (a wide pelvis, shorter limbs, larger lumbar lordosis etc.). When women walk, numerous 'automated habits' are applied, therefore the walk is more complicated and more varied between individuals. A woman's step is short, the sideways deviations of the centre of gravity and the rotations of the pelvis are large.

Although the quoted paragraphs on walk from the anatomical point of view deal with its variability, the main analysis refers to the so-called 'average walk'. To enable its cultivation on one hand and to utilise deviations on the other, we must examine the 'ideal walk':

---

*Translator's note

a walk which is ideal in regard to biomechanics, psychology and aesthetics, i.e. a walk that is harmonious and natural.

One can achieve grace and a natural manner within the framework of an individual disposition and temperament by seeking a harmonious interplay of movements. In the cultivated walk, the trunk and the head are carried smoothly forward so that there is less swaying sideways, upward and downward, less 'wobbly' movement than that described above. Nevertheless it is more mobile than the 'average walk' because it is comprised of very subtle nuances, which are inconspicuous, yet pass organically through the whole body.

Firstly, the movement stream passes through the spine, providing that it is not rigid or that it is not weighed down by a sunken chest, but mainly depending on the pelvis. Excessive lordosis, or the permanent 'tucked under' position of the pelvis, immobilises the centre of the body. The movement flow is then interrupted. If, on the contrary, the pelvis is lightened and lumbar arching is reduced (by a 'muscular girdle'), if the chest is lightened and the whole spine is 'drawn upward from the crown of the head', the pelvis will become slightly vertical during each step and return again to the basic position. The slower the walk the more obvious this becomes. During the correct functioning of the pelvic and abdominal muscles, a slight push backward of the upper crest of the pelvis helps to transfer the leg from the back to the front. Sideways swaying is moderated by the correct body posture. The chest is carried smoothly forward. The shifts and lifting caused by the spinal undulations (which are a reaction to the movement of the pelvis) are almost imperceptible and definitely not 'fabricated'. They occur involuntarily during a sensation of overall elasticity (providing the legs and the pelvis function correctly). Then the advance *is led* by the sternum. (When walking upstairs you can convince yourself about the mechanism of the pelvic movement while transferring the leg from the back to the front. This movement, in a moderated form, belongs also to the walk on flat ground.) The movement backward *is led* by the pelvis. When the pelvis is correctly engaged while walking, the abdomen is actually constantly 'massaged' by the activity of the abdominal muscles. When the body posture is slack, however, this does not happen. Slackening of abdomen and chest also hinders substantial breathing.

It stands to reason that in walking a lot depends on the proper work of the legs. If the trunk is lightened, the legs are as if 'suspended in the hip joints' underneath the trunk and they have full freedom. Even the legs' mobility needs to be practised. They tend to limit the movement in the ankle joints and not to extend completely the movement in the knees. The soles then touch the floor in front in almost the same shape as they pull away from the floor in the back. This causes a rigid walk.

The leg mechanism has been created in order to rebound elastically in each step in all joints. That is why it is best to practise walking bare-footed. The sole should cling neatly to the floor and then literally peel away from it. When stepping on the forefoot first, the sole moves more and is, therefore, more exercised than when starting with the heel. This way, it stretches and bends twice at each step. This technique is used in the dance and gymnastic walk. An actor, however, needs more variation in treading. All can be done sensitively, silently and without affectation, as naturally as possible. To these variations, it is necessary to adjust the length of the step, sometimes even the speed, and thus even the movement flow through the body. Footwear limits the movement of the sole to a certain degree (high heels most of all) and shoes, therefore, should be varied.

In the ideal walk the knees are constantly in motion; they softly link extension with slight bending but without locking during extension. The knee actually extends twice, just before the foot makes contact with the floor (especially in a longer step) and then in the phase when it carries the body weight. The knee of the back leg should be well extended at the moment the step rebounds (this is usually neglected). At the same time, taking advantage of this ability saves strength which is needed elsewhere. When putting the foot down, the knee bends slightly and during the transfer from the back to the front it bends a little more. In fast walking, the double movement in the knee is reduced to a minimum and occurs in the forward-backward direction rather than upward-downward.

There is, however, a more bouncy style of walk which can be seen, for example, in tourists marching with backpacks. The heavier the load, the more elastic bouncing is required. Tahitian women, who carry their loads either on their head or on their shoulder, naturally counterbalance the bouncing of their legs by rebounding their spine in such a way that the load (e.g. a vessel of water) is carried as smoothly as possible. While practising walking, objects like a rubber ring, small bean bags or bags filled with polystyrene granules, books or even upturned chairs (holding onto them lightly, without lifting your shoulder!) are of help. These are, however, only helpful when we know how to elongate our neck, and hold our back and head in a correct position (do not push out the chin!). Carrying loads on the head for its own sake is not a self-redeeming aid for developing a correct walk (some porters finish up with a damaged spine).

Turning the shoulders in a contra-direction towards the legs is not recommended in the ideal walk. It can, however, be utilised in certain characterisations (e.g. young ladies of the twenties and thirties with a handbag under the arm and on high heels used to turn their shoulders at each step with a slight affectation in their whole body, instead of swinging their arms. Some models still walk in this way today)*. In the ideal walk the shoulders are pulled downward (in their full width) and the arms hang freely (as if on one single thread) in the shoulder joints. In a slower and a medium-slow walk they swing naturally in a contra-direction towards the leg. It is just enough to loosen them (make use of their weight) and regulate their swing to limit excessive movement. When accelerating, it is possible to reduce the swing. In a fast walk the arms are carried almost without motion. During a very slow pacing the contra-directional swings do not occur at all. When the arms are really relaxed, they move in unison, i.e. during a transfer of the body weight they move slightly back and then they return. This movement is not led but is reactive, it originates during an ideal movement wave in walking led out of the sternum. This kind of walk has been mastered by French actresses in the roles of noble ladies who are devoid of affectation or of a petty self-possession and have arrived at a calm, naturally cultivated movement.

In the ideal walk we move in 'a narrower track'. If one drew a line on the floor, the slightly turned-out feet would make contact with the floor in such a way that they would touch the line with one point of the back part of the heel. In the dance walk this line passes through the centre of the heel. The body weight must be transferred in time so not to weigh down the heels, so that the feet 'do not walk ahead of the body' and so the abdomen does not 'push forward'. At the beginning of the exercise it is better to attain the feeling that the legs are always behind us and that the body weight

---

*Translator's Note: Excessive swinging from side to side in addition to forward displacement of the pelvis will cause strain on the spine segments, affecting the overall health.

is on the front leg, not on the back leg. It is more difficult in a slower walk than in a medium-fast walk. Ideally, one achieves an even progress of the body forward. A good exercise is to alternate two medium-speed steps with one slow step. These are connected in legato mode in a smooth forward movement. This we can control when following, out of the corner of the eye, the illusionary backward shift of the wall or surrounding objects. (All three steps are the same length. There are no breaks in the flow of the movement, as in the Russian dance Beriozka). The movement *is led* by the sternum and by the groins (be careful not to lead with protruding anterior rib arches and stomach as such a posture hinders the movement wave of the spine and leads to a faulty hold of the head).

Michael Chekhov used to recommend his students let the imaginary centre of the body out a few centimetres in front of their chest, in order to lead the movement by a forward pull.

During a walk backward the smooth progress in space is more difficult and that is why it is better to practise it before the walk forward.

While practising the ideal walk, a student can easily feel tangled up. There is a story that someone asked a centipede what method it used to place its fifty pairs of legs behind each other. It thought deeply and from that moment never moved again. Too many demands at once block the ability to move naturally. It takes a long time to gradually achieve the skills necessary for a controlled walk. Prerequisites for this work are formed only after long movement studies. Walk can then be analysed in detail and utilised in diverse ways. However, as long as we have to think about the detail, the acquired skills are not much use to us. We need to feel 'at home' with them with the help of associations or entering into the spirit of human characteristic features connected with the chosen kind of walk. While practising the ideal walk itself, rather than concentrating on detail we should concentrate more on the movement fluency or the rhythm which connects the movement. We should also concentrate on radiating into space, incorporating the details into a total movement intention.

An actor has to be able to take advantage of all faults and deviations from the ideal walk. There are many variations of making foot contact with the floor, many variations of knee function, variations in pelvic movements, turning or lowering of one's hips, in the bearing of the chest and shoulders, and in the hold of the neck and the head. There are very many variations of bending the arms and of the hold of the forearms and hands, in the length of steps, in the manner of transferring the body weight. Some of them are necessary to practise technically, to use in folk and period dances; in expressive improvisation, body language studies and in observing people in one's own environment. Studies with this theme belong to the tuition of stage movement. There are as many kinds of walks as there are different people. To understand them, it is essential to have the knowledge and skills of the ideal walk.

PHYSIOLOGICAL RHYTHM OF MOVEMENT

This term is used to define the movement course of an exercise in which rhythm is not given by outside influences (e.g. music, rhythmic beat or verbal commands). The rhythm is conditioned by a correct physiological and bio-mechanical function. Because body structure and personality are individual, so is the ideal tempo-rhythm of movement. For this reason, it becomes necessary to perform certain kinds of exercises from the beginning without musical or vocal accompaniment. Individual departures in tempo-rhythm are possible while searching for the ideal movement course. A typical example of respecting a natural rhythm is breathing exercises. Swings and acrobatic exercises are other examples.

SWINGING

Swings belong to a movement category which has its own characteristic 'tempo-rhythm' and dynamics. At the beginning of the swing, under the influence of gravity, the movement accelerates; but after the culmination point (in so-called 'true swings' this is the lowest part of the curve) it slows down until it reaches the point of natural immobility—at which point the direction changes. Together with its velocity, the dynamic curve rises to weaken and fade away at the moment of almost weightless suspension in space. Practice should not be accompanied by sound until the later stage of training and then only by carefully selected and relevant music. Otherwise, it can lead to a 'movement cliché' lacking in genuine emotional experience of a given movement course. The movement performed in the true 'swing manner', that is, with a quality which differs from the so-called 'led movement' by utilising the weight of a limb or some part of the body, is also conditioned by correct breathing. So-called pseudo-swings have the same rhythmic-dynamic course in any curve directed in space e.g. horizontal.

In swing movements most people do not make use of the momentary passivity of the swinging part of the body (the section in free fall) or retain the 'fading away' of the movement. In other words, the changeability of the movement's rhythmic-dynamic course is limited. Thus they lack the dynamic wave or the 'true feature' of the swing, which helps enliven the forgotten organic flow of a natural movement. A correct course of swing movement is beneficial for the nervous system thanks to its organic quality. Whoever penetrates the secret of the 'true swing' will discover new sensations in addition to new possibilities for movement expression.

Konstantin Stanislavski's concept of relaxation derives from the Russian: *osvobozhdenie* , meaning 'freeing oneself'. The word relax ation has several meanings: as an opposite to 'tension', as an opposite to 'contraction' or 'constriction', as an opposite to 'elongation' or 'pulling' and as an opposite to 'filling' or 'occupation'. According to Stanislavski none of these meanings properly correspond to the working concept we use in theatrical practice. We must define its content more exactly. Relaxation describes a 'psychosomatic state' which is necessary during various degrees of tension if it is to be appropriate to a relevant action.

When speaking about relaxation in acting (in a studio, on the stage, in front of the camera), we mean a state of a 'eutonic' or 'relaxed activity' *corresponding to the given circumstances of a dramatic situation*. In the studio this means an optimal activity for the correct execution of a given task in such a way that the movement appears free and natural. Relaxation must be 'adopted' perfectly and be capable of expressive change. General relaxation, therefore, presumes concentration on the task.

When speaking of slackening, loosening, spasm and stiffness, we mean either insufficient or exaggerated tension which are inappropriate to the task. It is possible, at the same time, to notice slackness in one part of our body and cramp in another. In both cases the result is inorganic expression and insufficient changeability, signifying a state of being 'outside' the game and connected to neither the stage nor the studio.

Psychosomatic relaxation is achieved by combining a correct economy of force with a balanced body posture and correct breathing. This ensures a certain movement quality while increasing fitness and good health. It is also a prerequisite for the refinement of movement or oral expression (including singing) and developing the ability to change expression. It is especially necessary during movement or voice deformation to prevent one's own health being affected. The ability to grade tension is connected with the ability to depict the stage life of a character through tempo-rhythm* which is incorporated into a purposefully built tempo-rhythmic form of staging.

Relaxation in this sense has nothing in common with passivity. *It is an organic concentration and an adequate rationing of force* which oscillates around the centre of its equilibrium. The force must not remain at this centre if an actor's performance is to be lively and alive.

Tempo-rhythm is the closest friend and co-worker of feeling because it very often becomes a direct, immediate, even automatic stimulator of the emotional memory and so of the inner experience (K.S. Stanislavski).

PREPARATORY EXERCISES

To properly understand swing movements and to be able to make full use of them in dance, it is appropriate to spend time at the beginning of practice searching for individual swing rhythm while putting in motion the centre of gravity of a certain body part. To give swings their correct rhythm it is necessary to enter into the spirit of our own body, to almost become absorbed in it and thus find our own laws of movement. A selection of swings follows:

---

*Tempo rhythm is a working term coined by Stanislavski for theatrical needs (i.e. in film, recitation and nowadays also in dance and TV performances). It signifies *one of the basic factors of a dramatic action*. Tempo rhythm denotes inner relationships between tempo, rhythm and dynamics during an artistic organisation of the elements of dramatic work (i.e. time, force, space). It is part of an artistic creation of a time-space dimension of performance.

The Stanislavski concept is not widespread in the dance world. That is why in the dancer's grounding the word relaxation is used mostly as an opposite to the concept of tension. It is, therefore, a matter of relaxation with passive or half-passive muscles. However, the psychological aspect of the sensation of relaxation is also included.

1. PENDULAR SWINGS

1(a) Pendular movements of the upper limb, fading to a standstill

Initial position: stand in first position, raise the right arm to the side with its palm facing downward, rest the left hand on the small of the back.

From the waist, tilt your trunk slightly forward. Let your arm fall down from the shoulder joint with its own weight and let it pendulate from side to side until the motion dies away to a standstill. Raise the trunk, the arm remains hanging along the body in a basic correct position (if the arm remains slightly away from the body it is not completely relaxed). Throughout this exercise, the shoulders stay established in their basic position and the arm becomes perceptibly heavier. Perform the same exercise with the left arm.

Mistakes:
- allowing one shoulder to slip downward in the course of the movement
- a slack thorax
- insufficient relaxation of the entire upper limb

Variations to exercise: perform the exercise with one leg (stretched in the knee) from a low forward-raising while standing at a support. The foot is in a dorsiflexion. Let the leg fall down from the hip joint in the same way as in the arm exercise. In this case, the swinging will occur in a forward-backward direction.

Perform the exercise with the head in a deep forward tilt of the trunk. Lift the head and let it fall until the motion stops by itself.

1(b) Coordinated pendulum movements

Initial position: stand in the first position with the right arm raised slightly forward and the palm facing downward.

Direct the free fall of the upper limb into a regular pendular movement which occurs in a backward and forward direction approximately at 45 degrees, while the muscles of the hand, forearm and the majority of the upper arm are absolutely passive. The pendular movements must be of the same height to both sides. Practise the same, from side to side, with a sideways lifted arm.

Mistakes:
- as in Exercise 1(a)

Variations to exercise: gradate the pendular movements from quite small to large with the limbs in the basic position and a relevant reduction of speed.

Perform the same from side to side with the head in a deep forward tilt.

Perform the same with one leg as in Exercise 1(a).

1(c) Pendular swings

Pendulous swings begin with a free fall with a maximal relaxation of muscles of the swinging body part and are finished by 'recapturing' the swing by the activity of some or all muscles of the relevant part. The swings differ from the regulated pendular movements partly spatially by a larger span, partly rhythmically by a fast beginning and slowed down ending, and partly dynamically by a vehement onset and moderate fading. We practise them in the last third of the movement by the prolongation of the muscles into distance, gradating the pendular movements which we 'capture' through prolongation of the muscles into distance.

Initial position: stand in the second position. Lift the right upper limb sideways with the palm facing downward and the back of the left hand resting on the sacrum.

Gradate the swings, gradually enlarge the arcs all the way to the ground and into torsion (rotate the trunk after the hand) with pulsing in the knees. First concentrate on the weight of the upper limb (as if we were holding weights which put our whole body, including the head, into a swinging motion). The eyes follow the hand. Next add the elongation of the arm and hand at the extreme points, consciously projecting into distance, followed again by their relaxation and the resulting free fall. Later, decrease the arcs (the body does not yield to the movement of the arm any more), but retain the same course in the upper limbs, i.e. alternate passivity with activity. Maintain a moderate pulsing in the knees and follow the hand with your eyes. Perform the same with the left upper limb, then with both upper limbs at the same time.

Variations to Exercise: stand in first position, perform the same movement forward and backward. Start with one arm, then use both arms in the same and opposite directions.

Perform the same forward and backward with the lower limb. Recapture the swing with the thigh muscle only (the limb remains slightly bent in the knee with a relaxed instep). This exercise is beneficial for relaxation of the hip joint.

In another variation, extend the lower limb along all its length into the distance.

Mistakes:

- as in Exercise 5 in SWINGS OF THE TRUNK FROM SIDE TO SIDE, p. 294.

Note: exercise with upper limbs at first as in Exercise 1(a) PENDULAR MOVEMENTS, Exercise 1(b) COORDINATED PENDULAR MOVEMENTS and Exercise 1(c) PENDULAR SWINGS. These can also be linked with circular swings of the arms, based on the same principle. Only then do we practise these exercises with the head and lower limbs. (It is better to divide these exercises into several lessons). All the following exercises (except for Exercise 4, RELAXATION OF THE TRUNK AND UPPER LIMBS, Exercise 8, SUSTAINED SWINGS OF LOWER LIMBS and Exercise 11, HORIZONTAL SWINGS OF THE UPPER LIMBS) contain free fall and must therefore be practised with a similar sensation and the same rhythmic and dynamic course as PENDULAR SWINGS.

In the beginning it is preferable to allow the students to retain their own individual slow tempo for at least three attempts at each new exercise. When they are urged to adjust too early to the given tempo, their movements lose their swing quality and can become 'led' or 'jerky.' In a given tempo, rhythm must be selected very sensitively with the appropriate delay in the culmination point, especially in circular swings which contain the so-called 'dead point' (or point of zero momentum) and a slow overflow which gathers speed.

Swings can be enriched by creating arcs of different sizes (even down to the ground), by torsion (turning the trunk after the arm), by pulsing in the knees as well as by different kinds of figures eight.

SWINGS OF THE TRUNK FROM A STRAIGHT FORWARD TILTED POSITION

2(a)

Initial Position: stand in the first position parallel, tilt the trunk forward with the arms raised until the palms rest at shoulder width on the support (barre, table, ladder). The trunk forms a right angle with the legs. Pulse, at medium speed, several times in the thoracic spine and shoulders during the downward movement.

Mistakes:

- slightly bent legs
- hunching in the lumbar region (due to insufficient flexion in the hip joints)

- contracted shoulders
- sunken-down head and neck (between the shoulders)
- slightly bent elbows
- bent wrists
- the body weight shifted excessively onto the hands
- feet too far from or too close to the support
- excessively large movements of the whole trunk (instead of small, intensive pulsing, especially in the thoracic section of the spine).

2(b)

Initial position: the same as before with hands on the support.

Swing with the upper limbs down and backward, knees bent, bounce once, spine relaxed, head hanging as low as possible. On the rebound, swing the arms down and forward, elongate the spine and extend the arms slightly above the support, then landing with their full weight on the support, with pulsing twice in the thoracic spine. The hands brush the floor during each swing. Combine Exercise (b) and Exercise (a) with a musical accompaniment of two bars at 6/8 time.

1st bar - pulse twice in the thoracic spine.

2nd bar - swing the arms down and backward bending in the knees. Bounce on the rebound continue the return swing to the initial position (as in 2(b)).

Mistakes:
- stooped back
- shoulders pulled together
- stiff arm movements
- rigid neck (the head is slightly raised) during the downward movement
- insufficient extension
- lifting the shoulders during the movement forward.

Variations to Exercise: perform the same with extended legs and without bending the knees; the same with hands folded on the small of the back to achieve the same quality of swinging but faster.

2(c)

Initial position: upright body, legs in the first position parallel, arms upward, palms facing forward.

Swing with arms in an arc forward, downward and backward through a forward tilted trunk similar to exercise (b). The spine hyperextends slightly for a moment before changing into a forward bend (the pelvis is tucked under in a folded position of the body). On the rebound, swing the arms together with the trunk, down, forward, upward; and follow the same arc as on the way down-backward (again, through a slightly hyperextended spine), finishing in the initial position in correct alignment. Make sure the pelvis is levelled into a basic position, The swing downward is more vehement and faster than the upward swing. Alternate exercises 2(b) and 2(c).

Mistakes:
- stiff movement
- insufficiently deep tilt due to rigid hip joints
- insufficient pulsing
- unlevelled lordosis on the end of recovery
- pulled-up shoulders
- as well as mistakes occurring in Exercise 2(b).

Variations to Exercise: perform the same with jumping up in the 'folded position' (pelvis tucked under) at the end of the first swing or with jumping up with an elongated body and legs and raised arms at the end of the second swing. The same with elongated legs (without jumping up).

2(d)

Initial position: wide second position with legs turned out, arms raised sideways, palms facing downward. The knees remain extended throughout.

Swing downward with the trunk and the arms into a suspended relaxed adduction of the arms crosswise (elbows slightly bent). The relaxed trunk and the head hang as low as possible. On the rebound of the trunk, swing with the arms into a hyper extended forward tilt of the trunk (the head rises slightly) while extending the arms wide sideways. Repeat the swing downward with the arms crosswise. On the rebound, do not stop in the hyper-extended tilt of the trunk forward but continue raising the body into the upright position while extending the arms to the sides. Make sure that the pelvis is shifted forward into the vertical and the hips are elevated as required by the correct body posture. The recovery into the initial position is slowed down.

Mistakes:
- In the downward movement they are the same as in 2(b) and 2(c)
- In the forward tilt of the trunk the shoulders are pulled together and the horizontal line of the arms is broken so that they point sideways-backward
- excessive lordosis in the lumber section
- narrowed shoulders
- the arms deviate backward from the initial horizontal line. See Diagram supplement.

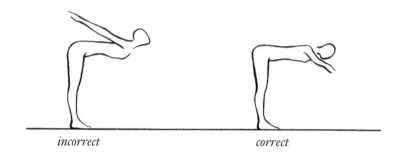

incorrect   *correct*

3. SWINGS WITH ROTATION OF THE THORAX

Preparatory exercises
Sit with the legs crossed and the heels in a straight line. Place the hands on the shoulders with the elbows drawn towards the waist.

3(a) Rotation of the trunk
Rotate the thorax to the right (diagonally) with an unchanged position of the head (the chin remains above the centre of the chest). Hold and recover into the initial position. Rotation is active, recovery is accompanied with the sensation of relaxation of oblique abdominal muscles (while pulling of the trunk upward remains). Repeat the same to the left.
   (i) Rotation of the thorax and head to the right: rotate both simultaneously. The chin moves approximately above the right shoulder.
   (ii) Rotation in opposite directions: thorax to the right, the head to the left. The chin moves approximately above the left shoulder.
Mistakes:

- insufficiently upward-elongated waist
- protruding anterior lower rib arches
- sternum not high enough
- impure movement (combined with a forward, backward or a sideways tilt, especially evident in the shoulder line).

Variations to exercise: perform with the hands on the back of the head, on the head, above the head, or with arms raised to the side: sitting on the heels requires a particularly well established 'tucked under' pelvis, kneeling with parallel legs, lying on the abdomen, thorax elevated, the hands clasped on the back of the head.

This exercise can be performed even lying on a table. One student lies prostrate with lower limbs on the table and trunk hanging down in a straight forward tilt (the trunk is in a right angle to the thighs). The other student holds his/her legs firmly above the ankles. Lift the trunk slowly into a horizontal line with the legs, as if lying on the abdomen. The whole trunk from the hip joints up to the head is in the air. Rotate the thorax to the right, recover to a straight line, rotate the thorax to the left, recover and lower the trunk through a hyperextended spine into the hanging position.

Perform the same while lying on the back, in a straight sitting position. To the slow rotation we can add two quick flickers in the extreme position of the rotation.

3(b) Swings with rotation of the thorax

Initial position: stand with the legs in a wide second position with the left side of the body to the support and arms raised above the head. The knees remain stretched throughout. Rotate the thorax towards the support (by turning in the waist, the pelvis remains frontal), tilt the elongated trunk into a horizontal forward-sideways stretch to the left with the palms resting on the support. The front arm is more stretched, the back one more bent and both are in front of the thorax. Pulse in the spine as in Exercise 2(a); on the rebound swing the hands downward-backward as in Exercise 2(b); the arms pass along the outer sides of the legs. The head and trunk bend forward-down in a relaxed manner. On the rebound, swing with hands downward and upward and continue with an active elongation until landing with the hands on the support (as in Exercise 2(b)). Repeat this exercise several times, then perform the same from the other side.

Mistakes:

- slightly bent knees
- inward rolling of the sole
- rotation of the hips towards the bar
- and other mistakes as in Exercise 2(b).

3(c)

Initial position: stand in a wide second position of the legs with the arms raised above the head and the thorax rotated to the right.

Swing downward-backward as in Exercise 3(b), on the rebound swing down and upward-right through an elongated forward-sideways tilt to the initial position with the arms above the head. Link the movement fluently with a rotation of the thorax from right to left. The swing downward is more vehement and shorter than the upward swing on the recovery, which is longer and is connected with a fluent rotation of the thorax to the other side. This transition must be executed with an intensively sensed and stressed elongation upward of the whole body, including the arms, while looking upward, with a slightly hyper-extended spine.

Mistakes:
- insufficient elongation to the sides of the forward-sideways tilted trunk during the recovery swing
- insufficient upward extension of the arms and trunk during the transition from the right rotation of the thorax to the left.
- lifting of the shoulders
- a narrowed position of the arms
- others, as in 3(b)

Variations to exercise: perform with a rotation of the thorax from right to left by a swift, brisk movement (without hyperextension of the spine and without looking upward), by pulling up in the waist. In this case the swing upward is equally as quick as the swing downward (extra time is given to the rotation of the thorax from side to side).

4. RELAXATION OF THE TRUNK AND ARMS

4(a) Into a forward bend

Initial position: legs in a wide second position, arms raised above the head, palms facing each other, a total elongation upward and looking up.

Gradually let the tension 'evaporate' from the fingers, palm, forearm and upper arm of the right limb. All relaxation is done step by step by starting slowly and building up speed until the entire arm falls down limply (the upward pull of the left arm and the whole spine remains). Perform the same with the left arm, perform the same with the head (as if there were a heavy object in the forehead which overweighs the head into a fall; the trunk remains erect) and perform the same with the trunk (as if the head overweighs the thorax as well) through a deep lateral bend passively into a forward bend. Hold in the deep forward bend, slowly and gradually erect the vertebrae one by one. Widen and establish the shoulders, gently straighten the head (on an elongated neck). The upper limbs remain hanging freely. Each phase of the exercise (except for the straightening) ends with a pendular movement fading to a standstill with an additional perception of weight in the relevant body part.

Mistakes:
- insufficient perception of weight
- allowing the fall of the upper limbs to pass through a forward elevation of the arms instead of collapsing along the axis
- insufficient 'folding' in the hip joints in the deep forward bend
- uneven straightening of the body.

Practise the same without the division into phases and with both upper limbs at the same time (falling down in one compact movement from an upward raising of the arms into a deep forward bend, picking up speed due to gravity.

4(b) Into a lateral bend:
Initial position: legs in a wide second position, upper limbs along the body, the spine pulled upward.

Let the head overbalance by tilting it sideways into a relaxed lateral bend. Perceive the weight due to gravity. Let the thorax overbalance and perceive the weight. Lift the opposite elongated arm through the side upward and let it fall over the head. The additional weight on the trunk increases the load even more. By relaxing the muscles, which until now have held the trunk in a frontal plane but bent sideways, 'roll' the trunk over with absolutely passive arms into a deep forward bend, then straighten gradually as in Exercise 4(a)

Mistakes:
- allowing the arm to fall in front of the face
- allowing the head to rotate sideways

- other mistakes as in Exercise 4(a).

Perform the same without the division into phases. Start with an active movement of the opposite arm (left arm when bending to the right) through the side into an upward raising; from here drop gradually into a lateral bend with an awareness of weight etc.

5. SWINGS OF THE TRUNK FROM SIDE TO SIDE EXTENDING THE ARMS IN AN ARC MOVEMENT ABOVE THE HEAD

5(a)

Initial position: stand in a wide second position with raised upper limbs and palms facing each other. The entire body is extended upward with eyes looking up.

Slowly bend the trunk and lifted upper limbs to the right into an extended lateral bend, reaching as far as possible. This movement is realised with intensive activity of the left arm which begins the pull over the head to the right. Continue in the same manner, from right to left, with the right arm initiating the pull over the head to the left. The trunk remains in a frontal plane throughout and is active at all times—unlike Exercise 4.

Mistakes:
- lifting the shoulders
- a narrowed position of the upper limbs
- an over-rotated thorax forward from the frontal plane
- dropping the upper arm in front of the head
- insufficient elongation into distance
- a sagging waist.

5(b)

Initial position: stand in a wide second position in a deep, relaxed forward bend. Fully relax the head and upper limbs. The shoulders remain established so that the arms hang from the shoulder joints.

Swing the trunk and arms into an elongated bend to the right; the eyes look to the right. Swing to the left via the lower arc through a relaxed forward bend. The fall of the swings is more vehement with a longer 'fading'. (Use a 3/4 time signature).

Mistakes:
- as in Exercise 5(a)
- stiff movement (insufficiently pliable trunk, arms and neck in the deep forward bend).

6. CIRCULAR SWINGS OF THE TRUNK—PREPARATORY EXERCISES

6(a) Hyperextension of the thorax (backward bend)

Initial position: sit cross-legged with the hands on the back of the head. Start by looking upward, while slowly bending the head, neck and shoulders backward (support the head very gently by the neck muscles). Hyperextend the thoracic spine. During a gradual and slow recovery the sternum leads the movement upward-forward, followed by a mutually balanced thorax, neck and head which are sensitively pulled upward all the way through. When reaching the vertical position ease the tension and elongate the spine from the coccyx upward into the initial position. The hyper-extension of the thoracic spine helps to turn out the shoulders.

Mistakes:
- excessive tension of the muscles in front of the neck
- head drops backward
- insufficient arching of the upper thorax
- pulling the shoulder blades together
- raising the shoulders
- not pointing the elbows sideways.
- movement is insufficiently arched.

Variation to exercise: perform with rotation of the head to the right or left, hands on knees, or arms in a forward lift, i.e. the elbows are bent so that the upper arms form a right angle with the forearms and trunk (forearms are on top of each other).

6(b) Hyperextension of the whole trunk

Initial position: straight kneeling position; the arms alongside the body or the hands on the back of the head.

To the hyperextension of the upper thorax add the hyperextension of the lowest part of the spine (the gluteal muscles are contracted). Lower the head as far as possible.

Recovery: slowly and gradually place the pelvis, waist, thorax, neck, and head into a vertical line, one vertebra after the other while sensing the upward elevation of the whole trunk.

Mistakes:
- a swollen neck
- a flat chest (the thorax does not form an arc)
- excessive shift of the pelvis forward and insufficient support of

the lumbar spine casuing an interrupted arc
- relaxed pelvic muscles.

6(c) The wave of the trunk
Initial position: straight kneeling position, (the thighs are parallel) the forearms folded in front of the thorax and elbows bent so that the upper arms and forearms form a right angle as in 6(a) Variation.

The movement occurs in a vertical axis. Tuck the pelvis under and lower it just above the heels (do not sit on them with your full weight). The lower spine is rounded, the neck and head are hyperextended. By contracting the gluteal muscles, press through the groins forward-upward (i.e. shift the pelvis forward-upward). From here the movement passes gradually through all vertebrae (one by one) until the hyperextension is completed, except for the head and neck, which are ti;ted forward. By contracting the abdominal muscles change the position of the pelvis to the tucked under; the neck and head start to hyperextend.. The head moves with delay, the arms are carried horizontally in front of the thorax throughout the movement.

Mistakes:
- excessive lordosis in the lumbar region
- a slack abdomen
- not allowing the movement to occur gradually (one vertebra after the other) and missing the thoracic section of the spine
- giving insufficient support to the posterior neck muscles leading to slackening of the neck spine
- slackening the muscles to effect recovery instead of passing through an arched thorax into an elongated trunk *led* by the sternum
- lifting the shoulders
- dropping the elbows.

Variations to exercise: perform with arms along the body, arms raised sideways, one or both arms above the head, head rotated right or left towards the shoulder.

6(d) Swinging into a deep forward bend of the trunk
This is a variation of Exercise 2(d). Swing with the trunk downward, arms swing into adduction crosswise (first swing). The final swing from down-upward is complemented at the end by a hyperextended thoracic spine forming an arc with a highly elevated

sternum. The arms swinging outward from the crosswise position do not finish in the sideways lift as the body reaches the upright position as in Exercise 2(d). Instead they continue to rise until they point diagonally upward-backward with the palms turned forward and the thorax and cervical spine arch actively backward.

Mistakes:
- 'flat chest' (insufficiently arched thorax)
- the head dropped backward
- insufficient support of the cervical spine
- inward rotation of the shoulders
- sinking the arms backward-downward
- insufficient support in the lumbar region.

6(e) Combined circular swings

Initial position: stand in a wide second position in a deep relaxed forward bend of the trunk. The head and upper limbs hang totally relaxed from the shoulder joints, the shoulder girdle is established.

Link two lateral swings of the trunk with a very actively executed circular swing starting from a relaxed forward bend and led through a lateral elongated bend to the left into a highly-arched backward bend of the spine. The arms and hands point upward-backward diagonally. Continue through an elongated lateral bend to the right into a relaxed forward bend.

Here, due to its relaxed fall, the trunk passes slightly beyond the midline to the left. On the rebound execute the swing sequence again, this time starting to the right. The movement *is led* with the eyes. The upper section of the circle is actively and strongly arched but becomes pliant in the lower section of the circle. Perform to four bars at 3/4 time:

left - right - whole circle - relax, rebound.
right - left - whole circle - relax, rebound.

Mistakes:
- as in Exercises 5(b) and 6(b).

Variations to Exercise: practise the same with the head only in the standing position and both hands resting on the small of the back (in the marginal points the head rotates to the sides, during the hyperextension the thoracic spine cooperates). Exercise the same with the whole trunk with hands on the small of the back. Pay attention to swing quality.

7. SWINGS OF THE LOWER LIMB—PREPARATORY EXERCISE

7(a)

Initial position: legs in the first position, moderately turned out, with the side of the body at the support, the inner hand at the support, the outer hand on the hip.

Transfer the body weight onto the well-extended and established inner leg and shift the outer leg slightly forward by loosening it. The abdominal and thigh muscles lift the thigh forward into a horizontal position, the lower leg together with the sole of the foot hang down (the weight-bearing leg is established and firm together with the pelvis, the body weight is on the forefoot). Let the lifted thigh fall down (the trunk remains elevated). Repeat several times. Practise the same with the other leg.

Mistakes:
- the calf and sole are insufficiently relaxed
- pointed toes are pulled under so that the lower leg and the thigh form an acute angle instead of a right angle
- the body weight is on the heel
- the knee of the weight-bearing leg is bent
- the hip of the weight-bearing leg shifts towards the support
- the instep arch of the weight-bearing leg is lowered
- a slack waist
- the elbow of the arm on the hip is twisted backward
- the leg is actively lowered into the initial position
- the trunk is slackened during the fall of the leg.

7(b)

Initial position: as in Exercise 7(a) first position, but the outer arm is raised to the side with the palm turned downward. Lift the fully turned-out thigh of the outer leg horizontally to the side with the lower leg hanging vertically down (the instep is passive).

7(c) Swings of a bent leg with a relaxed lower leg and instep

This exercise is a combination of Exercises 7(a) and 7(b).

Initial position: standing at a support as in Exercise 7(a) with the difference that the outer arm is lifted to the side with the palm turned downward. Raise the slightly turned-out outer thigh forward as in exercise 7(a) so that the lower leg is hanging vertically down with a passive instep.

Begin the swing by letting the leg drop down with its own weight and finish by lifting the thigh actively sideways, fully turned out. (The maximal rotation of the leg starts immediately after the foot touches the floor.) Lift the thigh to the horizontal (forward or sideways) only the lower leg hangs down vertically with a relaxed instep. Alternate a swing from the front to the side with a swing from the side to the front. In this kind of swing the leg always passes through a lower curve from one direction to another and the foot brushes the floor each time it passes the lowest point of the curve. Pay attention especially to correct relaxation of the entire leg. Use an accompaniment in 6/8 time.

Mistakes:
- rotating the pelvis in the direction of the sideways lift of the leg
- an unsteady or slack hold of the upper limb
- insufficient swing quality during the transfer of the lower limb from the front to the side and vice versa
- pulling the lower leg towards the thigh instead of letting it hang passively
- further mistakes as in Exercise 7(a).

7(d) Swings from bending to stretching
Initial position: as in Exercise 7(c). First position, slightly turned out, standing at a support with the outer arm lifted sideways.

The accompaniment has a 6/8 time signature (subdivided in two). On the upbeat, raise the thigh of the outer leg forward so that the relaxed lower leg and instep hang down from the knee (first swing). On the down beat (the accented first beat of the following 6/8 bar), the leg swings downward and finishes extended and turned out in a sideways lift (second swing). At the beginning of this swing, a short passive stretching of the leg (due to its fall) enables the foot to touch the floor and to slide through the first position. After passing the first position and during the sideways lift the entire lower limb (especially the instep) becomes actively extended and the leg rotates maximally outward. With a new swing return the leg forward into the bent position (the lower leg and instep hang down from the knee).

Mistakes:
- as in Exercise 7(c)
- slackening the trunk in the waist during the swing forward
- insufficient outward rotation of the leg while swinging sideways.

Variations to exercise: practise the same swing with a constantly extended instep (except while sliding through the first position). When the leg is bent the lower leg with the thigh forms an obtuse angle.

Alternatively, practise the same swing with an added rotation of the head sideways while the leg swings to the side.

Bend the leg forward, extend it backward raising the leg low above the ground and simultaneously rotating the head to the side.

Bend the leg sideways, extend it forward. The head turns forward.

7(e) Swings during a walk (i.e. swings combined with walking forward or backward).

Swing the bent leg forward, backward, forward, step forward in 4/4 time, simultaneously lifting backward the free leg. Swing with a relaxed lower leg and instep; try to move the thigh as high as possible and maintain an elevated body posture; complete the step on an elongated and established lower limb. Hold the arms sideways. Practise the same while walking backward.

In 3/4 time, the step and the swing forward occur simultaneously on the first beat.

Variation to exercise: in 2/4 time, swing the right leg backward, forward; step forward as the other leg swings backward simultaneously etc. Practise the same, this time with an extended leg swinging sideways, forward (leg is bent), step in front of the other leg in the third position as the other leg swings sideways etc.

8. SUSTAINED SWINGS (HELD-BACK SWINGS)

These swings of the leg are equivalent to all kinds of classical *battement tendu* extended *à terre* or *en l'air* (45 degrees, 90 degrees or more). Both the outward and inward sliding of the foot occurs actively, with force.

9. SWINGS WITH A WAVE INTO A BACKWARD BEND (HYPER-EXTENDED SPINE)

9(a) Circles of the upper limbs executed along the side of the body in the form of a swing

Initial position: legs in first position parallel, arms stretched and lifted forward, palms facing downward (in pronation).

The 'outward' circle: begin the swing of the arms by rotating them upward (supination) so that the elbows face downward and are slightly rounded. The course of the following swing is: downward (knees bend), backward (knees stretch), upward (zero momentum) and forward where the arms finish in the initial position with palms downward.

The 'inward' circle: in this swing it is best first to prepare the arms down-backward (slightly passing the plumb line), before starting the swing of the arms downward-forward (bending the knees), upward (stretching the knees and passing through the zero momentum), backward, downward (the speed increases) and forward. The arms are stretched and hands are in pronation both at the beginning and at the end. Before repeating the same swing, prepare the arms backward again.

To ensure that these movements are correct the shoulders must help by their downward pressure and rotation outward, together with a pressure of the shoulder blades towards the thorax, all of which create a support for the slightly hyper-extended spine during the movement upward. The cooperation of these factors ease the lifting of the arms during the execution of the back curve of the circle. The movement does not have to be exactly in the sagittal (lateral) plane (the arms are more apart when they are at the back than at the front) but must continue movement fluently without interruption. Practise first with one arm which is followed by our gaze, then with both (gazing upward). Finally, the movement is accompanied by a moderate pulsing in the knees. Emphasise the first third of the circle.

Mistakes:
• lifting the shoulders
• rotating the shoulders inward
• pressing the head forward
• a stiff back
• excessive lordosis in the lumbar and sacral region
• a slack pelvis
• a rigid movement during the back curve
• poor swing quality.

9(b) A small wave of the spine into a backward bend in a kneeling position

similar to exercises 6 (c) and 9 (a).

9(c) Pendular arm swings combined with a circular swing along the side of the body

Initial position: legs in first position parallel, both arms raised forward, see PENDULAR SWINGS Exercise 1(c).

Link four pendular swings of the arms (backward, forward, backward, forward while the knees pulse with each swing) with one 're-captured' circular swing along the side of the body started 'outward'. Knees gradually stretch with the upward movement of the trunk and arms. As the arms reach the shoulder level, start elevating the body on high demi-pointe (the gaze is directed upward). The body returns to the vertical. At the height of the movement (the 'dead point') the axis of the whole body slowly leans forward until it falls over into a few small steps forward terminated by a folded body (the pelvis is tucked under and the knees slightly bent). The arms finish their circle and fall downward and pendulate until the motion dies away. Raise the body into an upright position while the arm lifts forward and starts another swing. Practise with one arm at a time and then with both arms.

Mistakes:
- allowing the upward elongation in the 'dead point' to extend only from the arms and not from stretching out the whole body
- leaving the head hanging backward
- falling over too quickly
- being insufficiently supple in 'folding' the body
- lacking of control over the last few steps after the end of the 'fall-over'.

Variations to exercise: exercise with one arm at a time (the other arm rests on the small of the back) with the difference that the gaze follows the hand and the thorax rotates after the swinging arm so that the whole body is subordinated to the movement of the arm.

Exercise along a diagonal line in an individual tempo without music and concentrate on an organic course of movement.

9(d) A combination of a circular swing of the upper limbs with a wave of the body into a hyperextension of the trunk

Initial position: legs in the first position, stretched arms are raised forward with palms facing downward (pronation).

Begin the circular swing of the arms by rotating them 'outward' (supination), letting them immediately fall along the lower curve into an approximately downward-backward raised position. The knees bend. At this moment initiate the swing of the body by shifting the pelvis forward, followed immediately by a strong impulse from the hip joints. (Both of these actions result from a pressure of contracted buttock muscles.) The sudden pressure of the pelvic shift with the impulse from the hip joints causes a swing of the relaxed trunk so that the body reacts by a wave resulting in an hyperextended spine.

The backward fall of the swinging trunk is instantly recaptured by a simultaneous contraction of the abdominal muscles which starts the elevation of the trunk and arms. Upon reaching the level of the support point of the neck and head, the shoulder blades apply a strong pressure on the ribs (the hyperextension of the upper thoracic spine increases). Recapture the motion of the upper spine and complete the swing upward by 'carrying' the thorax with the arms, the cervical spine and the head along the upper curve into a highly elevated body posture (as if the whole body was growing from the ground to the sky).

The pressure of the shoulder blades, the hyper-extension and the pulled-down and turned-out shoulders enlarge the range of the movement and make easier the rotation of the arms during their lifting in the last section of the circle.

Mistakes:
- as in Exercise 9(a)
- excessive lordosis in the lumbar spine
- slack abdominal muscles
- dropping the head backward (insufficiently supported by the upper back muscles)
- lifting the shoulders
- not allowing the movement to occur gradually (due to an insufficient elevation of the sternum and therefore an insufficiently arched thorax); a flat back due to an insufficient involvement of the back, especially shoulder-blade muscles at the moment when the arms slant diagonally backward-upward
- lifting the heels off the floor.

An 'outward' circular swing of the arms with a wave into a hyper-extension of the trunk (spine bent backward) as in Exercise 9(d) combined with a forward swing of the straight runk completed by a circular swing of the arms 'inward'.

Initial Position: legs in first position, arms raised upward. After

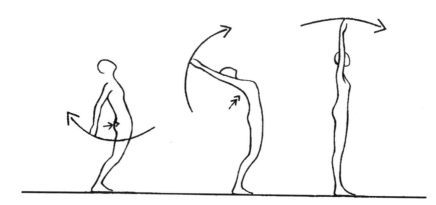

completing the circular swing with the wave add a forward swing of the trunk with the spine slightly hyper-extended on the way down. When the body reaches the 'folded' position (i.e. the pelvis is tucked under, the whole spine curves and the head is close to the bent knees; the arms are raised downward-backward). On the rebound start a circular swing of the arms 'inward'.

The swinging arms elevate the whole body into a maximal elongation where the 'dead point' occurs. From here an independent circle of the arms continues up into the initial position, while the trunk remains vertical. Every time the arms fall down with their own weight the knees bend.

10. HORIZONTAL SWINGS OF THE ARMS

Initial position: legs in a turned-out second position, both arms are prepared to the left closely under the shoulder level, the left arm is raised sideways (abduction), the right arm is crosswise left and slightly bent (adduction), palms are downward.

Transfer the body weight on the left leg (the knees of both legs are slightly bent) and swing the arms horizontally one after the other (the right and left almost simultaneously) to the right through an extended semi-circle with the accent on the elongation forward into distance (both legs stretch). Together with the swing dying away to the right, transfer the body weight to the right leg (legs bend slightly) swing back (i.e. to the left) first with the left, immediately followed by the right arm. The gaze follows the arms which extend one after the other. Together with the stretching and relaxing of the legs, the spine also slightly elongates and relaxes.

Mistakes:
- lifting and shifting the shoulders forward
- slackening the thorax
- too heavily accenting the beginning of the swing
- an insufficient spatial feeling
- an insufficient sense of the accent and of the fading away of the movement.

10(a) Horizontal swings of the folded arms

Initial position: first position parallel, arms in low adduction crosswise.

Lower the pelvis into a semi-squat, wrap the arms around the trunk (the right arm is bent in front of the body with the palm downward, the left arm is behind the body with its back resting on the sacrum). Rotate the thorax to the left, with the head tilted slightly to the right; the gaze is forward. With an active elongation of the whole body (actively stretch the knees) and of the elbows, the arms fly through a curve closely one after the other via a low forward raising to the opposite side; the thorax rotates to the right. The movement is completed by a drop in the knees, a momentary relaxation of the whole body, wrapping the arms around and tilting the head to the opposite side; the gaze is forward. The movement must be executed by a swing, i.e. with an accented beginning, a strong outreach and a subtle and sustained fading away.

Exercise to two 3/4 bars, bending the knees elastically twice. Close to the beginning of the accent, drop in the knees a little and start the accented swing on the rebound.

1st bar – a flight of the arms started by an accent, the legs stretch (on the rebound).

2nd bar – complete the movement of the arms, semi-squat, on the third count of the bar bend the legs and on the rebound in the following bar start a new swing.

Mistakes:
- making stiff movements of the arms instead of supple elongation and slight bending
- lifting the shoulders
- failing to maintain the swing rhythm and succession of both arms
- Omitting to tilt the head from side to side

- insufficient folding of the body into a spiral line at the closure of the movement
- a protrusion of the pelvis.

Note: all swings of the trunk are connected with an exhalation and an inhalation (the exhalation is during the downward movement). Bear in mind a development of spatial feeling and a relaxed 'fading away' of the movement. Otherwise the swings become oscillations or led movements.

11. CIRCULAR SWINGS OF THE ARMS ABOVE THE HEAD

Before beginning circular swings of the arms above the head and swings in the figure eight, it is advisable to revise all the movements of the thorax, head, shoulders and arms and all parts (within the possibilities of the joints), as well as waves and swings of the arms.

Initial position: sitting cross-legged, arms raised to the sides, palms downward (hands above the shoulder level).

Another swing is a horizontal one, with arms wrapped around the body (from the spot forward or backward) from a moderately turned out fourth position. At the onset of this swing, elevate the body into a high jump. While in the air, the back leg executes a small semicircle from the back to the front. Land on both feet in a fourth position with the back leg now in front. Alternate the legs. The same can be done in a backward motion. In that case, the front leg executes a semicircle from the front to the back.

Swing with the right arm forward to the left, above the head backward and finish the curve back into the initial position, the palm faces upward. Follow the hand with your eyes and cooperate

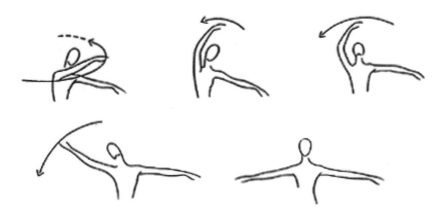

with your whole trunk (a sideways bend, a backward bend, a bend to the other side). The arm does not describe a regular circle, rather an oval path, but despite that we talk about a circle in order to achieve a larger roundness. The left arm can either stay in a controlled sideways lift or it can, at the beginning of the swing, move into a rounded position in front of the body (at the height of the stomach) and at the closure of the swinging arm it returns to the initial position. Perform the same swing with the left arm to the right.

Mistakes:
- a stiff movement of the arm
- insufficient work by the thorax, particularly by the shoulder-blades and sternum, especially during the hyperextension
- a slack neck
- an excessively bent elbow above the head
- insufficient 'accent' at the beginning of the swing and excessively fast 'fading away' of the movement.

Variations to exercise: perform the same with both arms from a parallel raised position and repeat several times in one direction. In this case it is a matter of a real circle (the movement is funnel-shaped with a centre in the waist). Here the trunk is more active than the arms.

12. SWINGS IN THE FIGURE EIGHT

Note: when the movement *is led* by the outer edge of the hand, a radial deviation of the hand occurs (towards the thumb) and with it always a slight bend of the wrist towards the index finger (inner side) in a contra-direction to the motion. When the movement *is led* by the inner edge of the hand there occurs an ulnar deviation of the hand (towards the little finger) and with it always a slight bend in the wrist towards the little finger side (outer) in a contra-direction to the motion.

12(a) 'Cutting' (preparatory exercise)
Initial Position: legs in the second position, the left hand resting on the small of the back, the right arm raised up with the palm facing inward, the fingers are elongated. Lead the arm along a vertical line down as if the little finger edge of the hand (outer side) were cutting the space in front of you. During the return movement of the arm 'cut' the space with the index finger edge (inner side). (The

partly relaxed thumb is outside the dividing line.) Change the direction to a diagonal right-downward (low abduction). This time leading with the little finger edge. From here, lead with the index finger edge (inner) horizontally to the left into adduction (cross-wise) and return upward to the initial position, 'cutting' with the outer edge of the hand. With every change in the direction of the 'cutting' action the hand's deviation also changes. The wrist is always slightly bent, as explained above.

Use various directions, later also altering the curves. Move always slowly with an intensive sensation in the corresponding edge of the hand. The wrist always bends slightly in the opposite direction, i.e. the hand 'cuts' with its slightly slanted longitudinal axis. Practise the same with the left upper limb. The trunk responds with its own activity.

Mistakes:
- a stiff movement of the arm lacking fluency
- lifting the shoulders
- a slack posture.

As mentioned earlier, there is a point of intersection between the upper and lower loops which is located in front of the waist.

12(b) Frontal figure eight led by the inner edge of the hand and started with a lower loop

Initial position: as in Exercise 12(a) with the difference that the right arm is in a low abduction sideways, the palm is facing backward.

Slowly 'carve out' a large vertical figure eight led by the inner edge of the right hand.

Begin with the lower loop by moving the hand downward-inward till reaching the floor in front of the body. Simultaneously with this movement lower the body to a *grand plié* (legs turned outward and the knees pointing to the sides). Continue with the arm to the left into a left adduction (crosswise). Together with the ascending motion of the body, the arm moves to the right and by the time the hand reaches the point of intersection it is in maximal supination (facing upward). Link up with the upper loop and on searching its culmination point (both legs are stretched, with the body weight distributed equally). The arm descends (adduction crosswise left) and moves to the middle with the hand passing through the point of intersection, maximally rotated inward (pronation) with the palm facing forward. Finish the figure eight in the initial position. The

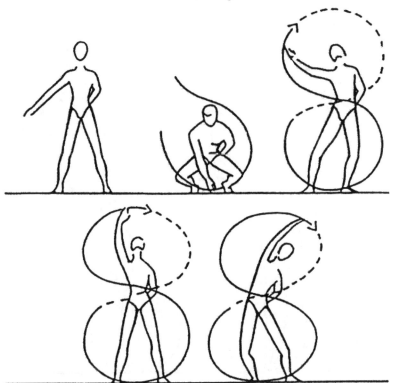

eyes follow the hand and the whole body cooperates in creating curves to the maximum extent. Perform the same with the left arm.

While ascending or descending, the knees partly bend or extend in succession due to a slight transfer of the body weight from one leg to the other (one leg is always weighted more than the other) with the exception of the highest and the lowest point. Practise the same in a swing, either with an accent downward or upward.

Mistakes:
- flattening the figure eight on one side (insufficient crossing)
- reducing of the upper half (the crossing is too high)
- lifting the shoulders
- turning the knees in during the grand plié
- an insufficient plié in the vertical axis and therefore an excessive forward tilt with the pelvis protruding backward
- an insufficient adjustment of the whole body.

Variations to exercise: Perform a sequence of exercises to 3/4 or 3/8 time.

(1) lower loop – 1 bar
     upper loop – 1 bar

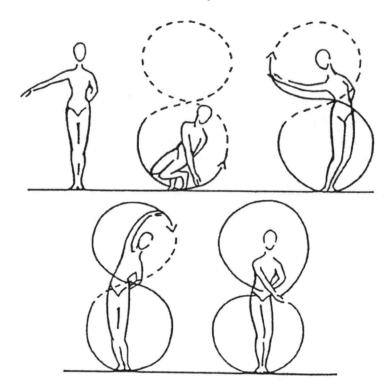

(2) lower loop – 1 bar
    upper loop – 2 bars
(3) lower loop – 1 bar
    upper loop – 3 bars

The accent is always on the shorter movement (i.e. the lower loop) and the longer movement (i.e. the upper loop) gradually becomes larger in space.

Practise the same but hold the legs together throughout the exercise in a parallel position with the knees together. The bent knees deviate from the midline to the right or to the left.

Lower loop: while descending into a squat the knees deviate diagonally forward-right into the opposite direction to the movement of the arm which is moving crosswise to the left (adduction).

Upper loop: while ascending the knees move into a left diagonal (opposite to the body and arm which moves in a right-upward direction). Both the knees and the hand pass at the same time through the midline in front of the body. At the culmination point of the upper loop the knees are elongated and the weight equally

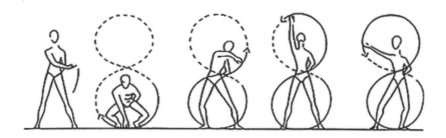

distributed on both legs. The body, together with the head and knees, moves in fluent curves.

12(c) Frontally located figure eight led by the outer edge of the hand

Initial position: legs turned out in second position, the left hand on the sacrum, the right hand in adduction crosswise to the left-forward with the palm facing backward.

Lower loop: while descending into a *grand plié* the hand leads downward, right, upward, through the point of intersection to the left adduction where the hand is in a maximal pronation with the palm facing forward.

Upper loop: while ascending, the arm continues left-upward. In the culmination point of the loop the knees are fully extended.

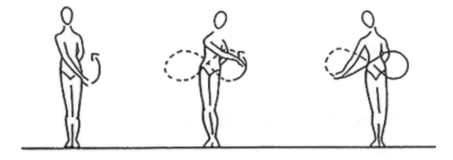

When reaching the point of intersection the hand is in a maximal supination with the palm facing upward.

Mistakes and Variations to exercise as in 12(b).

12(d) Frontally located figure eight executed with both arms

Initial position: stand with legs in a turned-out second position. Both arms are prepared on the same side of the body (on the right).

The right arm is in abduction-right with the palm facing backward (pronation), the left is slightly lower in adduction crosswise-right with the palm facing upward (supination). The right hand leads with the outer edge, the left one with the inner edge.

First variation: both hands proceed, parallel throughout, thus drawing two figures eight which cut through each other.

Second variation: the hands move one after the other, along the same line. In this case, the hands slightly cross each other at waist level. The distance between both hands is approximately 1/4 of the loop.

12(e) Frontally located figure eight with a horizontal axis

First revise pendular swings focusing on the 'free fall'. This figure eight differs from the vertical one by the fact that it is flatter (like the mathematical sign for infinity), both its halves are equally large and equally long lasting. Each one has its own accent.

Note: the figures eight are not only executed in a frontal plane with either a horizontal or a vertical axis. They can be differently located in space, e.g. slanted or bent (the lower loop in front of the body, the upper loop above the head with a hyperextended spine), large or small, adjusted to the needs of the following movement. In more complicated combinations they are connected with steps, skips, lunges and turns. The first essential is to master the basic exercises and to focus on the swing quality of the movement (the accent and 'fading away' to standstill), an organic involvement of the whole body in the rounded curves, sensitivity of hands (their edges) etc. Boys must practise the swings more robustly and energetically than girls. The girls' execution of the swings must be elastic but not too soft.

HARMONIOUS BREATHING

In teaching there are two golden rules:

(1) Correct body posture is essential to all breathing exercises

Human bone structure is such that it is almost impossible to achieve correct breathing if the skeleton is not purposefully structured against gravity. For us, this means that breathing can only be controlled to the extent that we can succeed indirectly in improving the organisation of the skeletal muscles. This allows the body to stand and move better (M. Feldenkrais, *Der Aufrechte Gang*, Frankfurt: 1968).

Before we start any breathing, voice, speech and singing exercise it is necessary to bring the body into the correct inter-relationship of all its parts. This inter-relationship is required by the rules of balanced and relaxed posture. (A barrier is often caused by a slight forward shift of the head and overtension in the wrong muscles, or by pushing forward the frontal rib arches to gain support from the diaphragm. Diaphragm support can be achieved without over-straining by a sideways extension of the ribs. It is also absolutely necessary to be in a positive, happy mood.) *At many drama schools, the conduct of breathing exercises is left to teachers of speech and singing. Here I recommend a method which acknowledge the fact that breathing is regulated by involuntary neuro-muscular systems and which, before drill, evoke sensory images and promote psychophysical relaxation to encourage cooperation between the involuntary and the motoric muscle centres. The most modern methods reject controlled breathing and evoke an involuntary deepening of the breath by massage and expert touches.*

(2) All movement exercises call for a free-flowing breath

It is physiologically wrong to hold back the breath or force it. This rule is sufficiently 'golden' to suffice without further instruction. There are, however, some movements that can be helped by con-trolled breathing, i.e. by a conscious coordination between the breath rhythm and the movement rhythm. Some exercises benefit from exha-lation during the active phase of the movement while certain awareness and relaxation exercises are helped by exhalation in the pas-sive phase. For example, in all true swings and exercises in which some parts of the body fall naturally with gravity, the downward movement is connected with an exhalation; and the subsequent return to the ini-tial position with an inhalation. There is a common tendency to connect each lift with an inhalation and each drop or downward movement with exhalation. This is faulty and not correct in general. Many methods, on the contrary, recognise that *flexors* tend to be spas-modic and to cramp and so emphasise and prolong movements of the erector and extensor muscles by an exhalation. Movements directed into space, including those aiming upward and strengthening move-ments, have better quality (not only in the physiological but also psychological sense) when connected with an exhalation. Thus we can adjust the rhythm accordingly if an exercise comprises a 'free-fall' phase and a strengthening phase each of which works better if con-nected with an exhalation.

One example is exercises for the oblique abdominal muscles while lying on the back with bent knees. While exhaling, drop the knees with their full weight to the right down to the floor until the pelvis turns right. At the same time push the left shoulder to the floor in a contra-movement and let the head 'fall' reactively into a small torsion to the left. Let the body rest for a little while so that after a small pause an unforced inhalation can take place. During the recovery movement, exhale again. In order to strengthen the abdominal muscles, we must have passive legs and start the recovery movement by pressing the left hip and sacrum towards the floor. The legs are heavier if we cross the right leg over the left leg from the beginning, as in a sitting position in an armchair. This is followed again by an inhalation in a resting position.

Take an example from breathing exercises, during which we often lift the arms sideways to enable the lungs to widen more during inhalation. It is recommended that after inhalation (with arms moving to the sides of the body) an exhalation with a conscious upward elongation of the spine (feeling slimmer) follows so that the exhalation is not associated with a passive feeling. Another reason is to make the inhalation more natural and relaxed (like a sponge reacts to squeezing by relaxing back to its original shape). *It is best that breathing is not an action, but a reaction.* (Agnes Schoch, *Gute-Haltung Schöner Gang*, Munchen, Basel: 1963).

Combining exhalation with a feeling of increasing passivity (in some cases necessary, e.g. for expression purposes) necessitates new, and therefore disproportionate, force during inhalation. (It is, however, good while exercising to exchange the inhalation and exhalation phases.) Only a few exercises should be accompanied by controlled breathing. In most it is best to leave it to the body to decide when it needs to inhale and when to exhale, under the condition that we maintain the muscles in elastic relaxation and parts of the body in the correct inter-relationship to leave sufficient space for the flow of the breath.

It is easier to breathe if the body weight is carried by the bone structure without unnecessary muscular strain. If we can breathe easily we will have a better body posture. Body posture and muscular activity which evokes deepened breathing stimulate psychological equivalents, i.e. readiness to be active; ability to make contact; as well as a disposition toward affectation. That does not concern deepened breathing at will, but rather breathing which evokes activity of our involuntary breathing regulators with the aid of imagery, whether it be smell, space or sound.

> *A restricted or unused movement ability, e.g. overstraining or slackness of certain muscle groups, can negatively influence breathing or blood circulation. On the other hand, restricted and incorrect breathing and blood circulation can have a negative impact on body posture and movement. Breathing, the function of which is conditioned by time and dynamics, has a natural, basic rhythm. The rhythm, however, varies in individuals according to their mental and physical state, action and experience. Conditioned by numerous mutual relationships, our state, action and experience can also be influenced by 'the form' of the breathing process. The way we control our breathing has also an influence on the movement expression, namely on the functioning of physical activity. We know from experience, in both senses, a receptive relationship between breathing and movement enables the whole body to organically take part in every movement.* (I. Loesch, *Sprechende Bewegung*, Berlin: 1974).

Our breathing rhythm should adapt to the body position within the field of gravity. The correct coordination of movement with breathing can best be observed in the state of psycho-physical relaxation, in a resting position and at first in slow tempo. Only then is it safe to increase the tempo of the movement. (Fast exercise is very often associated with incorrect breathing!)

> *Breathe in your usual rhythm, no deeper than usual, do not hold your breath. The main thing now is to give positive, joyful and enthusiastic attention to your breathing. Listen carefully to your breathing joy.*
> *No force, nothing artificial or affected. After a while, your breathing will slow down, deepen and become more regular. The muscles of the whole body will become more relaxed and it is possible that you will feel a slight warmth because your blood vessels will have also relaxed. Now you are relishing how freely you can breathe, you are almost getting intoxicated by the freedom of your breath. The heart gradually begins to have a concentrated and peaceful rhythm.* (V. Levi, *Umění Sebevlády*, Prague: 1981).

The necessity to be relaxed does not apply only in inactivity and during rest. It is most useful, particularly during strenuous exercise, to attain relaxed breathing to be able to cope with future stage work. During this relaxation, however, we must not slacken any parts of the body. The breathing muscles in particular must retain activity and maintain free space in the middle of the trunk to be able to send impulses for a more substantial breathing. The sensation is that of the so-called 'diaphragm support of breathing' if it is correctly understood and executed. In practice, this means that we must maintain a position of slight inhalation even when exhaling, with the aid of the voluntary breathing muscles.

So far we have been discussing exercises in which we should, in a natural way, enlarge our breathing capacity in order to reinforce our vitality through a larger supply of oxygen. (Careful, breathing too quickly prevents this!) In acting, however, one must also portray emotions that are not connected with free breathing. We know from our experience how the rhythm of breathing changes when we are surprised, scared, frightened, happy, in a hurry, hesitant, attentive etc. On the other hand, conscious changes of the breathing rhythm can, in reverse, influence our feelings to such an extent that we can re-live the experience. That is why these possibilities are utilised in the education of stage movement. Imagery of smell and scent, which aid natural reactions, is used also.

> *Breathing, regulated subconsciously by involuntary neuro-muscular centres, responds at the same time to our willpower, creating a bridge between the outside and the inside, between the 'I' and the 'It', between the soul and the body. Through breathing, our whole body and its functions may be put into chaos, or in order and harmony.*
>
> *There is more. Breathing can be a means of bodily expression and psychological and spiritual embodiment. This fact has been proven for a long time and has been recorded in theories on breathing introduced into the cult and philosophies of the East, as well as those of ancient Greece. (D. Jacobs, Die Menschliche, Ratingen: Bewegung, 1962).*

> *Inhalation connects and binds, everything that is true occurs in the pause, and exhalation relaxes and completes because it surmounts all limitations. (Zen).*

APPENDIX II

DIAGRAMS SUPPLEMENT

Head

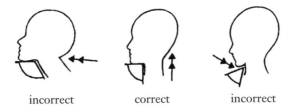

incorrect   correct   incorrect

Positions of the Head

Spine

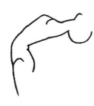

incorrect backward bend of the spine

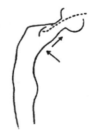

correct backward bend of the
spine (hyperextention)

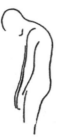

incorrect rounded forward
bend of the spine

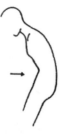

correct rounded forward
bend of the spine

Positions of the Spine

Shoulders

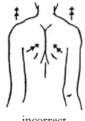 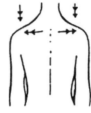 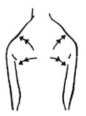

incorrect   correct   incorrect

Positions of the Shoulders

shoulder rotated outwards

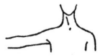

shoulder in its basic position

shoulder rotated inwards

Arms

Arms Raised Upward

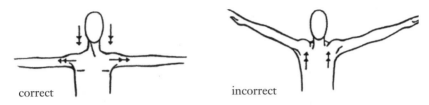

Arms Raised Sideways
Incorrect – the horizontal line of the arm is broken, arms shift backward-upward.

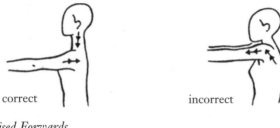

Arms Raised Forwards

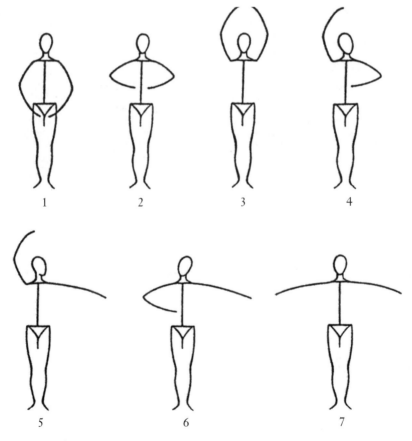

Positions of the Arms

Elbows

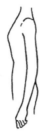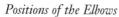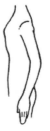

Positions of the Elbows

elbow rotated outwards

slightly bent elbow

elbow rotated inwards

Direction of Elbow Rotation

Hands

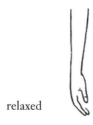

relaxed

Positions of the Hands

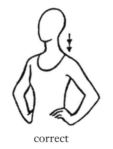

correct   incorrect

Hands on the Waist

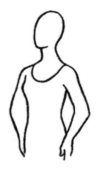

Hands on the Hips

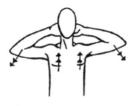

incorrect

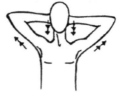

correct

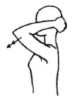

incorrect

Hands at the Back of the Head

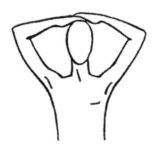

Hands on the Head

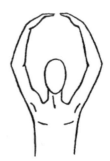

Hands above the Head

Knees

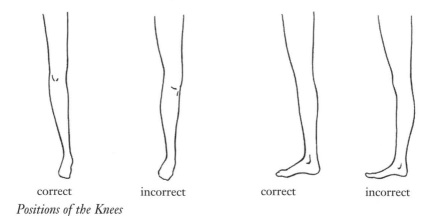

Positions of the Knees

Instep Arch

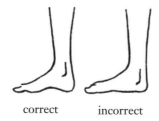

Positions of the Instep Arch

Feet

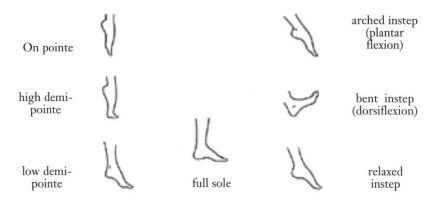

Positions of the Foot

Parallel position
(feet close together or apart)

1st position -   turned out   fully turned out   turned in
slightly turned out
(heels together)

2nd position -   2nd position -
feet apart   wide
turned out

3rd position -
the heel of one foot touches the
side of the arch of the other foot

4th position -
feet apart slightly crossed

5th position -
fully crossed

Positions of the Feet

About the Authors

JARMILA KRÖSCHLOVÁ (1893 - 1983) was a dancer, educator, choreographer, theoretician and an author of significant books on technical and artistic development. She grew up in Prague and after completing her studies in 1921 under Émile Jacques-Dalcroze, became a leading educator of movement theory and education in Hellerau, near Dresden. She initiated the expansion of the school by the addition of a new department which developed the study of contemporary dance and expressive dance technique.

Like other great personalities and outstanding dancers of the time such as Rosalia Chladek—who studied the movement fundamentals of Kröschlová—and the American Martha Graham, Jarmila Kröschlová recognised the need to place studies of movement on a proper technical basis. She began to create her own method, based on the anatomical and physiological laws that govern movement and integrated with the practical education of awareness and the projection of emotional experience. Kröschlová's method is enduring because it finds application in a wide range of creative movement styles. A dancer's correct body posture, the rules of which Jarmila elevated to an aesthetic principle governing the technical basis of expressive dance, became the keystone of her method. Using this principle, Jarmila directed her dancers to consciously control muscular work and, when necessary, their breathing. In particular, she enabled her budding artists to capture and consciously feel the emotional experiences associated with all the components that make up movement expression.

Jarmila's approach was ahead of its time. She realised that by combining kineasthetic awareness with an emotional involvement one could create movement forms infused with an inner tension which would endow movement with the power of artistic expression. Only in recent times have contemporary teachers of movement begun to consider as important a balanced body posture and a general knowledge of anatomy, as a means to achieve technical refinement with a substantial reduction of the risk of injury.

In 1924 Jarmila became choreographer of her own dramatic

dance group for which she created many works mainly to the music of contemporary Czech composers such as B. Martinu and Iša Krejcí. In 1932 she was awarded the bronze medal for choreography at the Association Internationale de Danse in Paris. Between 1926 and 1955 she choreographed many theatre productions in Prague and Brno and collaborated with the best Czech directors. In the years 1949 to 1958 she taught stage movement at the dance faculty of the Academy of Musical Art in Prague.

Jarmila collated her life-long experiences in three books, *Foundations of Movement Education of Dancers and Actors* (Prague : Orbis, 1956) which systematically classified her movement techniques; *Movement Theory* (Prague: Státní Pedagogické Nakladatelství, 1975, second edition, 1980) which describes the analysis and synthesis of movement; and *Expressive Dance* (Prague: Orbis, 1964).

EVA KRÖSCHLOVÁ was born in 1926 in Prague. She is a dancer, choreographer, educator and author of a number of specialised books such as: *Dynamika, Švihy* (Dynamics, Swings) Gottwaldov: OKS 1985, a co-author of *Pohybové Etudy* (Movement Etudes) Prague: Orbis 1963 and of *Czech Orff School Vol.1* Prague: Supraphon 1969; an author of *Tanecní Etudy* (Dance Etudes) Prague: UDLUT 1974; of *Kontratance Ruznych Koncin* (Counterdances of Various Regions), Ostrava: OKS 1979; and *Dobové Tance* (Period Dances) Prague: SPN 1981. At the Drama Faculty of the Academy of Arts in Prague, Eva also created an outstanding series of teaching texts, *Stage Movement - Movement Training for Actors*, which pertain to both stage movement and problems of education.

Eva, her mother Jarmila and her aunt Nada were the forerunners of the development of Czech expressive dance. She is a significant figure in the cultural movement that was and is *expressive dance*. This movement is concerned with changes in artistic attitudes and with philosophical and spiritual attitudes to movement.

After graduating at her mother's School of Movement and Dance Education, she started teaching there. As a choreographer, Eva cooperated with many directors of drama and opera in Prague. She is a member of many Czech and international panels and dance associations including the Choreological Group of the International Council of Traditional Music (ICTM), where she is a co-author of the syllabus for structural analysis of folk dances.

ZORA ŠEMBEROVÁ was born in Moravia. In the 1930s she trained with Eliska Blahova, a leading advocate of the principles of anatomy and music theory; and the dancer Rosalia Chladek, who included Kroschlova's principles of movement in her teaching. In 1938 Semberova attracted national attention by dancing Prokofiev's Juliet in *Rome and Juliet* without points. The performance was forbidden by the German occupational forces in 1939.

In 1943 she became a member of the National Theatre in Prague; and in 1945 was co-founder of the dance department of the Prague Music Conservatorium. As a soloist she created many roles, including the title role in *Vittorka*, choreographed by Sasha Machov, which won her a prestigious national prize. In 1957 she joined Alfred Radok, film director and founder of Laterna Magika, as a choreographer of his Dance Group.

In 1968 Šemberová left Prague for Flinders University, Adelaide, at the invitation of Drama Professor Wal Cherry. She became a staff member in 1970 and received an honorary doctorate in 1979 following her retirement. In Adelaide she corresponded with Jarmila and Eva Kröschlová, who became her mentors. 'Jarmila made me a better teacher', she says. Her Australian students include the stage director Gale Edwards, the film director Scott Hicks, the dancer Cheryl Stock and the designer Michael Pearce.

In 1993 former students Jiří Kylián and Pavel Smok gave her a gala performance at the National Theatre of Prague; and she received honorary membership for her choreography and for 'educating the best dance artists' in the former Czechoslovakia. In 1999 she received the Thalia Prize, the highest recognition of the Czech Republic. for a lifetime's achievement. The same year she received an award from SBS radio for her contribution to art in Australia.

OLGA MALANDRIS grew up in Prague where she studied languages at the Foreign Languages University. In 1968 she emigrated to Australia and continued her studies at Flinders University. She has a diploma of Early Childhood Eductaion from Kingston College of Education and is an accredited translator. She has been a pre-school teacher for over twenty years and has applied Kroschlova's principles of movement to the physical and emotional development of the children in her care.